MW01100213

Neuropharmacology
and Behavior

Neuropharmacology and Behavior

Edited by

Bernard Haber

The Marine Biomedical Institute
Department of Human Biological Chemistry and Genetics
and Department of Neurology
University of Texas Medical Branch
Galveston, Texas

and

M. H. Aprison

Institute of Psychiatric Research and
Departments of Psychiatry and Biochemistry
Indiana University School of Medicine
Indianapolis, Indiana

PLENUM PRESS · NEW YORK AND LONDON

Library of Congress Cataloging in Publication Data

Main entry under title:

Neuropharmacology and behavior.

Published in honor of H. E. Himwich.
"Bibliography of Harold E. Himwich": p.
Includes bibliographies and index.
1. Neuropsychopharmacology. 2. Neurochemistry. 3. Human behavior. I. Haber,
Bernard. II. Aprison, M. H., 1923-   III. Himwich, Harold Edwin, 1894-1975.
[DNLM: 1. Psychotropic drugs. 2. Behavior – Drug effects. QV77 N496]
RM315.N47   615'.78   77-14178
ISBN 0-306-31056-2

© 1978 Plenum Press, New York
A Division of Plenum Publishing Corporation
227 West 17th Street, New York, N.Y. 10011

Printed in the United States of America

Contributors

M. H. Aprison, Section of Applied and Theoretical Neurobiology, Institute of Psychiatric Research, Indiana University Medical Center, Indianapolis, Indiana

G. F. Ayala, Department of Neurology, University of Minnesota, Minneapolis, Minnesota. Present address: Department of Neurology, Baylor College of Medicine, Houston, Texas

Arvid Carlsson, Department of Pharmacology, University of Göteborg, Göteborg, Sweden

E. Costa, Laboratory of Preclinical Pharmacology, National Institute of Mental Health, Saint Elizabeths Hospital, Washington, D.C.

A. Guidotti, Laboratory of Preclinical Pharmacology, National Institute of Mental Health, Saint Elizabeths Hospital, Washington, D.C.

D. Johnston, Department of Neurology, University of Minnesota, Minneapolis, Minnesota

Seymour Kety, Department of Psychiatry, Harvard Medical School, Boston, Massachusetts and Mailman Research Centre, McLean Hospital, Belmont, Massachusetts

Lawrence F. Kromer, Department of Neurosciences, University of California at San Diego, La Jolla, California

Margit Lindqvist, Department of Pharmacology, University of Göteborg, Göteborg, Sweden

Arnold J. Mandell, School of Medicine, University of California at San Diego, La Jolla, California

Robert Y. Moore, Department of Neurosciences, University of California at San Diego, La Jolla, California

Ann Reifman, Laboratory of Clinical Psychopharmacology, Division of Special Mental Health Research, IRP, National Institute of Mental Health, Saint Elizabeths Hospital, Washington, D.C.

J. R. Smythies, Department of Psychiatry and the Neurosciences Program, University of Alabama in Birmingham, Birmingham, Alabama

K. Tachiki, Section of Applied and Theoretical Neurobiology, Institute of Psychiatric Research, Indiana University Medical Center, Indianapolis, Indiana

Ryo Takahashi, Department of Neuropsychiatry, Nagasaki University School of Medicine, Nagasaki, Japan

Kenneth M. Woodrow, Department of Psychiatry, Stanford University Medical School, Stanford, California

Richard Jed Wyatt, Laboratory of Clinical Psychopharmacology, Division of Special Mental Health Research, IRP, National Institute of Mental Health, Saint Elizabeths Hospital, Washington, D.C.

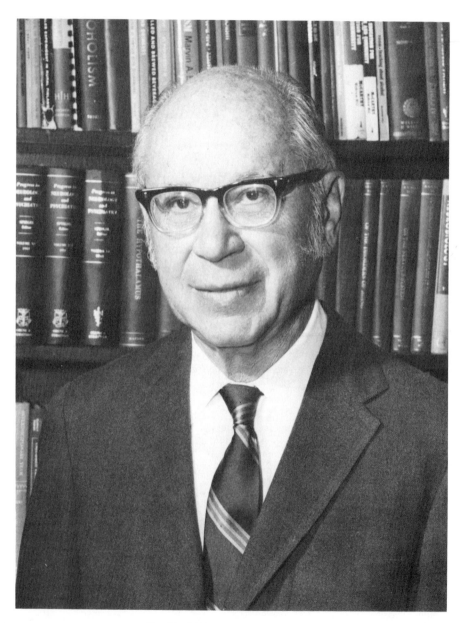

Dr. Harold E. Himwich, 1894–1975.

Preface

Science lost one of its distinguished researchers in the fields of biological psychiatry and neuropsychopharmacology on March 4, 1975, with the death of Harold Himwich. Some of his colleagues, friends, and former associates have expressed their esteem for this gentle person by the contribution of chapters in this book. Since this book can represent only an incomplete indication of Harold Himwich's influence, the editors have included his complete bibliography at the end of this volume.

Harold Himwich's research career was divided into several phases, some of which overlapped. Starting with his first paper on rhabdomyoma of the ovary in 1920, he was entranced by research as well as by the puzzles and results which it promised. During the period that he was a resident and house officer at Bellevue Hospital in New York, he studied the physiology of muscular exercise. This work led him into studies of exercise in various types of disease. With Meyerhoff in Kiel, Germany, he began studying the respiratory quotient of muscle, and after returning to this country, he produced a number of papers on respiratory quotients of various organs including the brain.

When his work led to the result that the respiratory quotient of the brain was one, his interest in the brain began to crystallize. These studies led him to carbohydrate utilization by the brain and problems of carbohydrate metabolism and diabetes in man. During this period of time, he was working at Yale Medical College and had access to a number of clinical patients. In this setting, he became interested in the effect of insulin, of diabetes, and of other diseases on the respiratory quotient of the brain and other organs. To some extent, this was followed by an interest in drugs, including alcohol, and culminated in the investigations of schizophrenia, first in the explanation of the hypoglycemic treatment and then in the use of anoxia in the therapy for schizophrenia. During this period, a number of drugs were studied for their effects on the brain, especially the respiratory quotient of the brain.

By 1941, Harold Himwich was well into his studies of developing brain, which were to continue as long as he was at Albany Medical College, that is, until the spring of 1946. Simultaneously, his research interest in cerebral blood flow, in cerebral metabolism, and in the effects of various agents on these parameters was increasing. He transferred to the Army Chemical Center at Edgewood, and while there became involved in the so-called "nerve gases" and published papers on acetylcholinesterase and the unclassified compound diisopropyl fluorophosphate. As a part of this work, Harold Himwich became engaged in recording the EEG in animals, and although he had used this technique previously, this period was really the beginning of his wide-ranging interest in the EEG as an effective technique to study the effects of drugs on the central nervous system.

In 1951, Harold Himwich was appointed Director of the Thudicum Psychiatric Research Laboratory at Galesburg, Illinois. This move brought about a greater interest in as well as a greater availability of patients. Harold Himwich began to follow by means of the EEG the effects on animals of the drugs he was using clinically for patients. Inevitably, this work led to studies of the biogenic amines and finally to attempts to define the biochemical errors in schizophrenia and in autism, a field in which he was still actively working at the time of his death.

Although his early research was done on organs all over the body, especially muscle, after 1929, the focus of his interest was the brain. One of the goals of his research was always to learn how to aid those who had problems of brain functioning from poor mental health or from epilepsy or similar diseases. It was inevitable, therefore, that he was drawn to the study of schizophrenia, which still remains one of the bigger mysteries, so clouded that no one has yet been able to piece together the various bits of the puzzle.

In a very real sense, Harold Himwich was a successor to Thudicum, after whom the very productive research laboratory in Galesburg was named. All those who had the pleasure of knowing Harold Himwich will miss him both as a great scientist and a kind human being. In the names of all those too numerous to list, the editors dedicate this volume to Harold Himwich.

B. Haber
M. H. Aprison

Contents

3 • The Organization of Central Catecholamine Neuron Systems

Robert Y. Moore and Lawrence F. Kromer

4 • Effect of Reserpine on Monoamine Synthesis and on Apparent Dopaminergic Receptor Sensitivity in Rat Brain

Arvid Carlsson and Margit Lindqvist

5 • The Induction of Tyrosine-3-monooxygenase in Rat Adrenal Medulla: A Model for the Transsynaptic Regulation of Gene Expression
A. Guidotti and E. Costa

6 • The Neurophysiological Effects of Diphenylhydantoin and Their Relationship to Anticonvulsant Activity
G. F. Ayala and D. Johnston

Amphetamine Psychosis—A Model for Paranoid Schizophrenia?

Kenneth M. Woodrow, Ann Reifman, and Richard Jed Wyatt

1. Introduction

Amphetamine psychosis is at times strikingly similar to paranoid schizophrenia. How closely the exogenous model fits the endogenous psychosis is of vital interest. If such a model is valid, it would have great potential for explaining paranoid schizophrenia. This chapter presents a review of the strengths and weaknesses of amphetamine psychosis as a model for paranoid schizophrenia.

The current interest in amphetamine psychosis evolved out of a zigzag history dating back to the mid-1930's, when the central excitatory effect of amphetamine was first documented (Prinzmetal and Bloomberg, 1935). Only three years later, in 1938, the initial reports linking amphetamines to paranoid psychosis were published. Although there was a question whether paranoia was directly attributable to amphetamine, the authors strongly inferred that amphetamine did bring latent paranoid trends to the surface (Young and Scoville, 1938).

Kenneth M. Woodrow, Ann Reifman, and Richard Jed Wyatt • Laboratory of Clinical Psychopharmacology, Division of Special Mental Health Research, IRP, National Institute of Mental Health, Saint Elizabeths Hospital, Washington, D.C. 20032. Dr. Woodrow's current affiliation is Department of Psychiatry, Stanford University Medical School, Stanford, California 94305

Clinical utilization of amphetamines to help soldiers continue functioning during periods of fatigue increased during World War II, and episodic reports of untoward psychological reactions trickled into the literature between 1945 and 1956. Connell (1958, pp. 16–26) examined 25 separate articles and noted not only that the case reports varied widely, but also that only a small number of patients were studied, the largest series consisting of seven patients. The primary picture of amphetamine psychosis that emerged from this group of papers was one of paranoid delusions and psychomotor agitation with excitement, euphoria, noisiness, and rambling conversation. The psychosis was characterized less often by confusion, disorientation, and formication (the feeling of insects crawling under the skin), which are more typical of toxic psychoses than schizophrenia.

These scattered reports thus indicated the possibility of paranoid reactions to oral, parenteral, and inhaled amphetamine. Although this amphetamine-induced paranoia was at times accompanied by manic excitement or toxic delirium, it also appeared at other times virtually indistinguishable from paranoid schizophrenia (Connell, 1958, p. 27).

Models of disease have been extremely important in the development of scientific medicine. If an exogenous substance, such as amphetamine, were capable of mimicking some aspects of schizophrenia, schizophrenia itself might be more easily understood. In the last ten years, there has been a growing consensus that schizophrenia has, at least in part, a biological base. Nevertheless, despite intensive investigations, nothing strong enough to be called a "cause" has been found. A biological model would certainly facilitate the study of causes of schizophrenia.

If a biological model for schizophrenia could be constructed, then biochemical efforts to inhibit synthesis of an offending substance or to block receptor sites of that substance could become focused. One example of a crucial use for such a model is in the screening of antipsychotic medications. At present, screening is carried out on animals by testing which drugs appear to alter crude animal behavior without putting the animal to sleep. Current animal models of psychosis are unrefined, however, and many potential antipsychotic medications may be missed. Clearly, an exogenous model for schizophrenia would be of vital use.

1.1. LSD as a Drug Model

First synthesized in a Swiss laboratory in 1938, LSD was found to have potent mind-influencing properties in 1943. On April 10th of that year, Albert Hoffman accidentally came under its powerful effects. It is unclear whether this first episode was the result of LSD absorption through his skin or transfer of trace amounts from his hands to his mouth. In either case, he experienced a by now well-known sequence of events that included "three characteristic types of symptoms: somatic, perceptual, and psychic" (Hollister, 1968*a*). His somatic symptoms consisted of dizziness, weakness, tremors, nausea, drowsiness, parasthesia, and blurred vision. He perceived altered shapes and colors, difficulty in focusing on objects, a sharpened sense of hearing, and synesthesias. His psychic symptoms included alterations in mood (happy, sad, or irritable at varying times), tension, distorted time sense, difficulty in expressing thoughts, depersonalization, dreamlike feelings, and visual hallucinations. His few physiological signs included dilated pupils, hyperreflexia, increased muscle tension, incoordination, and ataxia.

The spectrum of effects Hoffman experienced was striking, but was even more intriguing because of the minute doses required to achieve them. LSD administration in the range of 100 μg was capable of causing very powerful alterations in psychological function. Indeed, effective doses were as small as 20–30 μg. Could the human body produce a natural LSD-like substance that might be responsible for the clinical symptoms of schizophrenia? This question was of course posed, but to date remains unanswered (Gillin *et al.*, 1976).

How closely did this LSD-induced psychosis mimic schizophrenia? In discussing the similarities and differences between schizophrenia and LSD intoxication, Hollister remarked that while schizophrenics and LSD subjects have difficulty expressing their thoughts, schizophrenics do not seem as concerned about this problem as do the LSD subjects. Schizophrenics withdraw; drug subjects generally prefer to talk to someone—even though they may resent intrusive questions and psychometric tests. Schizophrenic hallucinations are primarily auditory, drug subjects' primarily visual (Hollister, 1968*b*). In short, Hollister found that the clinical symptoms of LSD intoxication and schizophrenia were so clearly differentiable that when 78 mental health professionals were asked to rate short taped interviews of 12 subjects, half of whom were schizophrenic and half of whom were hallucinogen subjects, their accuracy ranged from 85 to 96%. Hollister (1968b) concluded that "in schizophrenics the primary disturbance was in thinking, while the drug subjects' disturbance was in perception" (p. 119).

1.2. Amphetamine as a Drug Model

Amphetamine was first synthesized in 1887 (Kramer, 1969), but clinical effects were not reported until the 1930's. Its ability to raise blood pressure was noted in 1930 (Innes and Nickerson, 1970), and its bronchodilating qualities in 1933. In 1935, Prinzmetal and Bloomberg published a paper detailing the CNS-stimulating qualities of amphetamine in the treatment of narcolepsy. Two years later, Bradley (1937) reported the paradoxical use of amphetamine to calm hyperactive children with shortened attention spans, and in 1939, its appetite-depressing qualities came to light (Kramer, 1969, pp. 2 and 3).

But the two features of amphetamine that were destined to bring it to widespread public attention were its effectiveness in elevating mood and in dampening fatigue. By the late 1960's and early 1970's, amphetamines were being abused by students cramming for exams, athletes straining to break records, truck drivers pushing for more miles, race horses, astronauts, and speed freaks looking for the ultimate "high."

In the same way that cocaine first came into heavy abuse following the routine prescription to troops in World War I, so too, amphetamine abuse rose sharply after World War II. "American, British, German, and Japanese armed forces had issued amphetamines to their men to counteract fatigue, elevate mood, and heighten endurance (*Licit and Illicit Drugs,* 1972, p. 279).

After the war, amphetamine abuse was an increasing but relatively minor problem until the 1960's. Indiscriminant dispensing of amphetamine became highly publicized. Concomitantly, illicit manufacture of stimulants began, followed by intravenous injection of drugs previously used orally.

The shift of large numbers of users to the intravenous mode surfaced the paranoia problem to a previously unknown extent. The typical result was the injection of the drug "many times a day, each dose in the hundreds of milligrams; the 'runs' progressed with the user remaining awake continuously for three to six days, gradually getting more tense, tremulous, and paranoid. The runs were interrupted by bouts of very profound sleep (called 'crashing') which lasted a day or two" (Nathanson, 1939). The individual became progressively more irritable and suspicious, with delusions of persecution, reference, and grandiosity. Initially, the drug user would recognize these feelings as drug-caused, but later he would lose contact with reality. Indeed, because of his irritability, suspiciousness, and irrationality, the speed freak became an outcast, even within the drug community. Finally, with the emergence of overt paranoid delusions, the individual who had been injecting speed would, in many instances, be indistinguishable from a person diagnosed paranoid schizophrenic.

2.   Clinical Description

The amphetamine psychosis is "the almost inevitable result of long-term high-dose, intravenous injection" (*Licit and Illicit Drugs,* 1972, p. 11). The psychosis can sometimes be "precipitated by a single large dose, or by chronic moderate doses'' (Kramer, 1969, p. 6). But contrary to the impression widely quoted in the press that "speed kills," "very few deaths have been recorded in which overdose of amphetamines has been causal" (Kramer, 1969, pp. 9 and 10). In fact, if the individual can remain abstinent, even severe paranoid delusions and intellectual disorganization tend to clear over time. Based on this strong evidence linking amphetamine psychosis and paranoid schizophrenia, we decided to compare the two psychoses.

The first case report of paranoid psychosis associated with amphetamine use was published by Young and Scoville (1938). It is somewhat disconcerting to note that all three patients they recorded had paranoid ideation prior to taking amphetamines. One had been taking ephedrine for narcolepsy, a second had been frankly psychotic, and the third had not only a high serum bromide level on admission, but also "delusions of tumor" 3 years previously. In the same year, Waud (1938) reported on the symptoms experienced following the inhalation of amphetamine over a 6-hr period. Episodic clinical and experimental reports continued to appear in the literature, culminating in a comprehensive monograph by Connell (1958) entitled *Amphetamine Psychosis,* which reviewed all clinical cases reported up until 1956. Kalant (1966) summarized these data (Table I).

The spectrum was rather wide and the doses varied. *d*-Amphetamine, 55 mg, taken by a 29-year-old male was the smallest single dose reported in the literature to have induced a *de novo* paranoid psychosis (Wallis *et al.,* 1949), while 50 mg/day for a month (Delay *et al.,* 1954), and 10–30 mg/day over 4 years appear to be the lowest intermediate and long-term dosages reported to have caused amphetamine psychosis (Chapman, 1954).

*Table I.   Incidence of Symptoms in
Amphetamine-Induced Psychosis*

Symptom	Incidence (%)
Delusions of persecution	83
Visual hallucinations	53
Hyperactivity	41
Auditory hallucinations	40
Anxiety, fear, and terror	26
Hostility	22
Agitation	17
Depression	15
Ideas of reference	14
Tactile hallucinations	11
Disorientation	7
Olfactory hallucinations	6

2.1. Differences and Similarities

The similarities between amphetamine psychosis and paranoid schizophrenia are striking. While a number of early authors (Slater, 1959; Bell, 1965) lamented that not enough attention was being given specifically to those similarities, today most investigators would agree that at times, "amphetamine psychosis can be indistinguishable from schizophrenia" (Bell, 1965, p. 701).

What about the differences? If the differences are great, an amphetamine model for schizophrenia is not valid. Bell (1965) (who also saw a striking similarity between the two psychoses) noted that amphetamine psychosis can be distinguished from true schizophrenia on the basis of "the prominence of visual hallucinations in some cases and the absence of thought disorder* in all cases" (p. 706).

Snyder (1972) commented on the similarities and differences between amphetamine psychosis and paranoid schizophrenia. His text is summarized in Table II.

What about the differences?

1. The *strong sexual stimulation* in amphetamine psychosis presented by Snyder (1972) as a distinguishing criterion between the two psychoses does not rest on solid ground. While Connell (1958, pp. 16–26) did report an increase in sexuality in 7 amphetamine psychotics, sexuality was not affected in 5 of his patients and was decreased in another 5. Ellinwood (1967) also stated that "changes in libido were found to vary extensively" (p. 278). In addition, while an increase in sexual stimulation correlated with

*"By thought disorder is meant the splitting and loosening of associations, concrete and bizarre meanings in abstract thought, an impairment of goal-directed thought" (Bell, 1965, p. 704).

Table II.   Comparison of Amphetamine Psychosis and Paranoid Schizophrenia

Similarities	Differences
1. Clear sensorium. 2. High incidence of auditory hallucinations, 3. Phenothiazines (and other antipsychotics) are highly efficacious in treatment.	1. Strong sexual stimulation and stereotypic compulsive behavior in amphetamine psychosis. 2. Failure to display flattened affect in amphetamine psychosis. 3. Lack of a formal thought disorder in amphetamine psychosis.

the development of psychosis in some amphetamine addicts, according to Ellinwood (1967), "an increase in libido and polymorphous sexual activity most often preceded the psychosis" (p. 278). A distinguishing criterion based on the comparison of prepsychotic with psychotic individuals is not useful.

Stereotypic compulsive behavior exemplified by pacing back and forth and by movements of the mouth from side to side in a grimacing fashion was noted as a characteristic that distinguishes amphetamine psychosis from paranoid schizophrenia (Snyder, 1972). Experimental animals exhibit pronounced stereotypic behavior when injected with high doses of amphetamines (5–20 mg/kg). For example, following injection, rats became hyperactive, began sniffing, gnawing, and exhibiting strange posturing; some walked backward (Van Rossum, 1970). Stereotypic behaviors are probably species-specific (Randrup and Munkvad, 1967); in addition, human behaviors (such as sexual behaviors) are often much more complex than animal behaviors. Consequently, stereotypy in man may not be as strikingly pronounced as, for example, the gnawing of rats. However, stereotypy is seen in the intricately detailed and purposeless activity of taking apart clocks and making an inventory of the pieces exhibited by Swedish Preludin addicts (Snyder, 1972). Stereotypic behaviors are also noted in the nonpurposeful repetitive activities of rocking, tapping, and picking, clearly evident in some schizophrenic patients. Therefore, this does not seem to be a valid distinguishing marker between the two psychoses.

2. The *failure to display flattened affect* in individuals with amphetamine-induced psychosis at first glance appears to be a helpful discriminatory feature. Flat or inappropriate affect is a basic characteristic of schizophrenia and indeed one of Bleuler's "four A's." Paranoid schizophrenics, however, particularly acute paranoid schizophrenics, are often marked not by flattened affect, but on the contrary by strong affect—hostility, derision, and terror. Sometimes the delusional system is not all-pervasive and remnants of the patient's normal personality remain. Moreover, "although the evaluation of a schizophrenic patient's emotional reaction may serve as one of the most valuable diagnostic criteria, it is also frequently the least reliable of all observed data" (Lehmann, 1967). Consequently, this distinguishing feature between the two psychoses noted by some researchers rests on a shaky base.

3. *Lack of a formal thought disorder* in amphetamine-induced psychotics is one of the most frequently cited features capable of distinguishing the amphetamine psychosis from paranoid schizophrenia. Bell (1965) definitively states the differential diagnostic value of the absence of a thought disorder. Of the 14 patients he studied, 12 had no thought disorder, and the other 2 later developed "true" schizophrenia. The strength of his argument

is somewhat attenuated by a failure to study a similar control group of acute paranoid schizophrenics.

To discuss this category, it is essential to examine definitions. Is paranoia different from paranoid reactions, and are these in turn different from paranoid schizophrenia? Do paranoid conditions represent different points on a single continuum? Is the presence of a thought disorder (i.e., loose associations, blocking, and word salad) necessary for the diagnosis of schizophrenia? How is paranoid schizophrenia related to the schizophrenias in general? These questions are tied up in whether the lack of a formal thought disorder in amphetamine-induced psychotics is a valid distinguishing category.

3a. Is formal thought disorder part of paranoid schizophrenia? Snyder (1972) notes that "acute paranoid schizophrenics often fail to manifest an obvious thought disturbance" (p. 173) [although the reference he cites (Cameron, 1959) fails to support his statement]. The thought disturbance that does occur in acute paranoid schizophrenics seems to more often resemble the pressured speech of hypomania, in which there is a flight of ideas; like mania and unlike chronic schizophrenia, one can usually supply the connecting links and follow the chain of associations.

More recently, in a review of 200 process schizophrenics of which 31% were diagnosed as paranoid, only 20% of these had tangential thinking (Tsuang and Winokur, 1974). This particular study lends support to the notion that thought disorder is not a necessary correlate of paranoid schizophrenia. In addition, *DSM-II* (1968) states that in schizophrenia, paranoid type, there is not "the gross personality disorganization of the hebephrenic and catatonic types" (p. 34). Indeed, in practice in the United States, the presence of a thought disorder in a paranoid individual is probably not necessary for the diagnosis of schizophrenia.

A group at Vanderbilt (Griffith *et al.*, 1972) found that thought disorder was not part of the paranoid amphetamine psychosis experimentally induced in 9 subjects. They designated the syndrome as a "paranoid state." But even though such a diagnosis is described in the *DSM-II*, "psychiatrists find it is difficult to distinguish between schizophrenia and non-schizophrenic paranoid disorders" (Snyder, 1972, p. 173).

3b. Is paranoid schizophrenia different from other forms of paranoia and other forms of schizophrenia?

Cameron (1959), an authority on paranoid conditions, wrote in 1959 that "pure paranoid reactions . . . ones which show no hint of schizophrenic thinking . . . are seldom encountered." But in 1963, in an apparent reversal, Cameron (1963) wrote, "paranoid reactions seem to be common in the general population, but their number cannot be accurately estimated." Still later, in 1967, he (Cameron, 1967) noted that while "paranoia is extremely rare . . . paranoia and paranoid conditions together make up about 10% of hospital admissions." Nevertheless, in terms of model-building, where precision of definition is crucial, the amphetamine psychosis seems to fit the paranoid state more precisely than paranoid schizophrenia.

Snyder (1972) notes that "schizophrenias characteristically switch from one subtype of schizophrenia to another during their clinical history, and genetic studies indicate that a variety of different subtypes of schizophrenia may 'run' in families" (p. 171). The implication is that paranoid schizophrenia is not a distinct entity. On the other hand, there is an increasing clinical and research tendency to divide schizophrenic patients into two categories—paranoid and nonparanoid, implying that paranoid schizophrenia is a distinct entity (Wyatt *et al.*, 1977*a*).

The traditional separation of adult schizophrenia into the four subtypes of simple, catatonic, paranoid, and hebephrenic has been largely replaced in clinical practice by the following: acute and chronic undifferentiated schizophrenia, acute and chronic paranoid schizophrenia, schizoaffective schizophrenia, and borderline schizophrenia. Catatonic stupor, complete with waxy flexibility, appears to have genuinely decreased in incidence, while there are indications that "catatonic excitement," with its high mortality, may in fact be an acute viral infection (Penn *et al.*, 1972,. Hebephrenia is now regarded by some as a merely more deteriorated form of other types of schizophrenia; persons who would be diagnosed as simple schizophrenics usually do not enter the health systems. Consequently, the relative clarity of clinical presentation is precisely the reason that "paranoid schizophrenia" has maintained its utility as a diagnostic entity.

Finally, one other feature that has been used to distinguish amphetamine psychosis from schizophrenia is a high percentage of visual hallucinations (Ellinwood, 1972). Recently, however, there have been reports that the frequency of visual hallucinations in schizophrenic patients with hallucinations is higher than previously believed—in the range of 46–72% (Goodwin *et al.*, 1971).

Ellinwood (1972) noted that "chronic amphetamine reactions are much like syphilis in that they can mimic any number of psychiatric disorders, including hypomania, depression, emotional lability, and obsessive reactions; but the most constant and characteristic form, however, remains the paranoid schizophreniform syndrome."

2.2. Experimental Induction

In the previous section, we examined the fit between illicit self-induced paranoid episodes and endogenous paranoid schizophrenia; in this section, we will examine specific reactions to amphetamine administered in carefully controlled experimental settings and review its metabolism.

The experimental induction of amphetamine psychosis in humans has been limited by appropriate ethical considerations. To date, four studies (see Table III) have been published (Griffith *et al.*, 1970,* 1972*; Angrist *et al.*, 1971, 1972; Bell, 1973) that indicate that paranoid delusions of reference, control, and persecution can be regularly induced through either oral or intravenous administration.

A summary of the findings from experimental induction of amphetamine psychosis in humans indicates that:

1. The sequence of drug effects proceeds from variable *euphoria* (set-dependent), to *generalized depression* reflected by hypochondriasis, irritability, fault-finding, and dependent–demanding behavior. Next, a *prepsychotic phase* lasting several hours appears with associated withdrawal, negativism, abnormal interest in detail, and decreased verbal responsiveness. Transitory egodystonic ideas of reference occur, but can be put out of mind with effort. Finally, there is an abrupt onset of *acute paranoid psychosis* corresponding to Cameron's "crystallization." Subjects suddenly "understand" all their unusual perceptions. Paranoid ideation tends to clear in 1–3 days (Griffith *et al.*, 1970) after cessation of drug administration.

2. Amphetamine psychosis can be reliably induced in a little over 24 hr using a total oral dose of 400–540 mg (Angrist *et al.*, 1972). It has been induced over a 2-day period with oral doses as small as 100 mg *d*-amphetamine the first day and 20 mg the second day (Griffith *et al.*, 1970). Intravenous induction of psychosis can be achieved in under an hour in some patients, using doses of 120–360 mg methamphetamine (Bell, 1973) (prior amphetamine abuse in these subjects, however, confounds this finding). Furthermore, somatic side effects make the intravenous approach less desirable than the oral route.

The amphetamine psychosis is, at times, virtually indistinguishable from acute paranoid schizophrenia.

The frequently cited "lack of thought disorder" as a criterion to differentiate the amphetamine psychosis from paranoid schizophrenia is shaky. Loose association—the hallmark of thought disorder—is often missing in the endogenous psychosis, and has been occasionally reported present in the induced psychosis (Angrist *et al.*, 1972).

2.3. Metabolism

d-Amphetamine, 10 mg p.o., is maximally absorbed in about 2 hr with a serum concentration of 35 ng/liter. Half-peak values occur from 0.5 to 1 hr

*These two references describe the same study.

Table III. Experimental Effects of Amphetamines in Man

Study	Number of subjects	Drug	Dosage, route and format	Administration duration	Clinical findings
Grittith et al. (1970)	6	d-Amphetamine	120–700 mg total dose, oral and intravenous	1–5 days	5 of 6 subjects had a clear-cut paranoid psychosis.
Angrist et al. (1971)	3	d-Amphetamine l-Amphetamine d,l-Amphetamine	270–640 mg total dose, oral	17–30 hr	Similar doses of d- and l-amphetamine isomers caused equivalent behaviors.
Griffith et al. (1972)	9	d-Amphetamine	120–770 mg total dose, oral and intravenous	1–5 days	8 of 9 subjects had paranoia.
Angrist et al. (1972)	4	d,l-Amphetamine	450–565 mg total dose, oral	23–32 hr	2 of 4 subjects became psychotic; 2 of 4 had tangential associations.
Bell (1973)	16	Methamphetamine	50–640 mg total dose, intravenous	75 min	12 of 16 became psychotic in 1–90 hr; stayed psychotic 1–6 days.

on the way up and from 6 to 8 hr on the way down, with levels dropping to about 5% of the peak values at 10 hr (Van Rossum, 1970). The biological half-life is estimated at 12 hr (Van Rossum, 1970). One-half the ingested amount is metabolized by biotransformation (presumably in the liver), and one-half is eliminated through renal excretion (Van Rossum, 1970). Metabolic pathways are species-specific: in man, deamination or *p*-hydroxylation, followed by conjugation and oxidation to benzoic acid; in the rat, ring hydroxylation; and in the rabbit, dealkylation.

3. Speculation

Large gaps exist in our knowledge concerning how amphetamine and paranoia are actually linked. We present speculative arguments based on investigations of how amphetamine might work in the body to produce paranoia. In addition, we explore other potential conditions necessary to make an individual paranoid.

3.1. Mechanism

Amphetamine is thought to have at least three pharmacological actions: blocking the enzyme monoamine oxidase, inhibiting catecholamine neuronal uptake, and inducing the release of catecholamines from neurons. The last of these is thought to be most the significant (Schildkraut and Kety, 1967; Fuxe and Ungerstedt, 1968). Recent investigation has been directed at whether the dopamine (DA) or norepinephrine (NE) system is more important and whether or not the two catecholamines might play different roles in amphetamine-induced behavior. Coyle and Snyder (1969) found that the *d* isomer of amphetamine was 10 times as potent as the *l* isomer in inhibiting reuptake of NE into neurons, while the two isomers were equipotent in inhibiting DA uptake. The same group (Taylor and Snyder, 1970) found a similar relationship with regard to behavior; i.e., the *d* isomer of amphetamine was 10 times as potent as the *l* isomer in enhancing locomotor activity, but only twice as potent in producing stereotypy. They concluded that NE, which was most significantly affected by *d*-amphetamine, was responsible for locomotion, while DA was responsible for the production of stereotypy.

Unfortunately, the apparent importance of these findings has decreased because (1) the initial observations have not been confirmed (Ferris *et al.,* 1972; Thornburg and Moore, 1973; Harris and Baldessarini, 1973); (2) the group's investigations focused on reuptake, while release is now thought to be the more important process (Simpson, 1975); and (3) the two isomers may in fact be metabolized differently (Ross and Renyi, 1975). Despite new explorations, no differential effect with regard to neuronal release has been found between the two amphetamine isomers (Ferris *et al.*, 1972; Heikkila *et al.*, 1975).

While it remains unknown which catecholamine is primarily involved in increased locomotor activity, recent investigations show that a functional increase in DA in the corpus striatum (Creese and Iversen, 1975; Randrup and Munkvad, 1970*) is related to amphetamine-induced stereotypy.

Phenylethylamine, a compound structurally related to amphetamine, has been proposed as involved in schizophrenia and other psychiatric disorders (Fisher *et al.*, 1972; Schildkraut, 1969; Wyatt *et al.*, 1977*b*). Since it is present in man (Saavedra, 1974), its relationship to schizophrenia is closer than the exogenous substance, amphetamine.

In addition to the catecholamines (DA and NE), and their close relative, phenylethylamine, other neurotransmitters including acetylcholine have been proposed as being involved in the amphetamine psychosis. For example, in rats, anticholinergic drugs potentiate amphetamine-induced stereotypy (Costall *et al.*, 1972; Deffenu *et al.*, 1970). Another study along these lines showed that the stimulant methylphenidate made 24 acute and chronic schizophrenic patients worse, but physostigmine given to 9 of these patients reversed the methylphenidate effect. Unfortunately, physostigmine given in the same manner alone to these patients had no effect (Janowski *et al.*, 1973).

3.2. Anatomical Substrate

To determine the anatomical sites of amphetamine activity, it is essential to examine the tracts that mediate NE and DA, the neurotransmitters thought to be primarily involved in amphetamine psychosis. In all probability, however, the action is multifactorial, depending on several neurotransmitters and on a number of brain structures (Van Rossum, 1970).

On the basis of fluorescent histochemical work done primarily in Sweden, the major pathways have been outlined in the rat (Ungerstedt, 1971). For NE, there are two pathways: ventral and dorsal. The ventral pathway has cell bodies in the medulla oblongata and pons with terminals in the lower brain stem, midbrain, and hypothalamus. The dorsal pathway has cell bodies in the locus coeruleus (at the stalk of the cerebellum) with terminals in almost all parts of the brain—but particularly in the cerebral cortex, the cerebeller cortex, and the hippocampus.

---

*Nine cross references are given in this paper, with further references given in Munkvad *et al.* (1968).

Similarly, there are three dopaminergic systems outlined in the rat: (1) nigrostriatal, (2) mesolimbic, and (3) tuberoinfundibular. The most important of these, the nigrostriatal, has cell bodies in the zona compacta of the substantia nigra in the midbrain, with terminals in the compacta, putamen, and amygdaloid nuclei.

The mesolimbic system arises in the interpeduncular nucleus of the midbrain and terminates in three structures that together comprise the "limbic striatum": (1) the nucleus accumbens septi (just anterior to the head of the caudate), and the general area in which Heath found EEG spiking using depth recording in schizophrenia (Hornykiewicz, 1966); (2) the bed nucleus of the stria terminalis; and (3) the deep portion of the olfactory tubercle (Stevens, 1973).

The tuberoinfundibular system has a possible role in the regulation of trophic hormones produced by the pituitary, such as prolactin. This relatively short tract originates in the arcuate nucleus of the hypothalamus and terminates in the median eminence (Snyder, 1972).

Stevens (1973) stated that most of the symptoms of schizophrenia resemble changes that follow lesions of the amygdala and hippocampus of the mesolimbic system. Schizophrenia, she (Stevens, 1973) speculates, in contrast to temporal lobe epilepsy, represents a derangement that occurs in "amine regulations at a limbic striatal filter or gate." Despite the current enthusiasm for tracing the mechanism via subcortical fluorescent catecholamine pathways, radioactively labeled amphetamine concentrates selectively in the brain hemispheres, and distributes uniformly throughout other tissues, without preference for the cell nucleus (Benakis and Thomasset, 1970).

3.3. Stress

The role of stress in precipitating many somatic disorders (such as peptic ulcer, asthma, headache) and psychological disorders (such as depression after death or anxiety before giving a speech) is well recognized. Stress has been shown to increase the activity of tyrosine hydroxylase, thus facilitating the production of DA and NE (Axelrod, 1972). Moreover, stress has been shown to increase plasma dopamine-β-hydroxylase (the enzyme that converts DA to NE) and to decrease mitochondrial monoamine oxidase (MAO) (Welch and Welch, 1970).

Stress is particularly intriguing in relationship to paranoia. If a person has delusions of persecution (a central feature of paranoid schizophrenia), he creates major external threats from minor external or internal stimuli. In addition, if a paranoid person is hyperreactive, he may then use his own heightened physiological responsiveness to tell him that a threat is larger than it in fact is.

Altered environmental conditions have been shown to lower the body's ability to handle amphetamine. For example, amphetamine is much more lethal when given to rats crowded together in a small enclosure than when given to rats who are housed by themselves (Frey, 1970). Similarly, short-term stress has been shown to elevate rat brain NE, DA, and 5HT, but more prolonged stress tends to lower brain amine concentrations (Welch and Welch, 1970, p. 422). Thus, a biologically normal person may respond to unusual stress by becoming paranoid.

Changes in the periphery might affect the brain. Alterations in the gonadal hormones may be related to the onset of schizophrenia. Dementia praecox, Kraepelin's name for the insanity ofpuberty and adolescence, seems to develop at a time when the body is specifically punctuated by the greatly increased production of gonadal steroids. In addition, "the special binding properties of the associated limbic and hypothalamic structures for gonadal and adrenal steroids suggest that particular vulnerability of the limbic striatum complex will be associated with maturation and other, including stress-induced, endocrine change" (Stevens, 1973). The possible role of gonadal steroids has been given new support by Wilson *et al.* (1974), who found that the addition of 15 mg oral methyltestosterone to a regimen of 150 mg impipramine caused the onset of clearcut paranoid ideation in 4 of 5 men. Along these lines, it is of some interest that there is a much earlier onset of schizophrenia in males than females (Rosenthal, 1970). It is well known that pituitary hormones activate testosterone and estrogen production. Is it not also possible that these same gonadal steroids influence brain function in ways other than through the feedback loop to the hypothalamus and pituitary?

Recent evidence to support the influence of the peripheral system on the CNS was reported by Post (1973). While studying the catecholamine hypothesis of affective disorders (i.e., mania has higher NE levels, depression lower levels), Post wondered about the effects of physical activity on central biogenic amines. Much to his surprise, simulated manic hyperactivity in moderately depressed subjects caused elevations in CSF NE, DA, and 5-HT.

Since both casual and scientific observation suggest that there are large differences in the amounts of environmental stress various persons can handle, it stands to reason that there may be differences in biological vulnerability to mental disease. In 1973, Wyatt *et al.* (1973) reported on platelet MAO activity in monozygotic twins discordant for schizophrenia. Not only did the schizophrenic twin have platelet MAO activity lower than normal, but so did his discordant twin. This group postulated that reduced platelet MAO activity may be a genetic marker for vulnerability to schizophrenia. Since decreased MAO by itself does not produce schizophrenia (MAO inhibitors are used to treat affective disorders), if reduced MAO is related to the cause of schizophrenia, it would have to be in conjunction with another genetic or environmental trait. Stress is one candidate for an environmental factor.

3.4. Chronic–Acute Differences

Despite great variation in psychiatric nomenclature, the qualifying adjectives "acute" and "chronic" have retained their widespread use in clinical and research settings. These terms are particularly prevalent in the description of schizophrenia. The wildly delusional "acute" patient conjures up a far different mental picture than the burnt-out "chronic" patient.

Sharp differences also exist in the way amphetamines act acutely and with more extended administration. For example, the previously mentioned progression of amphetamine effects described by Griffith *et al.* (1970), from euphoria, to generalized depression, to withdrawal and negativism, and to acute paranoid delusions represents a time sequence of 1–5 days. No thought disorder was noted. In animals, acute amphetamine primarily depletes NE, whereas chronic administration depletes both NE and DA (Grunne and Lewander, 1967). The vital importance of seeing the amphetamine psychosis as an evolving sequence of behaviors was stressed by Ellinwood *et al.* (1973). Swedish workers also emphasized that "the duration of the amphetamine intoxication is of greater importance than the drug level (Anggard *et al.*, 1973).

3.5. Amine-Interaction Etiology

So far, we have dealt with quantitative or qualitative differences in neurotransmitters (transmitter depletion and false transmitters) for a single biogenic amine, such as DA. But there is also the possibility of varying balances of NE, DA, and 5-HT being responsible for differing symptomatology. Just using these three transmitters with combinations of elevation or decrease, there are eight permutations (Table IV), each of which may reflect a differing pattern, such as depression, loose associations, agitation, hallucinations, or delusions. Schildkraut (1969) noted that large doses of

Table IV.   Permutations with Combinations of Three Neurotransmitters

Drug	1	2	3	4	5	6	7	8
NE	↑	↑	↑	↑	↓	↓	↓	↓
DA	↑	↓	↑	↓	↑	↓	↑	↓
5-HT	↑	↑	↓	↓	↑	↑	↓	↓

amphetamine lower the brain NE in animals and also cause small elevations in serotonin levels.

Knoll (1973) found that small and medium doses of amphetamine enhance catecholaminergic tone, while with high doses, the serotonergic tone is dominant. Schildkraut (1972) also stated: "Almost invariably, drugs which affect one of these monoamines will alter the metabolism of one or another. It has been difficult to isolate these effects experimentally, suggesting that functionally important interactions of the biogenic amines may occur within the brain."

Prange *et al.* (1974) also stressed the concept of amine interactions in their "permissive hypothesis of affective disorders," which postulates that "a deficit in central indoleaminergic transmission permits affective disorder, but is insufficient for its cause; and changes in central catecholaminergic transmission, when they occur in the context of a deficit in indoleaminergic transmission, act as a proximate cause for affective disorders and determine their quality, catecholaminergic transmission being elevated in mania and diminished in depression." More simply, this is a restatement of the catecholamine hypothesis with the additional prerequisite of lowered serotonin activity. Although the interactional model described above was designed for affective illness, the same kinds of biogenic amine interactions may be operative in schizophrenia.

3.6. Other Conditions Associated with Paranoia

In addition to paranoid schizophrenia and amphetamine psychosis, there are a variety of conditions in which paranoid thinking becomes prominent. Among these are postcardiac surgery (particularly aortic valve repairs) (Layne and Yudofsky, 1971), uremia, and senile dementia. Furthermore, there are many drugs that induce paranoid ideation with varying degrees of regularity. These include: *stimulants* (amphetamine,* cocaine, methylphenidate, ephedrine*), *antidepressants* [nortriptyline,* imipramine,* tranylcypromine (Himmelhoch *et al.*, 1972)], L-DOPA,* *analgesics* (lidocaine,* indomethacin,* opium alkaloids,* pentazocine,* carbamazepine*), *tranquilizers* (chlorpromazine, trifluoperazine,* diazepam*), ethosuximide, prednisone,* amantadine, LSD, atropine,* digitalis,* bromide, nitrogen narcosis, and lithium.*

It is interesting that a number of these conditions or agents that produce paranoia are characterized by a hypermetabolic state. Some forms of senility, however, are characterized by decreased brain oxygenation.

*These drugs were computer-indexed to paranoia by the FDA adverse drug reaction data bank during the period October 1969 through September 18, 1972.

The very early work of Kety (1959) disputed the importance of oxygen insufficiency in schizophrenia. We propose, however, that perhaps metabolism and oxygenation are still important. Perhaps some paranoia is the result of relative cerebral oxygen insufficiency.

Amphetamine, cocaine, and marijuana are the clearest examples of drugs that elevate the pulse and are also capable of inducing paranoid ideation. The transformation from euphoria to irritability to paranoia is commonplace. Moreover, subjects often report an awareness of increased pulse prior to the onset of euphoria or paranoia.

4. Conclusion

The search for answers to the problem of schizophrenia has led some investigators to explore the use of exogenous models of the endogenous psychosis. Amphetamine-induced psychosis in man closely corresponds to paranoid schizophrenia. Amphetamine-induced behavioral changes in animals mimic behaviors of paranoid schizophrenics. Consequently, the model of amphetamine-induced psychosis has been used to further understand paranoid schizophrenia.

Whether animal models are appropriate for a primarily cognitive disorder is open to question. Whether the behavioral differences between the two psychoses (which we see as small) significantly hinder investigation remains debatable. Certainly, the use of a model to explore the disorder has great value. Other substances and situations have been shown to produce paranoid reactions. If studied adequately, perhaps some of these could provide excellent models for paranoid schizophrenia. At present, the amphetamine psychosis appears to most closely fit the naturally occurring paranoid schizophrenic state.

5. References

Anggard, E., Jonsson, L.-E., Hogmark, A.-L., and Grunne, L.-M., 1973, Amphetamine metabolism in amphetamine psychosis, *Clin. Pharmacol. Ther. 14*(5):870–880.

Angrist, B. M., Shopsin, B., and Gershon, S., 1971, Comparative psychotomimetic effects of stereoisomers of amphetamine, *Nature, (London) 234*:152–153.

Angrist, B., Shopsin, B., and Gershon, S., 1972, Metabolites of monamines in urine and cerebrospinal fluid, after large dose amphetamine administration, *Psychopharmacologia (Berlin) 26*:1–9.

Axelrod, J., 1972, Biogenic amines and their impact in psychiatry, *Semin. Psychiatry 4*(3):199–210.

Bell, D. S., 1965, Comparison of amphetamine psychosis and schizophrenia, *Br. J. of Psychiatry 111*:701–707.

Bell, D. S., 1973, The experimental reproduction of amphetamine psychosis, *Arch. Gen. Psychiatry* 29:35–40.

Benakis, A., and Thomasset, M., 1970, Metabolism of amphetamines and their interaction with barbiturates and SKF-525A, in: *Amphetamines and Related Compounds: Proceedings of the Mario Negri Institute for Pharmacologic Research, Milan, Italy* (E. Costa and S. Garattini, eds.), pp. 153–164, Raven Press, New York.

Bradley, C., 1937, The behavior of children receiving Benzedrine, *Am. J. Psychiatry* 94:577–585.

Cameron, N., 1959, Paranoid conditions and paranoia, in: *American Handbook of Psychiatry* (S. Arieti, ed.), Vol. 1, p. 510, Basic Books, New York.

Cameron, N., 1963, *Personality Development and Psychopathology—A Dynamic Approach,* p. 475, Houghton Mifflin Co., Boston.

Cameron, N. A., 1967, Psychotic disorders. II. Paranoid reactions, in: *Comprehensive Textbook of Psychiatry* (Alfred M. Freedman and Harold I. Kaplan, eds.), p. 666, Williams & Wilkins Co., Baltimore.

Chapman, A. H., 1954, Paranoid psychosis associated with amphetamine usage: A clinical note, *Am. J. Psychiatry* 111:43.

Connell, P. H., 1958, *Amphetamine Psychosis,* Chapman and Hall, London.

Costall, B., Naylor, R. J., and Wright, T., 1972, The use of amphetamine-induced stereotyped behavior as a model for the experimental evaluation of antiparkinson agents, *Arzneim.-Forsch.* 22(7):1178–1183.

Coyle, J. T., and Snyder, S. H., 1969, Catecholamine uptake by synaptosomes in homogenates of rat brain: Stereospecificity in different areas, *J. Pharmacol. Exp. Ther.* 170:221–231.

Creese, I., and Iversen, S. D., 1975, The pharmacological and anatomical substrates of the amphetamine response in the rat, *Brain Res.* 83:419–436.

Deffenu, G., Bartolini, A., and Pepeu, G., 1970, Effect of amphetamine on cholinergic systems of the cerebral cortex of the cat, in: *Amphetamines and Related Compounds: Proceedings of the Mario Negri Institute for Pharmacologic Research, Milan, Italy* (E. Costa and S. Garattini, eds.), pp. 357–368, Raven Press, New York.

Delay, J., Pichot, P., Lemperiere, T., and Sadown, R., 1954, *Ann. Med-Psychol.* 112(2):51.

DSM-II (Diagnostic and Statistical Manual of Mental Disorders), 1968, 2nd Ed., American Psychiatric Association, Washington, D.C.

Ellinwood, E. H., Jr., 1967, Amphetamine psychosis. 1. Description of the individuals and process, *J. Nerv. Ment. Dis.* 144:273–283.

Ellinwood, E. H., Jr., 1972, Amphetamine psychosis: Individuals, settings, and sequences, in: *Current Concepts on Amphetamine Abuse* (E. H. Ellinwood and S. Cohen, eds.), p. 144, National Institute of Mental Health, Rockville, Maryland.

Ellinwood, E. H., Jr., Sudilovsky, A., Nelson, L. M., 1973, Evolving behavior in the clinical and experimental amphetamine (model) psychosis, *Am. J. Psychiatry* 130(10):1088–1093.

Ferris, R. M., Tang, F. L. M., Maxwell, R. A., 1972, A comparison of the capabilities of isomers of amphetamine, deoxypipradol and methylphenidate to inhibit the uptake of tritiated catecholamines into rat cerebral cortex slices, synaptosomal preparations of rat cerebral cortex, hypothalamus and striatum and into the adrenergic nerves of the rabbit aorta, *J. Pharmacol. Exp. Ther.* 181:407–416.

Fisher, E., Spatz, H., Saavedra, M., Reggiani, H., Miro, A. H., and Heller, B., 1972, Urinary elimation of phenylethylamine, *Biol. Psychiatry* 5(2):139–147.

Frey, H. H., 1970, *p*-Chloroamphetamine—similarities and dissimilarities to amphetamine, in: *Amphetamines and Related Compounds: Proceedings of the Mario Negri Institute for Pharmacologic Research, Milan, Italy* (E. Costa and S. Garattini, eds.), p. 343, Raven Press, New York.

Fuxe, K., and Ungerstedt, U., 1968, Histochemical studies on the effect of (+)-amphetamine, drugs of the imipramine group and tryptamine on central catecholamine and 5-hydroxytryptamine neurons after intraventricular injection of catecholamines and 5-hydroxytryptamine, *Eur. J. Pharmacol. 4*:135–144.

Gillin, J. C., Kaplan, J., Stillman, R. C., and Wyatt, R. J., 1976, The psychedelic model of schizophrenia: The case of *N,N*-dimethyl-tryptamine (DMT), *Am. J. Psychiatry 133*:203–208.

Goodwin, D. W., Alderson, P., and Rosenthal, R., 1971, Clinical significance of hallucinations in psychiatric disorders: A study of 116 hallucinatory patients, *Arch. Gen. Psychiatry 24*:76–80.

Griffith, J. D., Cavanaugh, J., Held, J., and Oates, J. A., 1970, Experimental psychosis induced by the administration of *d*-amphetamine, in: *Amphetamines and Related Compounds: Proceedings of the Mario Negri Institute for Pharmacologic Research, Milan, Italy* (E. Costa and S. Garattini, eds.), pp. 897–904, Raven Press, New York.

Griffith, J. D., Cavanaugh, J., Held, J., and Oates, J. A., 1972, Dextroamphetamine: Evaluation of psychotomimetic properties in man, *Arch. Gen. Psychiatry 26*:97–100.

Grunne, E., and Lewander, T., 1967, Long-term effects of some dependence-producing drugs on the brain monamines, in: *Molecular Basis of Some Aspects of Mental Activity* (O. Wahaas, ed.), Vol. 2, pp. 75–81, New York.

Harris, J. E., and Baldessarini, R. J., 1973, Uptake of [³H]catecholamines by homogenates of rat corpus striatum and cerebral cortex: Effects of amphetamine analogues, *Neuropharmacology 12*:669–679.

Heikkila, R. E., Orlansky, H., Mytilineou, C., and Cohen, G., 1975, Amphetamine: Evaluation of *d*- and *l*-isomers as releasing agents and uptake inhibitors for ³H-dopamine and ³H-norepinephrine in slices of rat neostriatum and cerebral cortex, *J. Pharmacol. Exp. Ther. 194*:47–56.

Himmelhoch, J. M., Detre, T., Kupfer, D. J., and Byck, R., 1972, Treatment of previously intractable depressions with tranylcypromine and lithium, *J. Nerv. Ment. Dis. 155*:216–220.

Hollister, L. E., 1968*a*, Human pharmacology of lysergic acid diethylamide (LSD), in: *Psychopharmacology: A Review of Progress 1957–1967* (D. H. Efron, ed.), Public Health Service Publication 1836, pp. 1253–1261, U.S. Government Printing Office, Washington, D.C.

Hollister, L. E., 1968*b*, *Chemical Psychoses,* pp. 117–126, Charles C. Thomas, Springfield, Illinois.

Hornykiewicz, O., 1966, Dopamine 3-hydroxytryptamines and brain function, *Pharmacol. Rev. 18*(2):925–964.

Innes, I. R., and Nickerson, M., 1970, Amphetamine, in: *The Pharmacological Basis of Therapeutics* (Louis S. Goodman and Alfred Gilman, eds.), 3rd Ed., p. 501, Macmillan Co., New York.

Janowski, D. S., El-Yousef, K., Davis, J. M., Sekerke, H. J., 1973, Antagonist effects of physostigmine and methylphenidate in man, *Am. J. Psychiatry 130*(12):1370–1376.

Kalant, O. J., 1966, *The Amphetamines—Toxicity and Addiction,* p. 53, Charles C. Thomas, Springfield, Illinois.

Kety, S. S., 1959, Biochemical theories of schizophrenia, *Science 129*:1–12.

Knoll, J., 1973, Modulation of learning and retention by amphatamines, in: *Pharmacology and the Future of Man: Proceedings of the Fifth International Congress on Pharmacology, San Francisco 1972*, Vol. 4, pp. 55–68, S. Karger, Basel.

Kramer, J. C., 1969, Introduction to amphetamine abuse, *J. Psychedelic Drugs 11*(2):1–16.

Layne, O. L., Jr., and Yudofsky, S. C., 1971, Postoperative psychosis in cardiotomy patients: Role of organic and psychiatric factors, *N. Engl. J. Med. 284*:518–520.

Lehmann, H. E., 1967, Schizophrenia: Clinical features, in: *Comprehensive Textbook of*

Psychiatry (Alfred M. Freedman and Harold I. Kaplan, eds.), p. 629, Williams & Wilkins Co., Baltimore.

Licit and Illicit Drugs, 1972 (Edward M. Brecher & the Editors of *Consumers Reports* eds.), Consumers Union, Mt. Vernon, New York.

Munkvad, I., Pakkenberg, H., and Randrup, A., 1968, Aminergic systems in basal ganglia associated with stereotyped behavior and catelepsy, *Brain Behav. Evol. 1*:89–100.

Nathanson, M. H., 1939, The central action of beta-amino-aminopropyl benzene (Benzedrine): Clinical observations, *J. Am. Med. Assoc. 108*:528–531.

Penn, H., Racy, J., Lapham, L., Mandel, M., and Sandt, J., 1972, Catatonic behavior, viral encephalopathy, and death, *Arch. Gen. Psychiatry 27*:758–761.

Post, R. M., 1973, Simulated behaviour states: An approach to specificity in psychobiological research, *Biol. Psychiatry 7*:237–254.

Prange, A. J., Wilson, I. C., Lynn, C. W., Allsop, L. B., and Stikeleather, R. A., 1974, L-Tryptophan in mania: Contribution to a permissive hypothesis of affective disorders, *Arch. Gen. Psychiatry 30*:56–62.

Prinzmetal, M., and Bloomberg, W., 1935, The use of Benzedrine for the treatment of narcolepsy, *J. Am. Med. Assoc. 105*:2051–2054.

Randrup, A., and Munkvad, I., 1967, Stereotyped activities produced by amphetamine in several animal species and man, *Psychopharmacologia (Berlin) 11*:300–310.

Randrup, A. and Munkvad, I., 1970, Biochemical, anatomical, and psychological investigations of stereotyped behavior induced by amphetamines, in: *Amphetamines and Related Compounds: Proceedings of the Mario Negri Institute for Pharmacologic Research, Milan, Italy* (E. Costa and S. Garattini, eds.), pp. 695–713, Raven Press, New York.

Rosenthal, D., 1970, *Genetic Theory and Abnormal Behavior,* McGraw-Hill, New York.

Ross, S. B., and Renyi, A.-L., 1975, Inhibition of uptake of ^{3}H-dopamine and ^{14}C-5-hydroxy-tryptamine in mouse striatum slices, *Acta Pharmacol. Toxicol. 36*:56–66.

Saavedra, J. M., 1974, Enzymatic isotopic assay for and presence of β-phenylethylamine in brain, *J. of Neurochem. 22*:211.

Schildkraut, J. J., 1969, Neuropsychopharmacology and the affective disorders, *N. Engl. J. Med. 281*:302–306.

Schildkraut, J. J., 1972, Neuropharmacologically generated models of the affective disorders: Biochemical versus behavioral models, *Psychopharmacol. Bull. 8*(3):61–62.

Schildkraut, J. J., and Kety, S. S., 1967, Biogenic amines and emotion, *Science 156*(3771):21–30.

Simpson, S. I., 1975, Blood pressure and heart rate responses evoked by *d*- and *l*-amphetamine in the pithed rat preparation, *J. Pharmacol. Exp. Ther. 193*:149–159.

Slater, E., 1959, Amphetamine psychosis, *Br. Med. J. 1*:488.

Snyder, S. H., 1972, Catecholamines in the brain as mediators of amphetamine psychosis, *Arch. Gen. Psychiatry 27*:169–179.

Stevens, J. R., 1973, An anatomy of schizophrenia?, *Arch. Gen. Psychiatry 29*:177–189.

Taylor, K. M., and Snyder, S. H., 1970, Amphetamine: Differentiation by *d* and *l* isomers of behavior involving brain norepinephrine or dopamine, *Science 168*:1487–1489.

Thornburg, J. E., and Moore, K. E., 1973, Dopamine and norepinephrine uptake by rat brain synaptosomes: Relative inhibitory potencies of *l*- and *d*-amphetamine and amantadine, *Res. Commun. Chem. Pathol. Pharmacol. 5*:81–89.

Tsuang, M. T., and Winokur, G., 1974, Criteria for sub-typing schizophrenia: Clinical differentiation of hebephrenia and paranoid schizophrenia, *Arch. Gen. Psychiatry 31*:43–47.

Ungerstedt, U., 1971, Stereotaxic mapping of the monamine pathways in the rat brain, *Acta Physiol. Scand. 367(Suppl.)*:1–48.

Van Rossum, J. M., 1970, Mode of action of psychomotor stimulant drugs, *Int. Rev. Neurobiol. 12*:307–383.

Wallis, G. G., McHarg, J. F., and Scott, O. C. A., 1949, Acute psychosis caused by dextroamphetamine, *Br. Med. J., 2*:1394.

Waud, S. P., 1938, The effects of toxic doses of benzyl methyl carbinamine (Benzedrine) in man, *J. Am. Med. Assoc. 110*:206.

Welch, B. L., and Welch, A. S., 1970, Control of brain catecholamines and serotonin during acute stress and after *d*-amphetamine by natural inhibition of monamine-oxidase: An hypothesis, in: *Amphetamines and Related Compounds: Proceedings of the Mario Negri Institute for Pharmacologic Research, Milan, Italy* (E. Costa and S. Garattini, eds.), pp. 415–445, Raven Press, New York.

Wilson, I. C., Prange, A. J., Jr., and Laura, P. P., Methyltestosterone with imipramine in men: Conversion of depression to paranoid reaction, *Am. J. Psychiatry 131*(1): 21–24.

Wyatt, R. J., Murphy, D. L., Belmaker, R., Cohen, S., Donnelly, C. H., and Pollin, W., 1973, Reduced monamine oxidase activity in platelets: A possible genetic marker for vulnerability to schizophrenia, *Science 179*:916–918.

Wyatt, R. J., Potkin, S. G., Gillin, J. C., and Murphy, D. L., 1977*a*, Enzymes involved in phenylethyalmine and catecholamine metabolism in schizophrenics and controls in: *Psychopharmacology: A Review of Progress 1967–1976* (M. Lipton and A. DiMascio, eds.), Raven Press, New York (in press).

Wyatt, R. J., Gillin, J. C., Stoff, D. M., Moja, E. A., and Tinklenberg, J. R. 1977*b*, β-Phenylethylamine (PEA) and the neuropsychiatric disturbances, in: *Neuroregulators and Psychiatric Disorders* (E. Usdin, J. Barchas, and D. Hamburg, eds.), pp. 31–45, Oxford University Press. New York.

Young, D., and Scoville, W. B., 1938, Paranoid psychosis in narcolepsy and the possible danger of Benzedrine treatment, *Med. Clin. North Am. 22*:637–646.

2

Hypersensitive Serotonergic Receptors Involved in Clinical Depression—A Theory

M. H. Aprison, Ryo Takahashi, and K. Tachiki

1. Introduction

As many investigators will attest, developing and conducting a research program in the field of mental health is a very difficult task. It is only in the last 20 years that a few hints have appeared in the literature from animal research in the fields of neuropharmacology and neurochemical correlates of behavior that give the researcher any leads on which to base an active clinical–basic research program. These ideas have led to some important clinical studies that will be referred to below. It is interesting that some recent work with animal models of depression has again provided the research clinician with new insights for further experimentation.

To investigate the causes of abnormal behavior in man, the researcher is confronted with ethical as well as technical problems in designing such studies, i.e., how to study biochemical events in the brain and relate these events to normal or abnormal behavior in man. For this reason, many researchers have begun their research programs in this field by studying the

M. H. Aprison and K. Tachiki • Section of Applied and Theoretical Neurobiology, Institute of Psychiatric Research, Indiana University Medical Center, Indianapolis, Indiana 46202 *Ryo Takahashi* • Department of Neuropsychiatry, Nagasaki University School of Medicine, Nagasaki, Japan

role of key compounds in the CNS of animals. Thus, at least two general types of studies with animals emerge in the field of behavior–neurotransmitter research: (1) those that utilize pharamacological and/or nondrug manipulations of behavior in addition to neurochemical measures, and attempt to correlate these parameters on a continuing time base, and (2) those that utilize only psychopharmacological procedures, i.e., the measurement of drug effects on behavior, but infer changes in neurotransmitter levels.

In investigating the relationships between brain and behavior, one hopes that such studies will lead to an understanding of the neurobiological mechanisms that underlie both normal and abnormal behavior. Further, if one assumes that the brain is the source of events that finally govern the behavior of an organism, then impaired behavior may occur due to one or more "lesions" of a biophysical, biochemical, or anatomical nature (Aprison and Hingtgen, 1970). In the CNS, these lesions affect the most important function of neurons, namely, the transfer of information to other neurons. Since this transfer of information is mediated by the process of synaptic transmission within the mammalian nervous system, and since this process is mainly chemical, it is not surprising that researchers have chosen to study the effect of changing the level of putative neurotransmitters on behavior (Aprison, 1965; Aprison and Hingtgen, 1970, 1972; Aprison et al., 1975; Nagayama et al., 1972; Takahashi et al., 1974, 1975; Tateishi et al., 1975). Although these studies are performed on animals, the ultimate goal of such work is that the data will provide useful insights into the specific biochemical mechanisms that may cause certain types of abnormal behavior in patients.

The research groups of Aprison in the United States and Takahashi in Japan have shown that by quantitatively measuring the behavioral responses of an animal, criteria for typical and atypical behavior can be clearly established (Aprison and Ferster, 1960, 1961a; Aprison and Hingtgen, 1970; Hingtgen and Aprison, 1965, 1976; Nagayama et al., 1972; Takahashi et al., 1974, 1975; Tachiki et al., 1976). From such studies, it is evident that patterns of responding can be determined for many different behaviors, both learned and unlearned. Thus, the effects of manipulating the levels of various neurotransmitters in the intact organism can be assessed by reliable, sensitive, and reproducible behavioral procedures. When biochemical analyses of the CNS tissue from animals are made before, during, and after these manipulations, a more complete picture of neurochemical correlates of behavior can be developed. The relevancy and validity of data from animal studies with regard to human behavior must always be cautiously and critically appraised. In agreement with many investigators in this field, however, the authors feel that there are some general behavioral–neurochemical relationships applicable to a number of animal species as well as the human organism.

In this chapter, the authors will review two lines of research that have employed animal models of depression.* These studies led to the conclusion that increases in the level of free 5-hydroxytryptamine (5-HT or serotonin) in the clefts of some serotonergic synapses produces behavioral suppression in animals. We will briefly review some of the data reflecting the present status of our knowledge concerning the serotonergic system in man. A quick perusal of the early literature pertaining to the animal data and the clinical data might lead the reader to conflicting conclusions (i.e., that suppression of animal behavior is caused by an increase in the levels of 5-HT in the synaptic cleft, whereas depression in human beings is associated with a deficiency of 5-HT in the synaptic region). We will present, however, our current hypothesis, which explains these apparent difficulties. With this hypothesis, we now feel that the existing data are compatible, and what is even more important, it suggests new experiments that after being tested in the animal models may lead to important clinical trials in humans.

2. Two Serotonergic Models of Depression Based on Drug-Induced Atypical Behavior in Animals

2.1. A Tryptophan–5-Hydroxytryptophan Model

Interest in the role of 5-HT in brain developed when it was shown in pharmacological studies on smooth muscle that d-lysergic acid diethylamide, a compound that provokes schizophreniclike states in man, is an antagonist of 5-HT at certain doses (Gaddum, 1954), but acts synergistically at lower doses (Costa, 1956). The studies of Woolley and Shaw (1954a,b) on antimetabolites of 5-HT also added impetus for work in this area. Costa and Aprison (1958a), while in Dr. Harold Himwich's laboratories, studied the distribution of 5-HT in human brain and showed that there were marked differences in various discrete areas. These results were similar to those found in the brains taken from animals (Bogdanski et al., 1957; Garven, 1956; Paasonen et al., 1957; Costa and Aprison, 1958b). All these studies

---

*Two groups of investigators were involved in these different studies. One group did their experiments in the United States (Aprison and co-workers) and the other in Japan (Takahashi and co-workers). To bridge the work between these two groups, Dr. Tachiki went to Japan as a visiting assistant professor (1974–1975) and as a Foreign Research Fellow of the Japan Society for Promotion of Science in Dr. Takahashi's laboratories.

suggested to many investigators that 5-HT probably played an important role in brain function.

Approximately 16 years ago, Aprison and co-workers began to conduct a number of neurochemical–behavioral studies designed to test whether any temporal correlations could be found between changes in the serotonergic system in areas of the brains of animals whose behavior was disrupted by pharmacological means. These experiments were made possible because the main metabolic steps involved in the biosynthesis and enzymatic degradation of 5-HT were known and indicated that the level of cerebral 5-HT can be elevated by (1) injecting its precursor, 5-hydroxytryptophan (5-HTP), or L-tryptophan; (2) injecting an inhibitor of the catabolic enzyme MAO (such as iproniazid); or (3) injecting 5-HTP (or tryptophan) after pretreatment with iproniazid. In addition to these pharmacological manipulations and the measurement of the increase in cerebral 5-HT quantitative measures of the behavior of animals were also necessary.

These latter measures can be obtained in a number of ways. Aprison, Ferster, and Hingtgen chose to use operant conditioning techniques, since they are objective, reliable, and sensitive (Aprison and Ferster, 1961a; Hingtgen and Aprison, 1965; Aprison and Hingtgen, 1970). The operant behavior measured in the studies to be described was emitted under an approach schedule of reinforcement. White Carneaux cocks, 6 months old at the start of the experiment, were used in these studies. The pigeons were maintained at 80% of their free-feeding weight and trained to perform in a Skinner box (Ferster and Skinner, 1957). The performance recorded was that of pecking at a 1-inch disk commonly used in operant conditioning research with pigeons. The birds pecked because they were hungry and occasionally rewarded with food. The experimental session was 6 hr long or 55 reinforcements, whichever occurred first. When injected compounds disrupted the birds' performance, the session was prolonged to measure the recovery of the performance. A multiple fixed-ratio, fixed-interval schedule of reinforcement (multiple FR 50 FI 10) was used as the base line to determine the behavioral effects of injected 5-HTP, 5-HT, or tryptophan. For rats, the approach schedule of reinforcement was a variable ratio 40 (VR 40), in which lever-pressing was reinforced with chocolate milk.

The initial attempt to assess the behavioral changes resulting from increased levels of cerebral 5-HT consisted of establishing a dose–response relationship following injections of 5-HTP into pigeons working on a multiple FR 50 FI 10 schedule of reinforcement. Similar experiments were conducted with L-tryptophan. Intramuscular injections of doses of 25, 50, and 75 mg/kg D,L-5-HTP or of 100, 200, and 300 mg/kg L-tryptophan have increasingly disruptive effects on the pigeons' rate of responding (see Table I and Aprison and Ferster, 1960, 1961a; Hingtgen and Aprison, 1975). The

Table I. Duration of Behavioral Depression in
Pigeons Working on a Multiple FR 50 FI 10
Schedule of Reinforcement after Administration
of D,L-5-Hydroxytryptophan (D,L-5-HTP) or L-
Tryptophan (L-Try)[a]

Dose (mg/kg)		Behavioral depression (min)[b]
D,L-5-HTP	L-Try	
25	—	56 ± 14
50	—	133 ± 24
75	—	209 ± 33
—	100	27 ± 10
—	200	54 ± 9
—	300	123 ± 20

[a]All injections were intramuscular. There were 6 cocks in each group.
[b]Mean ± S.E.M.

duration of the effect was usually over before the 6-hr experimental session ended.

Since little 5-HT crosses the blood–brain barrier under normal physiological conditions compared with its precursor 5-HTP (Costa and Aprison, 1958b), a study was made to determine the behavioral effect of an intramuscular injection of 5-HT into pigeons performing on a multiple FR 50 FI 10 schedule. A behavioral effect comparable to that of 5-HTP was produced, but with a much smaller dose of 5-HT; this effect was thought to be due principally to the peripheral actions of 5-HT. Since small doses of 5-HT had large behavioral effects, one might argue that the behavioral effects of 5-HTP were also due to peripheral serotonin. The following evidence suggests, however, that even though 5-HTP acting peripherally may affect the animal's behavior, its major influence is through the CNS. Iproniazid, which is a much better central than peripheral MAO inhibitor *in vivo*, enhanced the behavioral effects of injected 5-HTP or L-tryptophan (Aprison and Ferster, 1961b,c; Hingtgen and Aprison, 1975).

When the same dose of 5-HTP was injected into iproniazid-pretreated pigeons at different intervals over a long period of time, both the behavior and the MAO activity in brain returned to normal levels in about 35 days, whereas the MAO activity in liver was back to normal in only 12 days. The return of the behavioral effect was readily correlated with the recovery of the brain MAO activity (Aprison and Ferster, 1961b,c). In studies in which the dose of 5-HTP was varied and the dose of iproniazid held constant, it was found that at any level of brain MAO activity (during the recovery period), the greatest behavioral effect was obtained at the highest 5-HTP dose injected. Even more important, these data show that at any given dose of 5-HTP, the greatest behavioral effect is obtained at the lowest brain MAO level during the recovery period (Aprison and Ferster, 1961b,c). The free 5-HT in brain, which apparently is involved in the production of the behavioral effect (as a transmitter or modulator), probably comprises the 5-HT found at any instant in the synaptic cleft. However, there probably exists a labile storage pool within the presynaptic nerve endings that is also very important. The latter pool can be thought of as a source of readily available 5-HT at a specific synapse, and is probably in equilibrium with a second pool of 5-HT, the firmly bound storage pool (Aprison and Hingtgen, 1972). Serotonin reentering the presynaptic nerve ending either enters the labile storage pool or is destroyed by MAO in the mitochondria. Since an identical amount of 5-HTP was injected at various times during the period that brain MAO activity was returning to normal in the experiments mentioned above, the observed behavioral change should be due to action of available cerebral 5-HT formed from its precursor and released at the appropriate synapses. As the MAO activity increased, more 5-HT was destroyed and less was available to produce physiological and behavioral effects.

If the behavioral changes seen in the pigeons is caused by the action of released 5-HT and the latter is controlled by the activity of its catabolic enzyme located in the mitochondria of the presynaptic nerve endings, important additional information can be obtained by studying the kinetic relationship between the 5-HTP- or tryptophan-induced behavioral disruption and the variation in the content of cerebral 5-HT in animals not given an MAO inhibitor. Such a study was conducted in 1962 (Aprison et al., 1962), and total serotonin was measured in four specific brain areas (telencephalon, diencephalon plus optic lobes, cerebellum, and pons–medulla oblongata), as well as in liver, heart, lung, and blood in pigeons sacrificed at various time intervals during the period of behavioral disruption following an injection of 50 mg/kg D,L-5-HTP (Hingtgen and Aprison, 1965). Since the time course of the behavioral effect in any given animal is relatively invariant with a constant dose of 5-HTP, while there is marked variation in the time course of response from animal to animal, a unique method of treating these data was developed by Aprison et al. (1962). The data on 5-HT were plotted against the percentage of the behavioral effect rather than the length of time after 5-HTP administration. In this way, the variation in behavioral effect of the same dose of 5-HTP in each pigeon was weighted, and the variability of the data was greatly reduced. The behavioral depression was temporally related to the three- to fourfold increase in 5-HT content in only the telencephalon and diencephalon (Fig. 1). Thus, the time

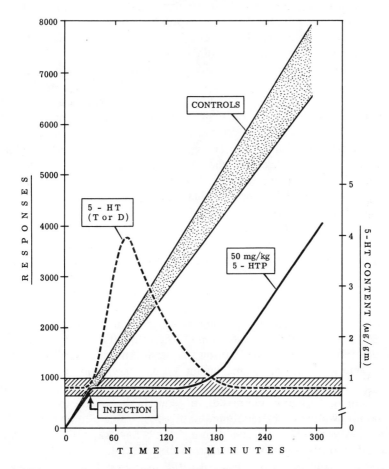

Fig. 1. Diagrammatic representation of the effect of an intramuscular injection of 50 mg/kg D,L-5-HTP on the approach response rate and the content of 5-HT in the telencephalon (T) or diencephalon plus optic lobes (D) of the pigeon. After the injection of 5-HTP, the level of 5-HT increases, passes through a maximum, and then decreases to normal. The behavior of the experimental animal was disrupted for a period of time and then returned to normal at approximately the same time as the levels of 5-HT returned to normal. The stippled band indicates the extreme range of response rates during control sessions (with or without saline injections). The hatched band at the bottom represents the range of the content of 5-HT in the telencephalon from control pigeons. The dashed line shows the change in content of 5-HT in this brain part at different times after the 5-HTP injection. Reprinted from Aprison and Hingtgen (1965) with permission. Copyright © 1965 by Pergamon Press, New York.

course of change in both parameters was remarkably similar, and confirmed the original explanation of the cerebral 5-HT–MAO–behavior correlation (Aprison and Ferster, 1961b,c; Aprison et al., 1962).

In 1965, the enzyme that synthesizes 5-HT, 5-HTP-decarboxylase, was thought to be the same as 3,4-dihydroxyphenylalanine (DOPA) decarboxylase, the enzyme that synthesizes dopamine (DA), the precursor of norepinephrine (NE). It therefore became imperative for Aprison and Hingtgen (1965) to measure DA and NE levels in a similar group of 5-HTP-injected pigeons. Consequently, another group of trained pigeons was given injections (intramuscular) of 50 mg/kg 5-HTP. The average period of depressed behavior following these injections was measured for each bird, and at various percentages of behavioral disruption, T, the pigeons were sacrificed by decapitation, and the four brain parts were assayed for DA and NE. No consistent significant changes were noted in the contents of DA and NE in the telencephalon and diencephalon. The levels of NE and DA in the pons–medulla oblongata and cerebellum appeared to change slightly with respect to normal levels; these changes did not appear to be correlated with the observed behavioral depression in the pigeons.

Aprison and Hingtgen (1966a) verified these data in another species by injecting 50 mg/kg 5-HTP into rats working on a VR 40 schedule of reinforcement. Similar correlations over the period of disruption were found between the changes in telencephalic 5-HT and changes in behavior. The elevated level of 5-HT in the brain stem returned to normal before the behavior returned to normal. During the period of behavioral disruption, the content of NE in the telencephalon did not vary from normal values, whereas after the behavior returned to normal, the content of NE in the brain stem was slightly depressed. In general, these data on rats agree remarkably well with the data found in pigeons. Using a third species, the monkey, Macchitelli et al. (1966) studied the behavioral effect of injecting D,L-HTP into these animals, which were working on food-reinforced approach schedules. As in the case of the pigeon and rat, the monkeys exhibited periods of behavioral depression.

Since increases in cerebral 5-HT are followed by disruptions in approach behavior, the question naturally arises: what behavioral changes would follow decreases in cerebral 5-HT? One method of reducing this amine in brain is to use drugs that deplete its bound stores in nerve endings. Since there are drugs, such as reserpine, tetrabenazine, and α-methyl-m-tyrosine (α-MMT), that can cause a fall in more than one transmitter, a differential fall in any one such compound over a reasonably long time period can be used to advantage by the researcher. Thus, Aprison and Hingtgen used α-MMT to produce a temporal differential depletion of cerebral 5-HT, NE, and DA, and then studied the relationship between the changes in these biogenic amines and the changes in behavior of the animals that were injected. At 3 hr after an injection of 100 mg/kg α-MMT, the behavioral response rates of pigeons working on a multiple FR 50 FI 10 schedule were lowered to about 20% of normal, and then gradually returned to preinjection levels after 9 hr (Hingtgen and Aprison, 1963). Another group of pigeons was decapitated at various times following α-MMT injection, and whole brain tissue was assayed for 5-HT, NE, DA, and the decarboxylation products of α-MMT, namely, α-methyl-*m*-tyramine (α-MMTA) and metaraminol (aramine). Amine levels varied as follows: (1) 5-HT was decreased 30% in 3 hr and returned to normal levels at about 9 hr; (2) NE was decreased 50% in 12 hr, and then returned to normal by 5–7 days; (3) DA decreased and remained below 50% of normal for 12 hr, returning to normal by 48 hr; and (4) α-MMTA increased and returned to normal by 2–4 days. The data indicated that the time course of the behavioral depression paralleled the time course of the changes in 5-HT content, but not that of the other amines measured (Aprison and Hingtgen, 1966*b*). The correlation of the changes in content of 5-HT and changes in behavior is seen in Fig. 2. Furthermore, it was noted that the increase in α-MMTA and metaraminol was best correlated with the fall in 5-HT plus NE

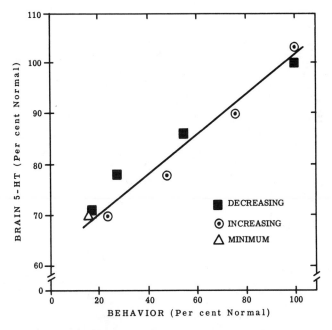

Fig. 2. Correlation between changes in the content of cerebral 5-HT and changes in the response rate of pigeons working on a multiple FR 50 FI 10 approach schedule of reinforcement after an intramuscular injection of 100 mg/kg α-MMT. Reprinted from *Federation Proceedings* 34:1813–1822 (1975).

plus DA (Fig. 3). Finally, an anorexic side effect for α-MMT was also ruled out, since pigeons working on the approach schedule as well as naïve birds consumed equivalent amounts of food after injections of saline or α-MMT (Hingtgen and Aprison, 1966). This also was true in the case of 5-HTP (Aprison and Hingtgen, 1965, 1966*b*).

2.1.1. *Hypothesis for Role of Serotonin in Depression of Approach Behavior and Some New Supporting Neurochemical Data*

After an injection of D,L-5-HTP, the levels of 5-HT in the brain increased, whereas after an injection of α-MMT, these levels decreased.

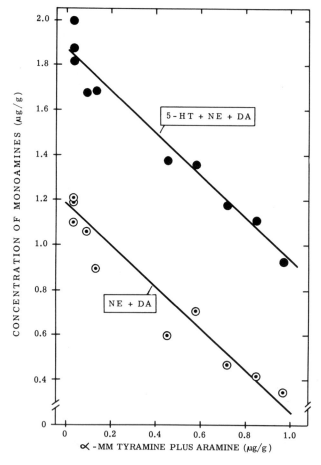

Fig. 3. Correlation between changes in levels of α-MMTA plus aramine and changes in levels of 5-HT plus NE plus DA in whole brain of pigeons following an intramuscular injection of 100 mg/kg α-MMT. Reprinted from *Federation Proceedings* 34:1813–1822 (1975).

Aprison's hypothesis to explain these two opposite biochemical states that result in the same type of behavioral change in the same animal species is that there is an increased release of 5-HT from nerve endings in both cases. It is these molecules of 5-HT that act on specific serotonergic receptors that cause the observed depression in the animal's behavior. Recent studies from Aprison's laboratories using isolated-nerve-ending preparations provided additional neurochemical evidence consistent with the theory that *in vivo,* both L-5-HTP and α-MMT could cause such an increased release of 5-HT.

Using preparations of nerve endings (P_2) isolated from the telencephalon and from the diencephalon plus optic lobes of pigeons and from the telencephalon of rats, McBride *et al.* (1974) studied the effects of 5-HTP on the content of 5-HT in nerve endings as well as the release of radioactively labeled 5-HT from nerve endings. The levels of 5-HTP, 5-HT, and 5-hydroxyindoleacetic acid (5-HIAA) were significantly higher in the nerve-ending fraction isolated from the telencephalon and from the diencephalon plus optic lobes of pigeons given intramuscular injections of 50 mg/kg D,L-5-HTP in comparison with control values (Fig. 4). These data provided direct biochemical evidence to indicate that the injected 5-HTP could accumulate within neurons and significantly raise the levels of 5-HT within the nerve endings.

Using amine concentrations (25 nM) that were supposed to label specifically serotonergic or catecholaminergic terminals, McBride *et al.* (1974) reported that L-5-HTP increased the release of tritiated 5-HT (5-[³H]HT) from serotonergic nerve terminals isolated from the telencephalon of the pigeon and rat (Fig. 5). Since this effect by L-5-HTP was blocked by *m*-hydroxy-*p*-bromobenzyl oxyamine (NSD-1055), a decarboxylase inhibitor, it would appear that it was not the L-5-HTP itself that caused the release of 5-[³H]HT, but instead was the newly synthesized 5-HT from the added L-5-HTP that resulted in the release of the labeled amine. Furthermore, L-5-HTP had no apparent effect on catecholaminergic terminals, since L-5-HTP, at a concentration of 1.5 mM, did not increase the release of [³H]NE or [³H]DA from nerve endings prepared from the telencephalon of the rat or the pigeon (see McBride *et al.,* 1974).

Studies similar to those carried out with L-5-HTP were also undertaken to determine the effects of α-MMT on the release of labeled 5-HT from isolated preparations of nerve endings (McBride and Aprison, 1973; McBride *et al.,* 1973). In the initial studies, it was determined that α-MMT itself had no apparent effect either on the uptake (McBride *et al.,* 1973) or on the efflux (Table II) of 5-HT. However, since the content of α-MMTA had also increased in pigeon brain after injection of α-MMT (Aprison and Hingtgen, 1966*b*), resulting in the relationship seen in Fig. 3, and since α-MMTA and aramine cause a release of NE in the heart and brain, these two amines were tested to determine whether they had any effects on the

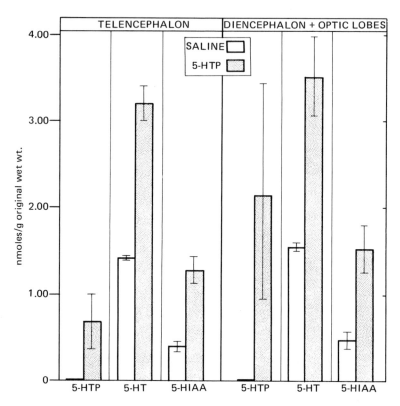

Fig. 4. Levels of 5-HTP, 5-HT, and 5-HIAA in a nerve-ending fraction (P₂) isolated from the telencephalon and diencephalon plus optic lobes of pigeons killed 60 min after intramuscular injections of saline or 50 mg/kg D,L-5-HTP in saline. The data represent the means ± S.E.M. of 4 animals in each group. All values for 5-HTP-treated pigeons were significantly higher ($P <$ 0.05) than control values. Reprinted from *Federation Proceedings 34*:1813–1822 (1975).

release of 5-[³H]HT from isolated nerve endings. In preparations from either the pigeon or rat, α-MMTA, at concentrations as low as 0.012 mM, caused a significant release of 5-[³H]HT from serotonergic nerve endings (Table 2). On the other hand, aramine at low concentrations had no apparent effect on the release of 5-[³H]HT. Therefore, on the basis of the combined (1) behavioral data, (2) correlation of *in vivo* neurochemical data, and (3) data obtained with isolated nerve endings, Aprison *et al.* (1975) drew the following conclusions concerning the mechanism of the involvement of 5-HT in producing depression in pigeons or rats working with specific learned behavioral tasks: In the case of studies in which total 5-HT levels increased, they believe that significant amounts of the injected 5-HTP were taken up by serotonergic nerve endings and there decarboxyl-

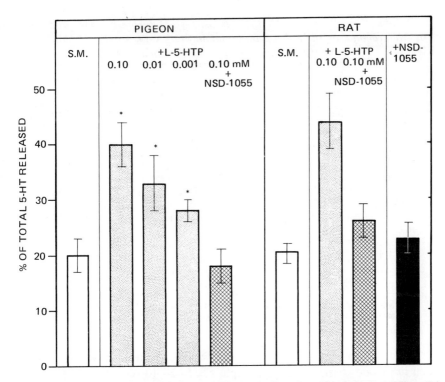

Fig. 5. Effects of L-5-HTP on the release of 5-[³H]HT from preparations of nerve endings (P₂) isolated from the telencephalon of the pigeon and rat. Efflux studies were carried out for 10 min at 37°C in the presence or absence of the aforementioned compounds. NSD-1055 is a decarboxylase inhibitor, and was used at a concentration of 0.20 mM. The data represent the means ± S.D. of at least 4 determinations each. In all cases in which L-5-HTP was present without NSD-1055, the amount of 5-[³H]HT released was significantly higher ($P < 0.05$) in comparison with control values. Reprinted from *Federation Proceedings 34*:1813–1822 (1975).

ated to 5-HT; the levels of 5-HT then increase in the nerve endings (Fig. 6). Although some of the 5-HT is converted to 5-HIAA by mitochondrial MAO, significant amounts of 5-HT are stored and some is released. Thus, in experiments involving the injection of a precursor, a finite storage capacity must be exceeded, and once this occurs, release (or spillover) is possible. Aprison and Ferster (1961*a*) showed that the injection of 15 mg D,L-5-HTP/kg did not produce behavioral depression, whereas larger doses did. In the case in which total levels of 5-HT decreases following injections of α-MMT, this amino acid is taken up and then decarboxylated; one of the decarboxylation products, α-MMTA, also causes an increased release of 5-HT (Fig. 6). The effect of this increased release of 5-HT is to decrease the tissue levels of this biogenic amine.

Table II. Effects of α-Methyl-m-tyrosine, α-Methyl-m-tyramine and
Metaraminol on the Release of Serotonin from Nerve Endings Isolated
from the Telencephalon of the Pigeon and Rat

Incubation conditions	Percentage of total released in 5 min (mean ± S.D.; $n = 4$)	
	5-HT	5-HIAA
Pigeon		
Control	1.94 ± 1.84	22.0 ± 0.44
+ 2.55 mM α-MMT	0	21.0 ± 1.00
Control	2.98 ± 0.25	14.3 ± 1.23
+ 0.012 mM α-MMTA	10.7 ± 1.50[a]	13.5 ± 1.55
Control	3.05 ± 1.49	16.0 ± 2.70
+ 0.012 mM metaraminol	3.78 ± 1.49	21.2 ± 1.28[a]
Rat		
Control	3.05 ± 2.15	11.9 ± 0.78
+ 0.012 mM α-MMTA	8.71 ± 0.63[a]	12.8 ± 0.70
Control	4.96 ± 0.29	10.9 ± 0.64
+ 0.012 mM metaraminol	5.37 ± 1.71	13.0 ± 0.52[a]

[a]Statistical significance of difference between control and drug-treated preparations is indicated
as follows: $P<0.05$. Adapted from McBride and Aprison (1973) and McBride et al. (1973).

The data presented above explain why the same behavioral effect is
seen in pigeons working on a multiple FR 50 FI 10 schedule of reinforcement when the levels of total 5-HT changed in opposite directions after an
injection of either 5-HTP or α-MMT. The data reviewed here support the
explanation of Aprison and Hingtgen (1966b, 1970, 1972) that in both cases,
5-HT in the synaptic cleft increased, and it was these molecules of 5-HT
acting on "key" receptors in specific areas of the brain that caused the
observed depression in the animal's behavior in their experiments.

2.2. A Tetrabenazine Model

Tetrabenazine (TBZ) is a drug that has long been known to have a
sedative effect on animals similar to that observed with reserpine, but of
shorter duration (Pletscher, 1957; Pletscher et al., 1958; Quinn et al., 1959;
Cahn and Herold, 1960; Leusen et al., 1959). After administration of TBZ,
the levels of 5-HT, NE, and DA decrease in brain (Pletscher, 1957; Quinn
et al., 1959; Pletscher et al., 1958, 1959, 1962; Pletscher and Gey, 1962;
Aprison and Hingtgen, 1966a). In addition, TBZ is known to precipitate
depression in some people (Ashcroft et al., 1961; Lingjaerde, 1963). An
interesting implication of the latter clinical observation is that the mechanism by which TBZ produces behavioral depression in animals may be

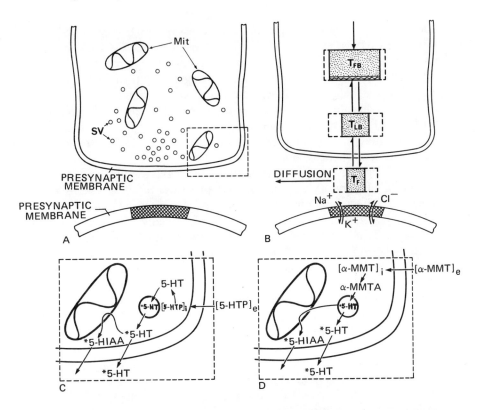

Fig. 6. (A) Simplified drawing of a nerve ending. (B) One hypothetical model of a typical synapse. A more complete description of a model serotonergic synapse was published by Aprison and Hingtgen (1972). (C) Simplified diagram of the proposed mechanism by which 5-HTP can cause an increased accumulation and release of 5-HT from serotonergic nerve terminals. (D) Simplified diagram of the proposed mechanism by which α-MMT can cause an increased release of 5-HT from such nerve terminals. Reprinted from *Federation Proceedings* *34*:1813–1822 (1975).

similar to the natural cerebral malfunction resulting in depressive illness in man. On the assumption that the idea stated above was correct, Takahashi and co-workers (Nagayama *et al.*, 1972; Takahashi *et al.*, 1974) developed an animal model of depression using motor activity and a conditioned-reflex technique (Dolin, 1951). In this experimental situation, a buzzer (conditioned stimulus) was paired with an intraperitoneal injection of 30 or 50 mg/ kg TBZ (unconditioned stimulus) for at least 11 trials. Once conditioning was established, the rats exhibited motionlessness after the presentation of the buzzer and an injection of saline. Unlike the behavioral effect produced by TBZ, the motionlessness occurring after the conditioned stimulus can be blocked by pretreatment with the antidepressant drug imipramine. Taka-hashi et al. (1974) suggest that the latter result displays a striking resemblance to a similar response to imipramine in human depressive illness.

In this section, the neurochemical changes in animals that are associated with the behavioral depression seen after treatment with TBZ are described.* In addition, some brief comments will also be made on the biochemical measurements reported to be associated with motionlessness after presentation of a conditioned stimulus to rats used in the studies of the animal model of depression.

The Sprague–Dawley rats used in the TBZ studies reported from Takahashi's laboratory were given food and water ad lib and were housed under controlled conditions of temperature (24 ± 2°C) and lighting (Tateishi et al., 1973; 1974; Takahashi et al., 1975). A daily light period was set between 7:30 P.M. and 7:30 A.M.. Since rats are nocturnal, the daily dark period was set between 7:30 A.M. and 7:30 P.M. so that their active hours would coincide with the daily work schedule of the Japanese investigators. All rats used in their experiments were allowed 3 weeks to accustom themselves to the lighting schedule.

Takahashi and co-workers monitored the behavior of each rat in a semi-soundproof chamber that was attached to an Animex DS apparatus (AB Farrand, two gain settings of 20 for recording large movements and 40 for total movements; sensitivity setting of 40). These investigators placed the rats into the behavioral apparatus between 4:30 P.M. and 8:30 P.M., and allowed the animals to accustom themselves to their new environment in the behavioral box during the next 13–18 hr.

Takahashi and his co-workers decided first to study the changes in 5-HT, 5-HIAA, NE, DA, and behavior after TBZ administration and note whether any of these parameters were temporally related during the experimental session. These data are shown in Fig. 7. After an injection of 50 mg/kg TBZ, there was a rapid decrease in the total levels of 5-HT, DA, and NE. These data are in agreement with the findings of earlier studies using other doses of TBZ (Pletscher, 1957; Pletscher et al., 1958; Quinn et al., 1959; Aprison and Hingtgen, 1966a). Only in the case of 5-HT, however, did the level in the telecephalon plus midbrain return to normal in conjunction with the resumption of motor activity. These data on cerebral 5-HT are similar to the data reported by Aprison and Hingtgen (1966a) for rats

---

*"Behavioral depression" is defined in this chapter as a significant lowering of rates of responding or motor activity by animals, and is not necessarily related to human depression as seen in psychiatric disorders. However, decreased rates of responding or reduced motor activity are seen in some patients who suffer from some types of depression. It may be that in certain types of depression, the biochemical lesions occurring in the brains of these individuals are similar to that seen in the two animal models presented here.

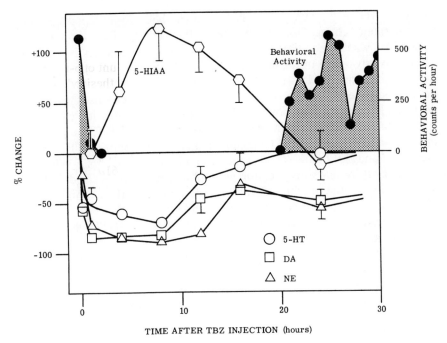

Fig. 7.   Behavioral activity and neurochemical changes in the brain of rats after an injection of 50 mg/kg TBZ. To reduce the effects of circadian rhythms, the time of injection was adjusted such that the time of sacrifice could be held constant (10:30 A.M.). Adapted from Tateishi *et al.* (1973).

working on an approach schedule of reinforcement and injected with 2 mg/ kg TBZ.

The data in Fig. 7 also show that changes in the levels of 5-HIAA correlate well with the period of behavioral disruption. These changes were in an increasing direction, passing through a peak at approximately 8 hr after the injection of TBZ. The cerebral level then decreased, reaching normal levels approximately 20 hr after the injection. What is extremely interesting is that the behavioral activity (see Fig. 7) was reduced to zero counts per hour until about 20 hr after the TBZ injection. This time point also correlates with the point at which 5-HT levels have returned to normal. On perusal of these data and those at the time of injection and shortly thereafter, one notes that the 5-HIAA curve appears to be shifted slightly to the longer time points. This phenomenon probably reflects the time for 5-HT to clear the synaptic cleft (i.e., uptake) and diffuse to the site of MAO, where it is oxidatively deaminated and subsequently oxidized further by a dehydrogenase to 5-HIAA. Thus, these data appear to support the concept that the 5-HT in the synaptic cleft caused the behavioral depression and that the rate of change of 5-HIAA reflects this activity. Takahashi and his co-workers wanted additional data to either support or refute this concept. They took advantage of the data reported by Aprison and Ferster (1961a), namely, that doses of less than 25 mg/kg D,L-5-HTP had little or no effect on the behavioral activity of pigeons, whereas higher doses caused a decrease in behavioral responding. If the behavioral depression caused by TBZ is due to a deficiency in the amount of functional 5-HT, the pretreatment of animals with L-5-HTP should antagonize the action of TBZ. If, on the other hand, TBZ causes and maintains an excess amount of 5-HT in the synaptic cleft by releasing the storage pool or newly synthesized 5-HT or both, the pretreatment with L-5-HTP should potentiate the action of TBZ. These ideas were tested behaviorally (Tachiki et al., 1974).

The results (Table III) show that when 9 mg/kg L-5-HTP was injected into rats, little or no apparent effect was observed on their motor activity. These findings are in agreement with earlier reports by Aprison and co-workers using pigeons and rats (Aprison and Ferster, 1961a; Aprison and Hingtgen, 1966a). When an intraperitoneal injection of 2 mg/kg TBZ was given, the motor activity also did not differ significantly from control data. When the rats were pretreated with a low dose of L-5-HTP 30 min prior to the injection of TBZ, a depression or inhibition of locomotor activity occurred for at least 6 hr (Tachiki et al., 1977). On the basis of these

Table III. Behavioral Data after Treatment of Rats with Low Doses of either L-5-Hydroxytryptophan or Tetrabenazine or Both Drugs

Treatment (n)	Motor activity (% of control)[a]
None[b] (4)	75.4 ± 17.0
L-5-HTP + solvent[c] (5)	63.1 ± 18.2
Saline + TBZ[c] (8)	63.9 ± 10.8
L-5-HTP + TBZ[c] (6)	17.8 ± 3.5

[a]Motor activity was measured in the Animex DS Apparatus. The means of the data from the rats injected with L-5-HTP plus TBZ are statistically different from the other means (P < 0.02).
[b]Rats were subjected to the same behavioral experiences as the experimental rats except that they received no injections.
[c]See Takahashi et al. (1974) for a description of the solvent (0.8 ml/kg.) L-5-HTP was given in a dose of 9 mg/kg i.p., and TBZ was given as a dose of 2 mg/kg i.p.

Table IV. Content of 5-Hydroxytryptamine, 5-Hydroxyindoleacetic Acid, Dopamine, and Norepinephrine of Brain Tissue from Rats 3 Hours after Treatment with either L-5-Hydroxytryptophan or Tetrabenazine or Both Drugs[a]

Treatment (n)	5-HT (nmol/g)[b]	5-HIAA (nmol/g)[b]	DA (nmol/g)[b]	NE (nmol/g)[b]
Controls[c] (10)	3.33 ± 0.16	3.09 ± 0.31	7.01 ± 0.57	2.25 ± 0.26
L-HTP + solvent[d] (4)	3.99 ± 0.45	3.16 ± 0.39	6.10 ± 0.31[e]	2.50 ± 0.18[f]
Saline + TBZ (4)	2.69 ± 0.61	2.49 ± 0.36	2.88 ± 0.47	1.74 ± 0.18
L-5-HTP + TBZ (4)	3.12 ± 0.45	4.19 ± 0.68[g,i]	2.33 ± 0.50[h]	1.13 ± 0.24[h]

[a]Adapted from Tachiki *et al.* (1977).
[b]Means ± S.E.M.
[c]Controls were not injected.
[d]The solvent is the carrier solution used to dissolve TBZ (Takahashi *et al.*, 1974).
[e-i]In these studies (Takahashi *et al.*, 1974; Tateishi *et al.*, 1974; Tachiki *et al.*, 1974), saline or a low dose of L-5-HTP (9 mg/kg) was injected at 10:00 A.M., followed 30 min later by TBZ (2 mg/kg) or the solvent used to dissolve this drug. When the L-5-HTP data are compared with the TBZ data, *e* represents $p < 0.01$ and *f* represents $p < 0.05$; when the TBZ data are compared with the L-5-HTP + TBZ data, *g* represents $p < 0.01$; when the L-5-HTP data are compared with the L-5-HTP + TBZ data, *h* represents $p < 0.01$ and *i* represents $p < 0.05$.

findings, it was concluded that L-5-HTP can potentiate the action of TBZ, and the latter appears to work through the serotonergic system.

Takahashi and co-workers reasoned that if the interpretation of the behavioral–neurochemical data presented above were correct, then comparing the levels of 5-HIAA in the brain of three groups of animals, i.e., those injected with 9 mg/kg L-5-HTP, those injected with 2 mg/kg TBZ, and those injected with both drugs, should show that the level of 5-HIAA was significantly higher only in the case of the third series of animals. To date, data are available from this research group for one time point, namely, for 3 hr after injection of TBZ (see Table IV). The data in Table IV confirm the suggestion that when using low doses of drugs that do not affect the absolute level of 5-HT (9 mg/kg L-5-HTP and 2 mg/kg TBZ), the injection of both drugs 30 min apart should show a marked increase in the levels of cerebral 5-HIAA in these animals. The changes in the levels of catecholamines did not correlate with the observed changes in motor activity.

Preliminary data of a biochemical nature concerning Takahashi's animal model of depression induced by conditioned stimulus support the data based on animal models of depression induced by drugs. Takahashi *et al.* (1975) now report the following interesting data in a rat exhibiting motionlessness after the sound stimulus: (1) a 50% decrease in total tryptophan in plasma; (2) a small increase in free tryptophan in plasma; (3) an increase in excess of 50% in the levels of tryptophan and 5-HIAA in the telencephalon and in the midbrain; (4) no major change in 5-HT in these brain areas; and

(5) no apparent changes in the activities of tryptophan pyrrolase and tyrosine transaminase of the liver.

In unpublished data, Takahashi and co-workers have additional supporting evidence. Preliminary results indicate that the pretreatment of rats with p-chlorophenylalanine (PCPA) has an inhibitory effect on the behavioral effects of TBZ. The duration of behavioral depression resulting from a dose of 30 mg/kg TBZ was reduced about 50% by pretreating rats 24 or 48 hr before with 300 mg/kg PCPA. This inhibitory effect of PCPA could be reversed by an injection of L-5-HTP. Furthermore, the sedative effects of TBZ are reversed by high doses of LSD-25 (1 mg/kg body wt.), an antagonist of 5-HT at the site of the serotonergic receptor. Bromo-LSD, which is a nonhallucinogenic LSD derivative, had no affect on the action of TBZ even at a dose of 10 mg/kg body wt.

These data support the idea that there is a greater turnover of 5-HT in the synapses of important neuronal pathways utilized by the animal during behavioral depression.

3. Selective Review of Clinical Studies Involving the Cerebral Serotonergic System and Depressive Illness in Man

A large literature of clinical papers has accumulated on the biochemical basis of depression and the serotonergic system. Since most of these papers have been reviewed or discussed previously (Coppen, 1971; Himwich, 1971; Goodwin and Post, 1974; van Pragg, 1974; Takahashi, 1975), this field will not be reviewed in detail; instead, selected papers dealing with the serotonergic system in human depression will be discussed.

In general, the concepts on which the current biochemical investigations of depressive illness are based can be traced from two lines of research: (1) neuropharmacological studies with either man or animals and (2) animal models dealing with suppression or depression of rates of responding. The data reported in the early papers from group (1) have led to the "serotonin deficiency" theory as the explanation of the cause of depression. The data reported in the papers from group (2) have led to the explanation that an increase in the concentration of free 5-HT in the synaptic cleft may be the cause of depression.

Although Brodie and Aprison had independently suggested in the early 1960's that increased levels of synaptic 5-HT were associated with depressed behavioral activity in animals, research clinicians were more impressed with the reports that reserpine (Bein, 1953; Shore, 1962) and

TBZ (Pletscher *et al.*, 1958, 1962) caused depression in animals whose tissue levels of total cerebral 5-HT were reduced. Furthermore, reserpine and TBZ can induce depression in man (Freis, 1954; Muller *et al.*, 1955; Schroender and Perry, 1955; Harris, 1957; Lingjaerde, 1963). When reserpine was administered to patients with hypertension, approximately 20% developed "depression" as a side effect. Data of this type prompted some clinicians to investigate the serotonergic system in patients with depression. It soon became apparent that some reports support the serotonin deficiency theory, while some contradict this idea. Clinical studies of the former type referred to above began to appear when Ashcroft *et al.* (1966) reported that 5-HIAA levels in CSF were low in depressed patients when compared with nondepressed controls. Similar data were reported by Dencker *et al.* (1966), van Pragg *et al.* (1970), Coppen *et al.* (1972), and McLeod and McLeod (1972). Three pieces of data suggest that the level of 5-HIAA in CSF cannot be used to support the serotonin deficiency theory of depression. First, Dencker *et al.* (1966) and Coppen *et al.* (1972) found reduced levels of 5-HIAA in the CSF from manic patients. Second, Coppen *et al.* (1972) reported that the level of 5-HIAA in CSF was also low in patients who recovered! Third, Bowers *et al.* (1969), Papeschi and McClure (1971), Sjöström and Roos (1972), and Goodwin *et al.* (1973) found no difference in this measurement between controls and depressed patients. All these data together weaken the serotonin deficiency theory.

Papers have appeared that report that the levels of 5-HT (Shaw *et al.*, 1967; Pare *et al.*, 1969) or 5-HIAA (Bourne *et al.*, 1968) were lower in the brain stem of depressed suicide patients. In addition, reduced 5-HT was also reported by Lloyd *et al.* (1974) in the raphe nuclei dorsalis and centralis inferior of the lower brain stem, but not in other areas, from depressed patients. Bourne *et al.* (1968), however, could not find any difference in the content of 5-HT in the brain stem from depressed suicides and controls. These data are shown in Table V. The question of postmortem changes was raised by Gottfries *et al.* (1974) and Beskow *et al.* (1976), and may account for conflicting reports in the literature. The present authors feel that there are not enough data available on the various components of the serotonergic system in man in which histories of the subjects, nature of depression, interval of time between death and proper handling of the tissue samples, and other details are known. These points were also discussed by Beskow *et al.* (1976) in a paper in which no differences were found between suicides and controls in whom 5-HT and 5-HIAA as well as DA, NE, and HVA were measured in several brain areas (data were corrected for postmortem changes). Cochran *et al.* (1976) also just published a paper in which they report no differences between the levels of 5-HT in 33 brain areas of controls and depressed suicides.

Table V.   Levels of 5-Hydroxytryptamine and 5-Hydroxyindoleacetic Acid in
         Several Areas of the Brain from Normals and Depressed Suicides

Investigators	Controls Mean ± S.E.M.	n	Depressed suicides Mean ± S.E.M.	n
	Content of 5-HT (ng/g) in brain stem			
Shaw *et al.* (1967)	307 ± 16	17	250 ± 19[a]	11
Bourne *et al.* (1968)	218 ± 13	13	211 ± 16	16
Pare *et al.* (1969)	350 ± 20	15	310 ± 10[a]	23
	Content of 5-HIAA (ng/g) in brain stem			
Bourne *et al.* (1968)	1698 ± 163	15	1271 ± 120[a]	16
	Content of 5-HT (ng/g) in raphe nuclei dorsalis			
Lloyd *et al.* (1974)	2.22 ± 0.13	5	1.55 ± 0.12[a]	5
	Content of 5-HT (ng/g) in raphe nuclei centralis inferior			
Lloyd *et al.* (1974)	1.32 ± 0.12	5	0.95 ± 0.07[a]	5

[a]Shows significant difference from control value.

Additional data pertaining to the serotonergic system and depression have appeared from studies employing probenecid, the inhibitor of the transport of metabolites of monoamines (i.e., 5-HIAA, HVA, etc.) from the CNS to the blood. In the studies involving the serotonergic system, the investigator is concerned with calculating the turnover of 5-HT by measuring directly the probenecid-induced accumulation of 5-HIAA in the CSF. A marked accumulation of 5-HIAA indicates a high rate of catabolism of 5-HT (or a high turnover of this biogenic amine). The data in Table VI show that in four of five studies, the probenecid-induced accumulation of 5-HIAA in the CSF was significantly reduced in depressed patients. From the reports of Sjöström (1973), Goodwin *et al.* (1973), and Goodwin and Post (1974), it would appear that the differences in probenecid-induced accumulation of 5-HIAA in CSF between the depressed patients and controls were not due to the difference in pharmakinetics of probenecid in these individuals. However, closer analyses of similar data in the literature (Sjöström and Roos, 1972) showed that probenecid-induced accumulation of 5-HIAA in CSF was lower not only in depressed patients, but also in manic patients, when compared with controls.

A highly significant piece of data has come from studies on patients during their treatment with the tricyclic antidepressants such as imipramine or amitriptyline. When compared with the pretreatment values, the level of 5-HIAA in the CSF or the probenecid-induced accumulation of 5-HIAA in the CSF of depressed patients was decreased significantly during the 1- to 3-week treatment with imipramine or amitriptyline (Papeshi and McClure, 1971; Bowers, 1974; Goodwin and Post, 1974). These data indicate that the metabolism of cerebral 5-HT in depressed patients is further decreased by antidepressants during the period when clinical improvement appears. This highly significant result strongly suggests that clinical improvement is associated with a reduction in 5-HT in the synaptic cleft. Since the tricyclic antidepressants are known to affect not only uptake of biogenic amines (5-HT, NE, DA), but also their synthesis, storage, release, and metabolism (Schanberg *et al.*, 1967; Corrodi and Fuxe, 1969; Reid *et al.*, 1969; Alpers and Himwich, 1972; Mandell *et al.*, 1972; Bruinvels, 1972; Murphy and Kopin, 1972), this conclusion or suggestion is reasonable. However, it is incompatible with the serotonin deficiency theory for depression, as supported by Coppen *et al.* (1972), Sano (1972), van Pragg (1974), van Pragg and Korf (1974), and Green and Grahame-Smith (1976).

One must look at still another type of experiment, i.e., the investigations of whether L-tryptophan and/or L-5-hydroxytryptophan, the immediate precursor of 5-HT, are effective in reversing depression in patients. Certainly one would expect these amino acids to be extremely useful in treating this type of mental illness if the serotonin deficiency theory is correct! When L-tryptophan and placebo were administered in a nonrandom design to depressed patients, the results did not support the serotonin deficiency theory, since no therapeutic effect was noted in most of the published papers (Carroll *et al.*, 1970; Bunney *et al.*, 1971; Murphy *et al.*, 1973; Gayford *et al.*, 1973; Mendels *et al.*, 1975). Coppen *et al.* (1972) reported that L-tryptophan was as effective as imipramine in depression. It

Table VI. Metabolism of Cerebral 5-Hydroxytryptamine in Human Depression

Study (probenecid dose)	Probenecid-induced accumulation of CSF 5-HIAA (ng/ml)			
	Control		Depression	
	Mean ± S.E.M.	n	Mean ± S.E.M.	n
van Praag *et al.* (1970) (5 g/3 days)	35 ± 5.4	11	22 ± 5.3[a]	14
van Praag and Korf (1971) (1 g/20 min i.v.)	27 ± 4.9	15	17 ± 3.1[a]	15
Sjöström (1973) (5 g/50 hr)	66 ± 3.3%[b]	13	27 ± 1.8%[a,b]	24
Goodwin *et al.* (1973) (160 mg/kg/9 or 18 hr)	112 ± 3.2	8	90 ± 3.9	6
van Praag *et al.* (1973) (1 g/20 min i.v. + 4 g/4 hr)	81 ± 12	12	49 ± 7.6[a]	28

[a]Shows significant difference from control value.
[b]Note that this value was expressed in terms of percentage increase.

is interesting to note that Murphy *et al.* (1974) and Prange *et al.* (1974) report that L-tryptophan is more effective in reducing hyperactive or manic behavior. The clinical efficacy of L-5-HTP in treatment of depression as reported by Sano (1972) was not confirmed in double-blind controlled studies reported by Brodie *et al.* (1973) and Matussek *et al.* (1974), nor by Kline *et al.* (1964) while using D,L-5-HTP.

The present authors must conclude that the serotonin deficiency theory is not presently supportable by the data in the literature. Some new hypothesis is necessary!

4. A Theory Suggesting the Presence of Hypersensitive Serotonergic Synapses in Clinical Depression

Let us assume that the following two sets of data are correct: (1) the probenecid-induced accumulation of 5-HIAA in the CSF in depressed patients is lower than that of proper controls, and (2) the probenecid-induced accumulation of 5-HIAA in the CSF of depressed patients was significantly decreased during the 1- to 3-week treatment with amitriptyline or imipramine when compared to the pretreatment values for these patients. These data suggest that (1) the turnover of cerebral 5-HT in depression is less than in normals, and (2) when the depressed patients receive one of the tricyclic antidepressants, and are improving clinically, there is a still lower turnover of cerebral 5-HT. If one also accepts the concept developed from basic research with animals, i.e., that the molecules of serotonin present in the synaptic cleft are the physiologically (functional) important pool (Aprison and Ferster, 1961*b*; Aprison and Hingtgen, 1966*a*), then one can offer the following new hypothesis to explain depression: Persons who are prone to become depressed release less 5-HT at serotonergic synapses than normal persons. Based on data from denervated preparations, the consequence of prolonged reduced release of 5-HT should result in a hypersensitive receptor in the postsynaptic membrane of the serotonergic synapse. During the developmental stages of the disease and prior to the onset of depression, the decrease in the level of released 5-HT is compensated for by an increase in sensitivity of the receptor (hypersensitivity). This type of person does not show any signs of depression. The hypersensitive receptor handles the information as though a normal amount of 5-HT had been released. Since this illness is predominantly one associated with adults, one could suggest that the process of reduced release probably occurs over a long period of time, or the patient inherits such a system from birth and it becomes critical only during stress. Thus, if a "psychiatric precipitating factor" occurs, and if this event causes more 5-HT than normal to be released, the impact on the hypersensitive receptor should be similar to that noted when the level of cerebral 5-HT within the synaptic cleft is increased dramatically as in the animal experiments (see Section 2). Thus, if the system in man is the same as that in animals, and as described in the two models given in Section 2, depression should occur.

With this hypothesis, one can now explain the following observations: (1) No improvement is seen with large doses of L-tryptophan or L-5-HTP because the administration of these amino acids would produce more 5-HT, not less, in the synaptic cleft. (2) Lower probenecid-induced accumulation of 5-HIAA in CSF from depressed patients is noted during chronic treatment with amitriptyline or imipramine because the major impact of the latter two tricyclic antidepressants is probably to reduce the synthesis of 5-HT, rather than only to block its uptake into neurons. (3) Further, if the mechanism in (2) is operative, it would explain why it takes 1 to 3 weeks of treatment with these tricyclic antidepressants; i.e., it would take that long for the reduction in the biosynthesis of 5-HT to result in less 5-HT in the synaptic cleft (Corrodi and Fuxe, 1969; Alpers and Himwich, 1972). (4) The depressive action of reserpine and TBZ in some patients is probably due *not* to the reduction of the level of total 5-HT in the presynaptic neurons in the brain, but to the inability of the continually synthesized biogenic amine to be stored in the nerve endings, thereby resulting in its continual release (the authors suggest that the free pool or 5-HT in the cleft becomes larger than the predrug administration level). (5) PCPA administration does not induce depression in normal (human) subjects (Cremata and Koe, 1966; Sjöerdsma *et al.,* 1970; Engleman *et al.,* 1967) because this drug causes a reduction in the level of 5-HT. (6) If depression is the "opposite" of mania, then the reports that methysergide aggravates symptoms of mania (Coppen *et al.,* 1969; Court and Mai, 1970) can be explained as the blockade by the drug of the postsynaptic action of 5-HT.

We would like to return to item (5) above, where we explain in terms of our theory why PCPA administration does not induce depression as would be required by the serotonin deficiency theory. In terms of our theory, however, this substituted amino acid should be tried as a therapeutic agent in treating some forms of depression, since it would cause a marked reduction in cerebral 5-HT. The investigator attempting this therapeutic approach should use a dose of PCPA that markedly reduces the level of both cerebral 5-HT and that in the cleft of key serotonergic synapses. If item (6) above is expanded, we can predict that if a drug that is a "pure" blocker of 5-HT uptake is given to patients, it will not help depressed persons, but only those who suffer from mania. Finally, our theory would support the suggestion that drugs that have proven antagonistic actions to 5-HT at the latter's synaptic receptor sites should be considered for antidepressive effects in man.

5. Final Comments

A current theory for depression, the serotonin deficiency theory, has been discussed and reasons the authors believe it is incorrect have been given. A new theory has been presented that is based on the two different biochemical studies of animal models of depression (as described in this chapter) as well as on reported studies that show that (1) the probenecid-induced accumulation of 5-HIAA in the CSF in depressed patients is lower than that of proper controls, and (2) the probenecid-induced accumulation of 5-HIAA in the CSF of depressed patients was significantly decreased during the 1- to 3-week treatment with amitriptyline or imipramine when compared with the pretreatment values for these patients. This theory stresses that in depression, there is an involvement of synaptic 5-HT with a hypersensitive receptor in the postsynaptic membrane, and suggests that depression is due primarily to an excess of free or functional 5-HT in the synaptic cleft. This new theory was used to (1) explain a number of observations in the literature and (2) predict possible experiments to test this hypothesis.

6. References

Alpers, H. S., and Himwich, H. E., 1972, The effects of chronic imipramine administration on rat brain levels of serotonin, 5-hydroxyindoleacetic acid, norepinephrine and dopamine, *J. Pharmacol. 190*:531.

Aprison, M. H., 1965, Research approaches to problems in mental illness. Brain neurohumor-enzyme systems and behavior, in: *Horizons in Neuropsychopharmacology* (W. Himwich and J. Schade, eds.), pp. 48–80, Elsevier, Amsterdam.

Aprison, M. H., and Ferster, C. B., 1960, Behavioral effects of 5-hydroxytryptophan, *Experientia 16*:159.

Aprison, M. H., and Ferster, C. B., 1961*a*, Neurochemical correlates of behavior. I. Quantitative measurement of the behavioral effects of the serotonin precursor, 5-hydroxytryptophan, *J. Pharmacol. Exp. Ther. 131*:100.

Aprison, M. H., and Ferster, C. B., 1961*b*, Neurochemical correlates of behavior. II. Correlation of brain monoamine oxidase activity with behavioral changes after iproniazid and 5-hydroxytryptophan administtration, *J. Neurochem. 6*:350.

Aprison, M. H., and Ferster, C. B., 1961*c*, Serotonin and behavior, in: *Recent Advances in Biological Psychiatry*, Vol. 3, Chapt. 12, (J. Wortis, ed.), pp. 151–162, Grune and Stratton, New York.

Aprison, M. H., and Hingtgen, J. N., 1965, Neurochemical correlates of behavior. IV. Norepinephrine and dopamine in four brain parts of the pigeon during period of atypical behavior following the injection of 5-hydroxytryptophan, *J. Neurochem. 12*:959.

Aprison, M. H., and Hingtgen, J. N., 1966*a*, Neurochemical correlates of behavior. V. Differential drug effects on approach and avoidance behavior in rats with related changes in brain serotonin and norepinephrine, *Recent Adv. Biol. Psychiatry 8*:87.

Aprison, M. H., and Hingtgen, J. N., 1966*b*, Neurochemical correlates of behavior. VI. 5-Hydroxytryptamine, norepinephrine, α-methyl-*m*-tyramines and 3,4-dihydroxyphenylethylamine concentrations in pigeon brain during the period of atypical behavior following the injection of α-methyl-*meta*-tyrosine, *Life Sci.* 5:1071.

Aprison, M. H., and Hingtgen, J. N., 1970, Neurochemical correlates of behavior, *Int. Rev. Neurobiol. 13*:325.

Aprison, M. H., and Hingtgen, J. N., 1972, Serotonin and behavior: A brief summary, *Fed. Proc. Fed. Am. Soc. Exp. Biol. 31*:121.

Aprison, M. H., Wolf, M. A., Poulos, G. L., and Folkerth, T. L., 1962, Neurochemical correlates of behavior. III. Variation of serotonin content in several brain areas and peripheral tissues of the pigeon following 5-hydroxytryptophan administration, *J. Neurochem.* 9:575.

Aprison, M. H., Hingtgen, J. N., and McBride, W. J., 1975, Serotonergic and cholinergic mechanisms during disruption of approach and avoidance behavior, *Fed. Proc. Fed. Am. Soc. Exp. Biol. 34*:1813.

Ashcroft, G. W., MacDougall, E. J., and Barker, P. A., 1961, A comparison of tetrabenazine and chlorpromazine in chronic schizophrenia, *J. Ment. Sci. 107*:287.

Ashcroft, G. W., Crowford, T. B. B., Eccleston, D., Sharman, D. F., McDougall, E. J., Stanton, J. B., and Binns, J. K., 1966, 5-Hydroxyindole compounds in the cerebrospinal fluid of patients with psychiatric or neurological diseases, *Lancet 2*:1049.

Bein, H. J., 1953, The pharmacology of reserpine, a new alkaloid from *Rauwolfia serpentina, Experientia 9*:107.

Beskow, J., Gottfries, C. G., Roose, B. E., and Winblad, B., 1976, Determination of monoamine and monoamine metabolites in the human brain: Post mortem studies in a group of suicides and in a control group, *Acta Psychiatr. Scand. 53*:7.

Bogdanski, D. F., Weissbach, H., and Udenfriend, S., 1957, The distribution of serotonin, 5-hydroxytryptophan decarboxylase, and monoamine oxidase in brain, *J. Neurochem. 1*:272.

Bourne, H. R., Bunney, W. E., Colburn, R. W., Davis, J. M., Davis, J. N., Shaw, D. M., and Coppen, A. J., 1968, Noradrenaline, 5-hydroxytryptamine, and 5-hydroxyindoleacetic acid in hindbrains of suicidal patients, *Lancet 2*:805.

Bowers, M. B., Jr., 1974, Lumbar CSF 5-hydroxyindoleacetic acid and homovanillic acid in affective syndromes, *J. Nerv. Ment. Dis. 158*:325.

Bowers, M. B., Jr., Henninger, G. R., and Gerbode, F., 1969, Cerebrospinal fluid 5-hydroxyindoleacetic acid and homovanillic acid in psychiatric patients, *Int. J. Neuropharmacol. 8*:255.

Brodie, H. K. H., Keith, H., Sack, R., and Siever, L., 1973, Clinical studies of L-5-hydroxytryptophan in depression, in: *Serotonin and Behavior* (J. Barchas and E. Usdin, eds.), pp. 549–559, Academic Press, New York.

Bruinvels, J., 1972, Inhibition of the biosynthesis of 5-hydroxytryptamine in rat brain by imipramine, *Eur. J. Pharmacol. 20*:231.

Bunney, W. E., Jr., Brodie, H. K. H., Murphy, D. L., and Goodwin, F. K., 1971, Studies of alpha-methyl-*para*-tyrosine, L-dopa, and tryptophan in depression and mania, *Am. J. Psychiatry 127*:872.

Cahn, J., and Herold, M. M., 1960, Etude pharmacologique du Ro 1-9569 (tetrabenazine), *Psychiatr. Neurol. Basel 140*:210.

Carroll, B. J., Mowbray, R. M., and Davies, B. M., 1970, L-Tryptophan in depression, *Lancet* 2:776.

Cochran, E. Robins, E., and Grote, S., 1976, Regional serotonin levels in brain: A comparison of depressive suicides and alcoholic suicides with controls, *Biol. Psychiatry 11*:283.

Coppen, A., 1971, Biogenic amines and affective disorders, *Adv. Ment. Sci. 4*:123.

Coppen, A., Prange, A. J., Jr., Whybrow, P. C., Noguera, R., and Paez, J. M., 1969, Methysergide in mania, *Lancet 2*:338.

Coppen, A., Prange, A. J., Jr., Whybrow, P. C., and Noguera, R., 1972, Abnormalities of indoleamine in affective disorders, *Arch. Gen. Psychiatry 26*:474.

Corrodi, H., and Fuxe, K., 1969, Decreased turnover in central 5-HT nerve terminals induced by antidepressant drugs of the imipramine type, *Eur. J. Pharmacol. 7*:56.

Costa, E., 1956, Effects of hallucinogenic and tranquilizing drugs on serotonin evoked uterine contractions, *Proc. Soc. Exp. Biol. (N.Y.) 91*:39.

Costa, E., and Aprison, M. H., 1958a, Studies on the 5-hydroxytryptamine (serotonin) content in human brain, *J. Nerv. Ment. Dis. 126*:289.

Costa, E., and Aprison, M. H., 1958b, Distribution of intracarotidly injected serotonin in brain, *Am. J. Physiol. 192*:95.

Court, J. H., and Mai, F. M., 1970, A double-blind intensive crossover design trial of methysergide in mania, *Med. J. Aust. 2*:526.

Cremata, V. Y., Jr., and Koe, B. K., 1966, Clinical–pharmacological evaluation of *p*-chlorophenylalanine: A new serotonin depleting agent, *Clin. Pharmacol. Ther. 7*:768.

Dencker, S. J., Malm, U., Roos, B., and Werdinius, B., 1966, Acid monoamine metabolites of cerebrospinal fluid in mental depression and mania, *J. Neurochem. 13*:1545.

Dolin, A. O., 1951, Uslovnoryeflektornoye katalyeptitseyeskoye sostoyaniye, *Pavlov J. Higher Nerv. Act. 1*:485.

Engleman, K., Lovenberg, W., and Sjöerdsma, A., 1967, Inhibition of serotonin synthesis by *para*-chlorophenylalanine in patients with the carcinoid syndrome, *N. Engl. J. Med. 277*:1103.

Ferster, C. B., and Skinner, B. F., 1957, *Schedules of Reinforcement,* Appleton-Century-Crofts, New York.

Freis, E. D., 1954, Mental depression in hypertensive patients treated for long periods with large doses of reserpine, *N. Engl. J. Med. 251*:1006.

Gaddum, J. H., 1954, Drugs antagonistic to 5-hydroxytryptamine in: *Ciba Found. Symp.: Hypertension, Humoral and Neurogenic Factors,* (G. E. W. Wolstenholme, M. P. Cameron, eds.), pp. 75–77, Little, Brown and Co., Boston.

Garven, J. D., 1956, The estimation of 5-hydroxytryptamine in the presence of adrenaline, *Br. J. Pharmacol. 11*:1.

Gayford, J. J., Parker, A. L., Phillips, E. M., and Rowsell, A. R., 1973, Whole Blood 5-hydroxytryptamine during treatment of endogenous depressive illness, *Br. J. Psychiatry 122*:597.

Goodwin, F. K., and Post, R. M., 1974, Brain serotonin, affective illness, and antidepressant drugs: Cerebrospinal fluid studies with probenecid, *Adv. Biochem. Psychopharmacol. 11*:341.

Goodwin, F. K., Post, R. M., Dunner, D. L., and Gordon, E. K., 1973, Cerebrospinal fluid amine metabolites in affective illness: The probenecid technique, *Am. J. Psychiatry 130*:73.

Gottfries, C. G., Roos, B. E., and Winblad, B., 1974, Determination of monoamines and monoamine metabolites in the human brain post mortem, Psihofarmakologija 3, in: *Proceedings of the Third Yugoslavian Psychopharmacological Symposium* (M. Mihovilovic, ed.), pp. 99–104, Opatija 1973, Medicinska Naklada, Zagreb.

Green, A. R., and Grahame-Smith, D. G., 1976, Effects of drugs on the processes regulating the functional activity of brain 5-hydroxytryptamine, *Nature (London) 260*:487.

Harris, T. H., 1957, Depression induced by *Rauwolfia* compounds, *Am. J. Psychiatry 113*:950.

Himwich, H. E., 1971, *Biochemistry, Schizophrenias and Affective Illnesses,* The Williams and Wilkins Co., Baltimore.

Hingtgen, J. N., and Aprison, M. H., 1963, The effect of alpha-methyl-*meta*-tyrosine on behavioral response rates in pigeons, *Science 141*:169.

Hingtgen, J. N., and Aprison, M. H., 1965, Interrelation between four measures of the behavioral response in pigeons with elevated serotonin levels, *Recent Adv. Biol. Psychiatry 7*:163.

Hingtgen, J. N., and Aprison, M. H., 1966, Food consumption in pigeons following the administration of α-methyl-*meta*-tyrosine during approach behavior and free feeding, *Life Sci. 5*:1249.

Hingtgen, J. N., and Aprison, M. H., 1975, Behavioral depression in pigeons following L-tryptophan administration, *Life Sci. 16*:1471.

Hingtgen, J. N., and Aprison, M. H., 1976, Behavioral and environmental aspects of the cholinergic system, in: *Biology of Cholinergic Function* (A. M. Goldberg and I. Hanin, eds.), pp. 515–566, Raven Press, New York.

Kline, N., Sacks, W., and Simpson, G. M., 1964, Further studies on one day treatment of depression with 5-HTP, *Am. J. Psychol. 12*:379.

Leusen, I., Lacroix, E., and Demeester, G., 1959, Quelques proprietes pharmacodynamiques de la tetrabenazine, substance liberatrice de serotonine, *Arch. Int. Pharmacodyn. Ther. 119*:225.

Lingjaerde, O., 1963, Tetrabenazine (Nitoman) in the treatment of psychoses. With a discussion on the central mode of action of tetrabenazine and reserpine, *Acta Psychiatr. Scand. Suppl. 170*:1.

Lloyd, K. G., Farley, I. J., Deck, J. H. N., and Hornykiewicz, O., 1974, Serotonin and 5-hydroxyindoleacetic acid in discrete areas of the brainstem of suicide victims and control patients, *Adv. Biochem. Psychopharmacol. 11*:387.

Macchitelli, F. J., Fischetti, D., and Montanarelli, N., 1966, Changes in behavior and electrocortical activity in the monkey following administration of 5-hydroxytryptophan (5-HTP), *Psychopharmacologia 9*:447.

Mandell, A. J., Segal, D. S., Kuczenski, R. T., and Knapp, S., 1972, Some macromolecular mechanisms in CNS neurotransmitter pharmacology and their physiological organizations, in: *The Chemistry of Mood, Motivation and Memory* (J. McGaugh, ed.), pp. 105–148, Plenum Press, New York.

Matussek, N., Angst, J., Benkert, O., Gmur, M., Papousek, M., Ruther, E., and Woggon, B., 1974, The effect of L-5-hydroxytryptophan alone and in combination with a decarboxylase inhibitor (RO4-4602) in depressive patients, *Adv. Biochem. Psychopharmacol. 11*:399.

McBride, W. J., and Aprison, M. H., 1973, Release of 5-hydroxytryptamine from serotonergic nerve endings by α-methyl-*meta*-tyramine, *Pharmacol. Biochem. Behavior 1*:587.

McBride, W. J., Aprison, M. H., and Hingtgen, J. N., 1973, Effects of α-methyl-*meta*-tyrosine, α-methyl-*meta*-tyramine and metaraminol on the serotonin content in preparations of whole tissue and synaptosomes from the telencephalon of the pigeon, *Neuropharmacology 12*:769.

McBride, W. J., Aprison, M. H., and Hingtgen, J. N., 1974, Effects of 5-hydroxytryptophan on serotonin in nerve endings, *J. Neurochem. 23*:385.

McLeod, W. R., and McLeod, M., 1972, Indolamines and cerebrospinal fluid, in: *Depressive Illness* (B. M. Davies, B. J. Carroll, and R. M. Mowbray, eds.), pp. 209–225, Charles C. Thomas, Springfield, Illinois.

Mendels, J., Stinnett, J. L., Burns, D., and Frazer, A., 1975, Amine precursors and depression, *Arch. Gen. Psychiatry 32*:22.

Muller, J. C., Pryor, W. W., Gibbons, J. E., and Orgain, E. S., 1955, Depression and anxiety occurring during *Rauwolfia* therapy, *J. Am. Med. Assoc. 159*:836.

Murphy, D. L., and Kopin, I. J., 1972, The transport of biogenic amines, in: *Metabolic Transport* (L. E. Hokin, ed.), pp. 503–542, Academic Press, New York.

Murphy, D. L., Baker, M., Kotin, J., and Bunney, W. E., Jr., 1973, Behavioral and metabolic effects of L-tryptophan in unipolar depressed patients, in: *Serotonin and Behavior* (J. Barchas and E. Usdin, eds.), pp. 529–537, Academic Press, New York.

Murphy, D. L., Baker, M., Goodwin, F. K., Miller, H., Kotin, J., and Bunney, W., 1974, L-Tryptophan in affective disorders: Indoleamine changes and differential clinical effects, *Psychopharmacologia 34*:11.

Nagayama, H., Kido, A., and Takahashi, R., 1972, Utsubyo no dobutsu moderu, *Igaku To Seibutsugaku 84*:163.

Paasonen, M. K., MacLean, P. D., and Giarman, N. J., 1957, 5-Hydroxytryptamine (serotonin, enteramine) content of structures of the limbic system, *J. Neurochem. 1*:326.

Papeschi, R., and McClure, D. J., 1971, Homovanillic and 5-hydroxyindoleacetic acid in cerebrospinal fluid of depressed patients, *Arch. Gen. Psychiatry 25*:354.

Pare, C. M. B., Yeung, D. P. H., Price, K., and Stacey, R. S., 1969, 5-Hydroxytryptamine, noradrenaline, and dopamine in caudate nucleus of controls and of patients committing suicide by cool-gas poisoning, *Lancet 2*:133.

Pletscher, A., 1957, Release of 5-hydroxytryptamine by benzoquinoline derivatives with sedative action, *Science 126*:507.

Pletscher, A., and Gey, K. F., 1962, Drug-induced alterations of the metabolism of cerebral monoamines, in: *Monoamines et système nerveux central* (J. de Ajuriaguerra, ed.), pp. 105–115, Georg & Cie SA, Genève.

Pletscher, A., Besendorf, H., and Bächtold, H. P., 1958, Benzo(a)chinolizine, eine neue Körperklasse mit Wirkung auf den 5-Hydroxytryptamine- und Noradrenaline-Stoffwechsel des Gehirns, *Arch. Exp. Pathol. Pharmakol. 232*:499.

Pletscher, A., Besendorf, H., and Gey, K. F., 1959, Depression of norepinephrine and 5-hydroxytryptamine in the brain by benzoquinolizine derivatives, *Science 129*:844.

Pletscher, A., Brossi, A., and Gey, K. F., 1962, Benzoquinolizine derivative: A new class of monoamine decreasing drugs with psychotropic action, *Rev. Neurobiol. 6*:275.

van Praag, H. M., 1974, Towards a biochemical typology of depression?, *Pharmakopsychiatr. Neuro-Psychopharmakol. 7*:281.

van Praag, H. M., and Korf, J., 1971, Endogenous depressions with and without disturbances in the 5-hydroxytryptamine metabolism: A biochemical classification?, *Psychopharmacology 19*:148.

van Praag, H. M., and Korf, J., 1974, Serotonin metabolism in depression: Clinical application of the probenecid test, *Int. Pharmacopsychiatry 9*:35.

van Praag, H. M., Korf, J., and Puite, J., 1970, 5-Hydroxyindoleacetic acid levels in the cerebrospinal fluid of depressive patients treated with probenecid, *Nature (London) 225*:1259.

van Praag, H. M., Korf, J., and Schut, D., 1973, Cerebral monoamines and depression. An investigation with the probenecid technique, *Arch. Gen. Psychiatry 28*:827.

Prange, A. J., Jr., Wilson, I. C., Lynn, C. W., Alltop, L. B., and Stikeleather, R. A., 1974, L-Tryptophan in mania. Contribution to a permissive hypothesis of affective disorders, *Arch. Gen. Psychiatry 30*:56.

Quinn, G. P., Shore, P. A., and Brodie, B. B., 1959, Biochemical and pharmacological studies of RO 1-9569 (tetrabenazine), a non-indole tranquilizing agent with reserpine-like effects, *J. Pharmacol. Exp. Ther. 127*:103.

Reid, W. D., Stefano, F. J. E., Kurzepa, S., and Brodie, B. B., 1969, Tricyclic antidepressants: Evidence for an intraneuronal site of action, *Science 164*:437.

Sano, I., 1972, L-5-Hydroxytryptophan-therapie, *Folia Psychiatr. Neurol. Jpn. 26*:7.

Schanberg, S. M., Schildkraut, J. J., and Kopin, I. J., 1967, The effects of psychoactive drugs on norepinephrine-^{3}H metabolism in brain, *Biochem. Pharmacol. 16*:393.

Schroender, H. A., and Perry, H. M., 1955, Psychosis apparently produced by reserpine, *J. Am. Med. Assoc. 159*:839.

Shaw, D. M., Camps, F. E., and Eccleston, E. G., 1967, 5-Hydroxytryptamine in the hindbrain of depressive suicides, *Br. J. Psychiatry 113*:1407.

Shore, P. A., 1962, Release of serotonin and catecholamines by drugs, *Pharmacol. Rev. 14*:531.

Sjöerdsma, A., Lovenberg, W., Engelman, K., Carpenter, W. T., Jr., Wyatt, R. J., and Gessa, G. L., 1970, Serotonin now: Clinical implications of inhibiting its synthesis with *para*-chlorophenylalanine, *Ann. Intern. Med. 73*:607.

Sjöström, R., 1973, 5-Hydroxyindoleacetic acid and homovanillic acid in cerebrospinal fluid in manic-depressive psychosis and the effect of probenecid treatment, *Eur. J. Clin. Pharmacol. 6*:75.

Sjöström, R., and Roos, B. E., 1972, 5-Hydroxyindoleacetic acid and homovanillic acid in cerebrospinal fluid in manic depressive psychosis, *Eur. J. Clin. Pharmacol. 4*:170.

Tachiki, K. H., Takagi, A., Tateishi, T., and Takahashi, R., 1974, Utsubyo no dobutsu moderu ni okeru tetrabenazine no sayokijo—III, *Bull. Jpn. Neurochem. Soc. 13*:29.

Tachiki, K. H., Takagi, A., Tateishi, T., Kido, A., Nishiwaki, K., Nakamura, E., Nagayama, H., and Takahashi, R., 1977, Animal model of depression. III. Mechanisms of action of tetrabenazine, *Biol. Psychiatry*, in press.

Takahashi, R., 1975, Cerebral amine metabolism in manic-depressive illness—Present status and reconsideration of amine theory, *Jpn. J. Clin. Chem. 4*:124.

Takahashi, R., Nagayama, H., Kido, A., and Morita, T., 1974, An animal model of depression, *Biol. Psychiatry 9*:191.

Takahashi, R., Tachiki, K., Nishiwaki, K., Nakamura, E., Tateishi, T., and Nagayama, H., 1975, Biochemical basis of an animal model of depressive illness, *Bull. Jpn. Neurochem. Soc. 14*:13.

Tateishi, T., Nakamura, E., Nagayama, H., Sakurai, Y., and Takahashi, R., 1973, Tetrabenazine-moderu ni yoru utsubyo no seikagaku-teki kenkyu—II, *Annu. Rep. Pharmacopsychiatr. Res. Found.*, No. 5, p. 82.

Tateishi, T., Tachiki, K. H., Nakamura, E., Takagi, A., and Takahashi, R., 1974, Tetrabenazine-moderu ni yoru utsubyo no seikagaku-teki kenkyu—III, *Annu. Rep. Pharmacopsychiatr. Res. Found.*, No. 6, p. 83.

Tateishi, T., Tachiki, K., Nakamura, E., Takagi, A., Nagayama, H., Sakurai, Y., and Takahashi, R., 1975, Behavioral sedation in animals and associated biochemical changes—study of a model of depression induced by tetrabenazine in rats, *Bull. Neuroinformation Laboratory Nagasaki University No. 2*:96–105.

Woolley, D. W., and Shaw, E., 1954a, A biochemical and pharmacological suggestion about certain mental disorders, *Proc. Natl. Acad. Sci. U.S.A., 40*:228.

Woolley, D. W., and Shaw, E., 1954b, Some neurophysiological aspects of serotonin, *Br. Med. J. 2*:122.

3

The Organization of Central Catecholamine Neuron Systems

Robert Y. Moore and Lawrence F. Kromer

1. Introduction

In the late 1900's, three phenomena gave great impetus to the study of the morphology of the nervous system: first, the evolution of the neuron doctrine; second, the development of powerful techniques for the analysis of neural structure; third, the prominence of the concept of localization of function. A natural consequence of the development of the neuron doctrine was the concept of the synapse, which, in turn, required that some mechanism be established by which information is transmitted from one nerve cell to another or from a nerve cell to an effector cell. The history of the development of the concept of chemical transmission at the synapse is too well known to be recounted here. Of particular importance for this review was the establishment of noradrenaline as the sympathetic neurotransmitter by von Euler (1946). This was followed by the landmark work of Vogt (1954) demonstrating that noradrenaline and adrenaline are present in brain with a distinct regional distribution that is independent of the sympathetic innervation of the CNS. Numerous subsequent studies have refined these observations, but it was not until the development of a specific and sensitive histochemical method for the intracellular demonstration of catecholamines (Falck *et al.*, 1962; Falck, 1962; Carlsson *et al.*, 1962; for a review,

Robert Y. Moore and Lawrence F. Kromer • Department of Neurosciences, University of California at San Diego, La Jolla, California 92092

cf. Corrodi and Jonsson, 1967) that a precise analysis of central catechol-amine (CA) neuron systems could be carried out. This was initiated by Hillarp and his colleagues in Stockholm (Andén *et al.*, 1964, 1965, 1966*b*; Dahlström and Fuxe, 1964, 1965; Fuxe, 1965*a,b*; Hillarp *et al.*, 1966; Fuxe *et al.*, 1970; Ungerstedt, 1971) and formed the basis for our current understanding of central CA neuron systems. The analysis of the organization of these systems has recently been greatly facilitated by the develop-ment of new, more sensitive modifications of the original Falck–Hillarp histochemical methods (Hökfelt and Ljungdahl, 1972; Lindvall *et al.*, 1973; Lindvall and Björklund, 1974a; Lorén *et al.*, 1976) and by the application of newly developed anatomical methods for the analysis of central CA neuron systems, such as immununohistochemistry (Hökfelt *et al.*, 1973, 1974*a*; Hartman, 1973; Swanson and Hartman, 1975), the autoradiographic tracing technique (Pickel *et al.*, 1974; Jones and Moore, 1977), and the retrograde transport method (Llamas *et al.*, 1975; Freedman *et al.*, 1975; Kuypers and Maisky, 1975). Since the original demonstration of CA neurons in the mammalian brain (Carlsson *et al.*, 1962), the organization and function of the systems comprised by these neurons has been of considerable scientific interest. The purpose of this review is to summarize briefly what is cur-rently known of the organization of central CA neuron systems, since this provides one key to the understanding of their function. The importance of these systems is already evident in work that has demonstrated their contribution to the central mechanisms participating in motor control, regulation of pituitary secretion, feeding and drinking behavior, and arousal.

2.   Dopamine Neuron Systems

2.1.   Nigrostriatal System

The nigrostriatal system was the first central CA neuron system to be identified in the mammalian brain. Following the demonstration by Bertler and Rosengren (1959) that dopamine was present in the mammalian brain and in highest concentration in the neostriatal nuclei, Ehringer and Horny-kiewicz (1960) demonstrated that dopamine was nearly absent from the neostriatal nuclei of persons suffering from Parkinson's disease, and that this was associated with a loss of dopamine in the substantia nigra, pars compacta, an area known to be the site of the primary pathology of that disease (Greenfield, 1963). These observations were in accord with the view that a direct projection from substantia nigra to the neostriatal nuclei was present (Ferraro, 1928), and that this projection was dopamine-producing. In subsequent studies, Andén *et al.* (1964, 1965), using the Falck–Hillarp method, provided histochemical evidence for a nigrostriatal pathway. Using this methodology, however, it is not possible to visualize the preterminal portions of the axon, so that definitive evidence for the projection was lacking. This was subsequently provided by a series of studies. Moore *et al.* (1971) demonstrated that using the Fink–Heimer technique, axonal degeneration could be traced from a lesion in the substantia nigra to a pathway ascending ventrally and medially to the red nucleus in the ventral tegmental area above the cerebral peduncle, mammillary peduncle, and fasciculus retroflexus. At the level of the mammillary bodies, the fibers of this pathway come together in a compact bundle lying ventrolaterally in field H of Forel, dorsal and medial to the subthalamic nucleus, and at the level of the premammillary nuclei, the bundle of degenerating axons becomes more elongated in a dorsal–ventral direction, with some axons present at the lateral hypothalamic area. Rostrally, the bundle of degenerating axons is located in the ventromedial zona incerta, in the lateral hypothalamus, and in the adjacent medial portion of the internal capsule. At rostral tuberal levels of the hypothalamus, the fibers run entirely in the medial internal capsule and adjacent lateral hypothalamus. As the entopeduncular nucleus and globus pallidus appear within and adjacent to the internal capsule, degenerating axons leave the main bundle to run laterally through the entopeduncular nucleus and globus pallidus to enter the caudal putamen. There are scattered, degenerating terminals in the entopeduncular nucleus and globus pallidus. Similarly, there are only scattered degenerating terminals evident in the caudal putamen, but the rostral three-fourths of the nucleus shows dense terminal degeneration. At the level of the expansion of the tail of the caudate nucleus into the head, the degenerating axons of the main bundle spread dorsally and laterally along the medial border of the internal capsule. As in the putamen, there are relatively few degenerating terminals caudally in the caudate nucleus, but the rostral three-fourths of the nucleus exhibits dense terminal degeneration. The distribution of degenerating terminals is homogeneous in the putamen, whereas in the caudate nucleus, more terminals are evident laterally than medially. This pattern of degenerating axons of the nigrostriatal pathway has been demonstrated following lesions in the substantia nigra in the rat (Shimizu and Ohnishi, 1973; Maler *et al.*, 1973) and in the monkey (Carpenter and Peter, 1972). In the study of Moore *et al.* (1971), lesions within the ascending nigrostriatal pathway produce significant decreases in caudate nucleus dopamine, tyrosine hydroxylase, and DOPA decarboxylase that conform closely to the amount of the nigrostriatal pathway transected as determined by the exact localization and size of the lesions analyzed histologically and with the extent of retrograde degeneration in the substantia nigra, pars compacta. In another study, Hökfelt and Ungerstedt (1969) demonstrated a loss of dopamine fluorescence as demonstrated by the Falck–Hillarp method in the caudate nucleus following substantia nigra lesions. This was accompanied by the appearance of degenerating terminals in the caudate–putamen of lesioned rats demonstrated by ultrastructural analysis in the immediate postoperative period and a loss of terminals with the capacity to take up α-methyl-noradrenaline *in vitro*. A subsequent ultrastructural study (Hattori *et al.*, 1973) demonstrated autoradiographic evidence for transport of tritiated protein from the substantia nigra to the caudate–putamen terminals as well as degeneration of terminals following 6-hydroxydopamine administration in the substantia nigra. With the development of the glyoxylic acid fluorescence histochemical method (Lindvall and Björklund, 1974a), it has been possible to follow the dopamine-containing axons of the nigrostriatal pathway in the rat from its origin in the substantia nigra to its termination in the caudate–putamen complex (Lindvall and Björklund, 1978). This has confirmed that the topography of the projection is essentially as described above for the cat and other species.

It is clear from each of the descriptions that there is a topographic arrangement of the axons making up the nigrostriatal pathway. Fibers terminating in the caudal portions of the caudate–putamen complex originate from the more lateral cells of the substantia nigra, pars compacta, whereas those going to the rostral and ventral regions lie more medially in an organized pattern. That the nigrostriatal pathway is topographically organized was previously suggested by Bedard *et al.* (1969), Ungerstedt (1971), Moore *et al.* (1971), and Carpenter and Peter (1972). In a recent study using the retrograde transport–horseradish peroxidase method, Fallon and Moore (1976b) confirmed the topography of this projection in the rat.

The elegant histochemical studies of Lindvall and Björklund (1974b, 1978) demonstrated the pathway using the fluorescence histochemical method, and in partially denervated specimens, they showed the remarkable axonal branching that takes place in this projection. Hökfelt (1968) and Hökfelt and Ungerstedt (1969) estimated that the dopamine-containing terminals in the caudate–putamen complex constitute about 12–16% of the total terminals innervating the nucleus. It should be noted that this is not the only area innervated by cells of the substantia nigra, pars compacta. There is significant evidence for a dopamine innervation to the globus pallidus (Moore *et al.*, 1971; Lindvall and Björklund, 1974b, 1978) and to the frontal and cingulate cortex (Lindvall *et al.*, 1974a). Nevertheless, if one restricts calculations only to the projection to the neostriatum, it has been calculated that each substantia nigra neuron has an axon 55–77 cm in length containing 500,000 terminals (Andén *et al.*, 1966a).

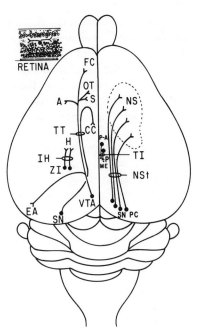

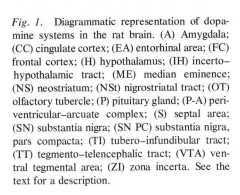

Fig. 1. Diagrammatic representation of dopamine systems in the rat brain. (A) Amygdala; (CC) cingulate cortex; (EA) entorhinal area; (FC) frontal cortex; (H) hypothalamus; (IH) incerto–hypothalamic tract; (ME) median eminence; (NS) neostriatum; (NSt) nigrostriatal tract; (OT) olfactory tubercle; (P) pituitary gland; (P-A) periventricular–arcuate complex; (S) septal area; (SN) substantia nigra; (SN PC) substantia nigra, pars compacta; (TI) tubero–infundibular tract; (TT) tegmento–telencephalic tract; (VTA) ventral tegmental area; (ZI) zona incerta. See the text for a description.

A schematic diagram of the dopamine systems in the rat brain is shown in Fig. 1. Photomicrographs of fluorescence histochemical preparations of the dopamine cells of the substantia nigra, pars compacta and their terminals in the caudate–putamen complex are shown in Figs. 5A and B.

2.2. Mesocortical System

Ungerstedt (1971) coined the term "mesolimbic system" to describe the dopamine innervation arising from cells within the ventral tegmental area (cell group A10 of Dahlström and Fuxe, 1964) and, probably, in part the adjacent substantia nigra to basal forebrain areas that were felt to contribute to the so-called "limbic" forebrain. Subsequent work originating from the laboratories of Glowinski and his collaborators (Thierry *et al.*, 1973a,b) indicated that this projection was much wider than previously suspected and involved significant portions of neocortex. Consequently, since all the areas innervated by this dopamine system are either archicortical, paleocortical, or neocortical, this will be referred to as the "mesocortical system" in its entirety. This nomenclature is also preferable on the grounds that the concept of a "limbic system" is based on a less than secure foundation (Brodal, 1969).

As noted above, the dopamine cell bodies giving rise to the mesocortical dopamine projection are located, for the most part, in the ventral tegmental area. Embryologically, they derive from the same primordium as the cells of the substantia nigra, pars compacta (Seiger and Olson, 1973). They are located medial to the cells of the substantia nigra, pars compacta, and throughout most of their extent form a cap over the interpeduncular nucleus, although they extend rostrally beyond it. More rostrally, some extend dorsally toward the periaqueductal gray. As with the nigrostriatal projection, the projection of these neurons is probably topographically organized, but has not as yet completely been elucidated. The projection is shown schematically in Fig. 1. Following their origin from the cells of the ventral tegmental area, the fibers of the mesocortical system ascend along the medial forebrain bundle in a position ventral and medial to the fibers of the nigrostriatal pathway. They continue unbranched in this position to the level of the tuberal hypothalamus, where some fibers turn laterally into the complex of fibers made up by the ansa peduncularis–ventral amygdaloid bundle system. These fibers give rise to a dense innvervation of the central amygdaloid nucleus, the intercalated amygdaloid nuclei, and a less dense innervation of the lateral and basolateral amygdaloid nuclei (Fallon and Moore, 1976*a*). Some continue through the amygdaloid complex to provide a sparse innervation to piriform cortex (Fallon and Moore, 1976*b*) and a dense innervation to the second and third layers of the ventral entorhinal cortex (Hökfelt *et al.*, 1974*b*; Lindvall *et al.*, 1974*a*).

The mesocortical axons ascending in the medial forebrain bundle have a widespread distribution within the basal forebrain and neocortex. One group, arising from ventral tegmental neurons immediately adjacent to the substantia nigra, turns dorsally and medially from the medial forebrain bundle to terminate in the nucleus accumbens. In this nucleus, it gives rise to a pattern of innervation identical to that observed from nigrostriatal axons in the neostriatum. That is, once the axons have reached the nucleus, they undergo an immense collateralization with numerous, closely approximated, small varicosities. A second group of fibers turns ventrally and distributes throughout the olfactory tubercle in a pattern of innervation also identical to that of the nigrostriatal system. The innervation is present throughout the olfactory tubercle, with the exception that occasional islands of Calleja are devoid of innervation (Fuxe, 1965*b*). At the same level, fibers turn further medially into the interstitial nucleus of the stria terminalis, where there is a dense dopamine innervation in the dorsal portion (Fuxe, 1965*b*), but there is also a smaller innervation to the ventral portion that is overshadowed by the dense noradrenaline innervation of that component of the nucleus (Lindvall and Björklund, 1974*b*, 1978; Moore, 1977). Fibers of the mesocortical system continue from the region of the nucleus accumbens and the interstitial nucleus of striä terminalis to enter the lateral septal nucleus. In this nucleus, there are two distinct patterns of termination. One is constituted by a very dense plexus of small axons and densely packed terminals in a thick band adjacent to the medial septal nucleus (Lindvall, 1975; Moore, 1977). The appearance of this plexus of dopamine fibers is nearly identical to that in the nucleus accumbens, the olfactory tubercle, or the neostriatum, with the exception that it is somewhat less dense. Scattered along the lateral border of this plexus and extending to the ventricular surface are scattered neurons that are heavily innervated by a different form of dopamine fiber. These fibers are thicker than those described above, and they run for long distances along the proximal dendrites and cell bodies of scattered, lateral septal nucleus neurons (see Fig. 6D). As they pass over the neurons, collaterals leave the parent axon and give rise to varicosities that are larger than those evident in the other dopamine terminal area. Occasionally, such fibers traversing the neuropil will also drop off a collateral with a terminal not in evident proximity to a cell body or proximal dendrite. For the most part, however, these fibers form dense, basketlike pericellular arrays about the lateral septal nucleus neurons, which are most striking in appearance (see Fig. 6D). Further fibers of of this system continue rostrally to leave the medial forebrain bundle at the level of the rostral septum. The fibers appear to sweep as a broad band along the medial and medioventral aspects of the nucleus accumbens, where the band then separates into four primary branches. The first, and largest, branch runs rostrally and dorsally into the external capsule to innervate the medial portion of the frontal cortex (Lindvall *et al.*, 1974*a*; Lindvall and Björklund, 1978; Berger *et al.*, 1976). The innervation in the frontal cortex is most dense in the second to sixth layers, but some extends into the molecular layer as well. The second branch turns dorsally to pass around the corpus callosum and ramify into a dense dopamine terminal system in the anterior cingulate cortex (Lindvall *et al.*, 1974*a*; Lindvall and Björklund, 1978). In the cingulate cortex, the dopamine innervation is most heavily concentrated in the second and third layers, with some fibers extending into the molecular layer. The third branch turns laterally into the external capsule to form a broad band of dopamine fibers in the transition cortical area between the piriform cortex and the neocortex above the rhinal fissure. The terminals of this dopamine system are largely confined to the fifth and sixth layers of the cortex (Berger *et al.*, 1976; Lindvall and Björklund, 1978). The fourth branch continues rostrally to join the medial olfactory tract and presumably terminates within rostral olfactory structures, but the site of termination has not yet been determined (Lindvall and Björklund, 1978).

The extensive projection of this system was not appreciated until recently, and there are many details that remain to be worked out. As noted previously, it does appear to be topographically organized, but with some significant overlap with the substantia nigra projection. The origin of the neurons giving rise to this system and its distribution and overlap of projections with the substantia nigra system strongly suggest that these should probably be viewed as a single dopamine system innervating telencephalon.

2.3. Tubero–Hypophysial System

The existence of catecholamines in the median eminence and infundibular stem of mammals was first observed by Fuxe (Fuxe, 1963, 1964; Fuxe and Hökfelt, 1966), using the Falck–Hillarp technique. These studies demonstrated the existence of cell bodies within the arcuate component of the periventricular nucleus of the hypothalamus, with some fluorescent cell bodies extending into adjacent components of the periventricular nucleus. Within the median eminence, a dense, nearly confluent innvervation comprised of very fine varicosities was found in the zona externa, with similar fibers intermingled among larger, coarser varicose fibers in the internal and subependymal layers. Subsequent studies indicated that the coarser, varicose fibers in the internal and subependymal layers of the median eminence are axons of noradrenaline-producing neurons the cell bodies of which are located within the brain stem (Björklund et al., 1970, 1973; Jonsson et al., 1972). The fine terminal plexus in the zona externa, and the cells in the arcuate and periventricular nuclei, were determined to be dopamine-containing on the basis of microspectrofluorimetry, and remained following complete deafferentation of the hypothalamus (Björklund et al., 1970). This strongly suggested that the dopamine innervation of the zona externa of the median eminence originated from the cells of the arcuate and periventricular nuclei. In a very elaborate lesion study, Björklund et al. (1973) demonstrated that the arcuate dopamine neurons, like the dopamine neurons described previously, are topographically organized within the arcuate nucleus–periventricular complex. Cell bodies in the rostral portion of the nucleus give rise to a diffuse projection extending along the entire median eminence and pituitary stalk. The remaining dopamine neurons of the arcuate nucleus project directly to the median eminence at the same level beneath them (Fig. 2). The ultrastructure of this projection was studied by Hökfelt and co-workers (Hökfelt, 1967; Ajika and Hökfelt, 1973, 1975). With the use of in vitro administration of 5-hydroxydopamine, terminals containing small, dense-core vesicles, about 50 nm in diameter, are observed in the external zone of the median eminence. These are most frequent in the lateral part of the external zone, where they comprise 33%

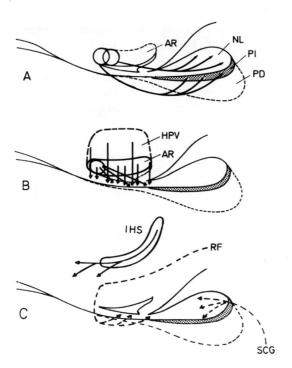

Fig. 2. Diagrammatic representation of the catecholamine innervation of the median eminence–pituitary region. The diagram is represented in the sagittal plane. (AR) Arcuate nucleus;
(HPV) periventricular nucleus of the hypothalamus; (IHS) incerto–hypothalamic system; (NL)
neural lobe; (PD) pars distalis; (PI) pars intermedia; (RF) reticular formation; (SCG) superior
cervical ganglion. See the text for a description.

of all terminals. In contrast to this, in the medial portion of the external
zone, they comprise only 13% of all terminals. In the adjacent internal
layer, such boutons comprised 17 and 7%, respectively, in the lateral and
medial portions of the median eminence. Further evidence that these
vesicles arise from cell bodies in the arcuate nucleus is provided by the fact
that the percentage of boutons with small granular vesicles decreases from
approximately 32% in control animals to 4% in animals with lesions of the
arcuate nucleus (Ajika and Hökfelt, 1975).

In addition to this component of the tubero–hypophysial dopamine
neuron system, there is also a direct innervation of the pituitary. This is
made up of a rich innervation of both the neural lobe and the pars
intermedia of the pituitary in the rat that originates from cell bodies located
in the anterior part of the arcuate nucleus (Fig. 2). The cell bodies innervating the pars intermedia lie just rostral to those innervating the neural lobe

(Björklund *et al.*, 1973). In a combined electron-microscopic and fluorescence histochemical study, Baumgarten *et al.* (1972) found that dopamine terminals make close contacts with neurosecretory axons and pituicytes in the neutral lobe and with endocrine cells of the pars intermedia. This suggests a possible role for these dopamine neurons in the regulation of hormone secretion from both the neural lobe and the pars intermedia.

2.4. Incerto–Hypothalamic System

Although several catecholamine-containing cell groups were identified in the diencephalon with the use of the Falck–Hillarp method (Dählstrom and Fuxe, 1964; Fuxe *et al.*, 1970; Ungerstedt, 1971; Björklund and Nobin, 1973; Jacobowitz and Palkovits, 1974), it was not until the introduction of the glyoxylic acid method (Lindvall and Björklund, 1974*a*) that an extensive group of cell bodies with low fluorescence intensity was identified in the medial portion of the zona incerta. In an extensive study using the glyoxylic acid method, Björklund *et al.* (1975) demonstrated that the dopamine-containing neurons forming this cell group in the zona incerta have a short, intrahypothalamic projection system (Figs. 1 and 2). The axons of the incerto–hypothalamic system are very delicate and have a low fluorescence intensity. These fine axons have regularly spaced, fine varicosities, and even in excellent preparations, the intervaricose segments are difficult to observe. On the basis of their studies, Björklund *et al.* (1975) divided the incerto–hypothalamic system into two topographic components: a rostral periventricular–preoptic part and a caudal diencephalic part.

The rostral part of the system is located in the anterior periventricular nucleus in association with neurons of the rostral periventricular dopamine cell group (A14 of Björklund and Nobin, 1973). This group is composed of scattered, small round or oval cells with an average diameter of approximately 10 μm. The cells are located medially in the rostral hypothalamus approximately from the level of the anterior commissure to the rostral border of the median eminence. Most of the cells are located within the anterior periventricular nucleus and somewhat lateral to it in the preoptic area. The axons of this system are particularly evident in the medial preoptic area, where they form dense patterns surrounding nonfluorescent perikarya. In addition, fibers extend rostrally into the periventricular and medial hypothalamic area, but not into the suprachiasmatic nucleus. Some of these fibers are believed to extend in a rostral and dorsal direction along the diagonal band to distribute into the most caudal portion of the lateral septal nucleus.

The caudal part of the incerto–hypothalamic system arises from the caudal thalamus, zona incerta, and adjacent posterior, dorsal hypothalamic area. The densest group of cells is located in the most medial portion of the zona incerta, just ventral and medial to the mammilothalamic tract and dorsal to the dorsomedial hypothalamic nucleus. The fine, varicose fibers of this caudal, incerto–hypothalamic system form a loosely arranged bundle that runs rostrally into the dorsal and anteriorhypothalamic areas, where the fibers form basketlike arrangements around neuronal perikarya (Björklund *et al.,* 1975). The location of the terminal innervation of the incerto–hypothalamic system is such as to suggest that it may well participate in neuroendocrine regulatory functions.

2.5. Retinal System

In the retina, a special type of dopamine-producing neuron has been described in a number of mammalian and nonmammalian forms (Malmfors, 1963; Ehinger, 1966*a*–*c*; Laties and Jacobowitz, 1966). This dopamine neuron, in most instances, lies among the amacrine cells of the inner nuclear layer of the retina. In most mammalian species (including the rat and the human), the terminals of these retinal dopamine neurons are located exclusively in the inner plexiform layer in a band at its outer border. In other species, notably New World monkeys and teleost fish, there is a second terminal plexus found in the outer plexiform layer (Laties and Jacobowitz, 1966; Ehinger and Falck, 1969; Ehinger *et al.,* 1969).

In the goldfish and in the Cebus monkey, Dowling and Ehinger (1975) showed that the dopamine neurons form synapses with amacrine cells in the inner plexiform layer and with bipolar and horizontal cells in the outer plexiform layer. The retinal dopamine neuron is of interest in that in some instances, it is postsynaptic to processes from amacrine cells in the inner plexiform layer and in other instances is presynaptic. Thus, it is probably best to view this catecholamine neuron as one that is an interneuron lacking an axon (Dowling and Ehinger, 1975).

2.6. Periventricular System

This system of dopamine neurons is not illustrated in Fig. 1. In the strict sense, it is not a dopamine neuron system. The axonal components of the system are probably comprised of dopamine-, noradrenaline-, and adrenalline-producing fibers, but the cell bodies comprised within the periventricular gray are largely, if not exclusively, dopamine-producing. This system, identified by Lindvall and Björklund (1974*b*, 1978), has cell bodies that are predominately distributed along the periaqueductal gray of the mesencephalon and the periventricular gray of the caudal thalamus. These are continuous with other components of the system that extend along the mesencephalic raphe ventral to the nucleus dorsalis raphe and scattered cells in the periventricular gray adjacent to the fourth ventricle.

The fibers of the periventricular catecholamine system are distributed along the periventricular and periaqueductal gray from the caudal medulla to the rostral diencephalon. Those in the brain stem, termed the "dorsal periventricular system" by Lindvall and Björklund (1974b, 1978), can be viewed as a component of the dorsal longitudinal fasciculus. These authors also identify a ventral periventricular system that extends along the periventricular region of the hypothalamus.

Caudally, the periventricular system lies within the periventricular gray of the fourth ventricle at the level of the nucleus of the solitary tract and the dorsal motor nucleus of the vagus. It probably receives fibers from the CA neurons of those dorsal tegmental cell groups that ascend in the periventricular gray. At the level of the locus coeruleus, the system increases considerably in the number of fibers within it, probably representing the locus coeruleus projection into the periventricular and periaqueductal gray. By autoradiographic analysis (Jones and Moore, 1977), it would appear that these fibers ascend along the periaqueductal gray into the periventricular nucleus of the hypothalamus. Rostrally, this system within the dorsal longitudinal fasciculus gives rise to the diencephalic periventricular system. This includes projections to the periventricular nucleus of the hypothalamus, the midline nuclei of the thalamus (nucleus rhomboideus and nucleus paraventricularis).

The ventral periventricular system, as described by Lindvall and Björklund (1974b, 1978), is first observed caudally in the region immediately dorsal and lateral to the interpeduncular nucleus. The fibers run rostrally and pass above the medial mammillary nucleus ventral to the caudal extension of the third ventricle. Fibers leave the system to innervate the mammillary complex and, at that level, receive collaterals from fibers ascending in the medial forebrain bundle system. The pathway ascends in a periventricular position to innervate the dorsomedial hypothalamic nucleus and the periventricular nucleus. More rostrally, it provides some innervation to the paraventricular hypothalamic nucleus, and then continues rostrally through the lateral and dorsal periventricular hypothalamus to terminate in the interstitial nucleus of the stria terminalis. According to Lindvall and Björklund (1974b, 1978), this system is very difficult to visualize in normal fluorescence histochemical preparations, but is quite evident in glyoxylic acid material. It is their view that in addition to the long projections noted above, there are numerous short axon projections within the periventricular and periaqueductal gray from the diencephalon to the medulla.

3. Noradrenaline Systems

3.1. Locus Coeruleus System

The locus coeruleus is a prominent nucleus located in the brain stem reticular formation at the level of the isthmus. Its existence has been known for a number of years, and an extensive review of its cytoarchitecture in a number of mammalian species was provided by Russell (1955). Until the development of the Falck–Hillarp method, however, very little was known of the connections or significance of this nucleus. The early work of Dahlström and Fuxe (1964) demonstrated that the locus coeruleus is composed virtually entirely of noradrenaline-producing cells (see Fig. 5C), and this being the case, it is the largest noradrenaline neuron nucleus in the mammalian brain. In the rat, for example, Swanson and Hartman (1975) indicate that it includes approximately 45% of all the noradrenaline-producing neurons of the rat brain. Early studies of the locus coeruleus indicated that it has widespread projections throughout the neuraxis (Andén *et al.*, 1966*b*; Olson and Fuxe, 1971; Ungerstedt, 1971). It was the work of Ungerstedt (1971), in particular, that demonstrated an extensive telencephalic innervation by locus coeruleus neurons. This work has subsequently been confirmed and extended using a variety of techniques, and the review of locus coeruleus anatomy and projections to follow is based on all this work. Since there is now an extensive literature on the projections of the locus coeruleus, no attempt will be made to review it in its entirety here.

The neurons of the locus coeruleus form a distinct, compact cell group largely contained within the central gray of the isthmus, medial to the mesencephalic nucleus of the trigeminal nerve (Russell, 1955; Swanson, 1976). There are few exceptions to this, but it is worth noting that in the cat, the nucleus is much more widely dispersed than in most mammalian species, and occupies a large portion of the dorsolateral tegmentum at the isthmic level (Chu and Bloom, 1974; Jones and Moore, 1974). The locus coeruleus has been studied using the Falck–Hillarp method in several primate species (Hubbard and DiCarlo, 1973; DiCarlo *et al.*, 1973; Felten *et al.*, 1974; Garver and Sladek, 1975). The nucleus is quite homogeneous in primates, and its size and appearance in these species conforms to that of most other mammalian species. Since nearly all the work on the projections

of locus coeruleus has been done on the rat, the remainder of this review
will be directed toward observations in that species. The locus coeruleus in
the rat is comprised of approximately 1500 neurons on each side (Swanson,
1976). In Nissl preparations, these cells are deeply staining, medium-size
neurons that appear fusiform or bipolar in shape. Swanson (1976) described
two components of the nucleus, a large dorsal component and a smaller
ventral component. In Golgi preparations (Swanson, 1976), locus coeruleus
neurons appear to be predominately multipolar with three to five large,
rather thin dendrites that radiate from the soma and typically branch once
or twice. Many of the secondary and tertiary branches of the dendrites
extend well outside the limits of the nucleus into the surrounding neuropil.
After emerging from the soma, the axon of locus coeruleus neurons typically gives off two or three fine collaterals within the nucleus and further
collaterals beyond it.

The evidence currently available indicates that locus coeruleus neurons give rise to descending axons into the spinal cord and brain stem,
ascending axons into the brain stem, diencephalon, and telencephalon, and
a further group of axons projecting into the cerebellum (Fig. 3). There is no
evidence at present that the projection of locus coeruleus neurons is
topographic to any of these areas. Indeed, the available evidence indicates

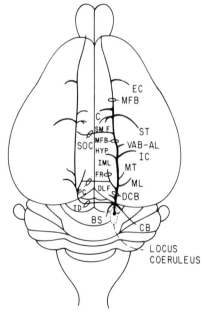

Fig. 3. Diagrammatic representation of locus coeruleus projections in the rat as seen from the horizontal plane. (AL) Ansa lenticularis; (BS) brain
stem; (C) cingulum; (CB) cerebellum; (DCB) dorsal
CA bundle; (DLF) dorsal longitudinal fasciculus;
(EC) external capsule; (F) fornix; (FR) fasciculus
retroflexus; (HYP) hypothalamus; (IC) internal capsule; (IML) internal medullary laminae; (MFB)
medial forebrain bundle; (ML) medical lemniscus;
(MT) mamillothalmic tract; (PC) posterior commissure; (SM) stria medullaris; (SOC) supraoptic commissure; (ST) stria terminalis; (TD) tegmental decussation; (VAB) ventral amygdaloid bundle. See the
text for a description.

that each locus coeruleus neuron provides innervation to more than one of the regions noted above.

The following description of the pathways of locus coeruleus neuron axons is derived from studies using the fluorescence histochemial method (Olson and Fuxe, 1971; Ungerstedt, 1971; Maeda and Shimizu, 1972; Lindvall and Björklund, 1974*b*, 1978) and studies using the autoradiographic tracing technique (Pickel *et al.,* 1974; Jones and Moore, 1977). In a preliminary study, Jones *et al.* (1977) demonstrated that tritiated proline injected into the locus coeruleus is taken up into locus coeruleus neurons and incorporated into protein, which is then transported along the axons to terminal sites. Injection of tritiated L-DOPA gave a pattern of transport identical to that with tritiated proline. Pretreatment of animals with 6-hydroxydopamine gave a pattern of distribution that was totally different in that transport to many areas known to receive locus coeruleus projections was not evident. These experiments formed the basis for an autoradiographic study.

In the autoradiographic material, the major ascending pathway originating from the locus coeruleus projects rostrally into the mesencephalic tegmentum as the dorsal CA bundle described by Ungerstedt (1971). In addition, there is a significant projection into the periventricular gray that ascends along the periaqueductal gray of the mesencephalon. The fibers of the dorsal CA bundle pass rostrally through the subcoeruleus area and then take a position in the midbrain lateral and ventral to the periaqueductal gray. At the level of the fasciculus retroflexus, the bundle turns ventrally to traverse the prerubral field of Forel and the medial portion of the zona incerta before joining the dorsal portion of the medial forebrain bundle complex at the level of the caudal, tuberal hypothalamus. This projection will be referred to as the "dorsal pathway." In addition to the fibers ascending in the periaqueductal gray, there is another ascending pathway, much smaller than either of the pathways described above, that turns ventrally to the tegmentum in the central tegmental bundle and enters the mammillary peduncle and ventral tegmental areas as a compact group. Two descending projections are evident. One enters the superior cerebellar peduncle to innervate the cerebellum (Pickel *et al.,* 1974). The other descends in the central tegmental bundle to innervate some cranial nerve nuclei and brain stem reticular formation before entering the spinal cord in the ventral white matter.

As the dorsal pathway crosses the fasciculus retroflexus in the rostral tegmentum, fibers are given off that descend along that tract to terminate in the parafascicular nucleus and habenula. Some fibers arising from the fasciculus retroflexus continue dorsally over the superficial zone of the thalamus, and others enter the medullary laminae of the thalamus, giving rise to the majority of the dorsal thalamic innervation. The ascending fibers of the locus coeruleus projection that enter the medial forebrain bundle give rise to several distinct groups of fibers innervating telencephalon and hypothalamus. A portion of the hypothalamic innervation, that to the periventricular and dorsomedial nuclei, appears to arise largely from ascending fibers in the periventricular system. Other fibers leave the medial forebrain bundle to terminate in the paraventricular hypothalamic nucleus. As the fibers ascend in the medial forebrain bundle system through the diencephalon, there are numerous fascicles of fibers that leave the main bundle to turn laterally and enter the ventral amygdaloid bundle and ansa peduncularis system. Part of these enter basal telencephalic areas (amygdala, entorhinal cortex, and hippocampus), and others continue into the external capsule. As the medial forebrain bundle system ascends, locus coeruleus fibers leave it at the level of the caudal septum in several groups. One group turns medially into the diagonal band of Broca to innervate the septum, and then enters the fornix. The second enters the stria medullaris, turning caudally and continuing along its length through the habenular nuclei. The third enters the stria terminalis and follows its path to the amygdaloid complex. The fourth group of fibers continues in the medial forebrain bundle as it enters the basal telencephalon. A portion of this continues rostrally into the external capsule, whereas other fibers are given off to deep layers of the olfactory tubercle and anterior olfactory nucleus. A final group of fibers traverses the diagonal band and Zuckerkandl's bundle to turn around the rostrum of the corpus callosum and run caudally within the cingulum.

In addition to these ipsilateral projections of the locus coeruleus, there are a number of commissures in the system giving rise to contralateral projections (Fig. 3). The first of these occurs just rostral to the locus coeruleus in the isthmic tegmentum. The fibers cross ventral to the medial longitudinal fasciculus adjacent to the commissure of Probst. These fibers then join the contralateral dorsal pathway. A second commissure is in the posterior commissure. Fibers leaving the dorsal pathway and ascending the fasciculus retroflexus course over the periaqueductal gray and enter the posterior commissure. They take an identical path on the contralateral side to form a component of the contralateral dorsal pathway. The third commissural pathway arises from the ipsilateral dorsal pathway fibers that run laterally into the internal capsule and collect on the ventral, lateral surface of the optic tract. At rostral, tuberal hypothalamic levels, these turn medially to cross in the dorsal supraoptic commissure and enter the contralateral forebrain bundle. A fourth commissure is present in the anterior commissure at the level of the interstitial nuclei of the stria terminalis. Last, there is a small, fifth commissure that crosses in the rostrum of the corpus callosum.

The terminal projections of the locus coeruleus are best seen in fluorescence histochemical material. As noted by Lindvall and Björklund (1974*b*, 1978), preterminal locus coeruleus axons are thin, with fusiform varicosities that are not of intense fluorescence. When a terminal field is reached, however, the preterminal fibers break up into a highly collateralized network that has many features common to all areas innervated. The primary feature is the axonal morphology. Axons of the locus coeruleus system in a terminal area are typically fine with regularly spaced, round, intensely fluorescent varicosities approximately 1–2 μm in diameter (Figs. 5D and 6B). Frequently, these form a plexus of apparently randomly arranged axons, but the pattern varies from area to area. The gray matter of the spinal cord contains a plexus of catecholamine-containing axons (Dahlström and Fuxe, 1965), and the recent work of Kuypers and Miasky (1975), utilizing the horseradish peroxidase–retrograde transport method, indicates that the locus coeruleus innervates all segments of spinal cord. There is also a clear locus coeruleus innervation in brain stem nuclei such as the cochlear nucleus (Kromer and Moore, 1976). The pattern of innervation in various brain stem areas may differ significantly; e.g., within the cochlear nucleus complex, there are areas in which locus fibers are found predominantly in the neuropil, presumably terminating on or around dendrites, whereas in in other areas, there are varicosities around proximal dendrites and neuronal somata.

A second area in which the innervation from locus coeruleus has been described in detail is the cerebellum (Olson and Fuxe, 1971; Bloom *et al.*, 1971; Mugnaini and Dahl, 1975). The work of Bloom *et al.* (1971) on the rat demonstrates a fairly sparse innervation of cerebellar cortex. Some fibers are present in the granule cell layer, but the major innervation appears to be to the molecular layer of the cerebellar cortex. The majority of this innervation is present in the vicinity of the proximal dendrites of Purkinje cells, where some fibers appear to run in a longitudinal direction along the Purkinje cell layer and others in a vertical direction toward the surface of the follium, along the Purkinje cell dendrites.

The major CA innervation of the thalamus originates from locus coeruleus (Lindvall *et al.*, 1974*b*). As noted above, the majority of these axons ascend in the dorsal pathway and enter well-known thalamic fiber groups. There is a typical locus coeruleus, plexus-type innervation within the geniculate nuclei, both medial and lateral. In the dorsal lateral geniculate nucleus, the innervation is quite dense as compared with that in the ventral lateral geniculate. The ventral thalamic nuclei, the lateral thalamic nuclei, and the midline–intralaminar complex exhibit a moderate to sparse innervation. There is a very dense innervation to the anteroventral and anteromedial nuclei, forming an extremely dense plexus. The dorsomedial nucleus receives a sparse innervation. The characteristic of all the thalamic innervation is that it is of the typical, plexus-type locus coeruleus form.

The telencephalic innervation exhibits a greater variability. This can be exemplified by describing three typical types of telencephalic innervation. In the septal nuclei, there is a sparse innervation of the medial septal nucleus and nucleus septofimbrialis by locus coeruleus fibers in a plexus-type arrangement. Similarly, the lateral septal nucleus and the interstitial nucleus of the stria terminalis exhibit a sparse, plexus-type innervation that, in both cases, is intermingled with innervation from brain stem noradrenaline cell groups and from dopamine cell groups in the rostral midbrain. Consequently, the septal nuclei represent a combination of pure locus-coeruleus-type innervation in the medial septal nucleus, with a mixed CA innervation in the lateral septal nucleus. In contrast to this, the hippocampal formation receives a pure noradrenaline innervation of locus coeruleus origin. Nevertheless, it differs from the innervation of thalamus in that it has a precise distribution within the hippocampal formation. In the hippocampus proper, there is dense innervation of the stratum moleculare and stratum lacunosum of CA1, with fibers leaving the predominantly longitudinally oriented fiber plexus of these layers in a radial direction along the apical dendrites of the CA1 pyramidal cells within the stratum radiatum. At the tip of the apical dendrite, many fibers branch longitudinally along the base of the pyramidal cell. There do not appear to be pericellular contacts on the pyramidal cells, and the stratum oriens is sparsely innervated. In CA3, the innervation of stratum radiatum is much more dense than in CA1, and this continues into the hilar zone of the area dentata. In the hilar zone, the innervation is most dense along the base of the granule cell layer, and there is only a sparse plexiform arrangement of fibers within the molecular layer.

This can be contrasted further with the innervation of neocortex. Neocortical innervation is similar in all areas of cortex and conforms, in many respects, to the descriptions of nonspecific cortical innervation as given by Lorente de No' (1949) and Scheibel and Scheibel (1957). Preterminal fibers leave the external capsule and turn radially toward the pial surface of the cortex. Shortly after leaving the white matter, they branch profusely and form a plexus in the deep layers that is continuous with a less dense plexus in the intermediate cortical layers (layers III and IV). Despite the plexiform arrangement, there continue to be numerous radial fibers that ascend through the second layer to enter the molecular layer, where they branch longitudinally with division extending for as long as a millimeter in either direction (see Fig. 5D). The innervation of the molecular layer is more dense than that of any other layer of neocortex. The noradrenaline innervation of neocortex is heaviest in the frontal and cingulate areas, and less dense in the somatosensory, auditory, and visual areas. However, there are no striking differences among the patterns of innervation in any of these areas.

A striking aspect of the locus coeruleus innervation to neocortex was recently described by Descarries *et al.* (1977). In a detailed electron-microscopic autoradiographic study of locus coeruleus noradreneline terminals within neocortex, Descarries and his associates found that only a minor proportion of these terminals (about 5%) make synaptic contacts with postsynaptic elements. This is in contrast to all other terminals in the cortex save for the serotonin terminals (Descarries *et al.,* 1975), which make many more synaptic contacts (approximately 50%). The serotonin terminals are quite similar to the noradrenaline terminals in number of synaptic contacts, and these observations suggest that the relationship of these monoamine-producing axons with postsynaptic elements in cortex differs significantly from that of other forms of cortical innvervation.

3.2. Lateral Tegmental System

The projection pattern of the lateral tegmental noradrenaline neuron system is shown diagrammatically in Fig. 4. This system originates from a scattered group of noradrenaline neurons that are located in the lateral tegmentum extending from the medulla to the caudal midbrain. They were described by Dahlström and Fuxe (1964) as cell groups, A1, A3, A5, and A7. Subsequent descriptions of these cell groups have been given in the rat by a number of investigators (Ungerstedt, 1971; Palkovits and Jacobowitz, 1974; Swanson and Hartman, 1975; Dupin *et al.,* 1976; Lindvall and Björklund, 1978). With minor distinctions among the descriptions, the overall pattern described is quite similar. There are two major accumulations of lateral tegmental neurons. The first is in the caudal medulla in the vicinity of the lateral reticular nucleus. The cells occasionally are found in the lateral reticular nucleus, but for the most part are present in the lateral tegmental field dorsal and lateral to the lateral reticular nucleus. Rostral to this, scattered cells are found along the lateral tegmental field to the level of the emerging route of the seventh nerve, where more numerous cells are present medial to the nerve fibers. This is a scattered group of cells that is continuous rostrally to the level of the rostral portion of the superior olivary complex. At the greatest extent of the superior olivary complex, these cells

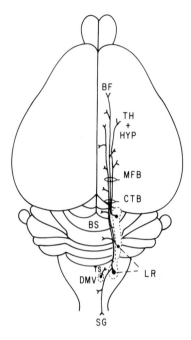

Fig. 4. Diagrammatic representation of the lateral tegmental noradrenaline cell group projections. (BF) Basal forebrain; (BS) brain stem; (CTB) central tegmental bundle; (DMV) dorsal motor nucleus of the vagus; (HYP) hypothalamus; (LR) lateral reticular formation; (MFB) medial forebrain bundle; (SG) spinal gray; (TH) thalamus, (TS) tractus solitarius. See the text for a description.

occupy a portion of the lateral tegmental field dorsal and lateral to the lateral superior olivary nucleus. At that level, they are ventral to the motor trigeminal nucleus and to the locus coeruleus, and there is a scattered group of multipolar, noradrenaline-containing neurons through the lateral tegmental field extending from the ventral part of the locus coeruleus to the cell group adjacent to the superior olivary complex. This group has been termed the "subcoeruleus" group (Ungerstedt, 1971), and it is continuous rostrally with a group of cells in the dorsal lateral tegmental field that extends rostral and lateral to the compact portion of the locus coeruleus. These cells lie in the lateral tegmental field adjacent to, and partly within, the dorsal portion of the ventral nucleus of the lateral lemniscus. In essence, however, the lateral tegmental group is a nearly continuous group of scattered neurons in the lateral tegmental field from the rostral isthmus to the caudal medulla. In addition, there is a dorsal medullary group of CA neurons that lies predominantly within the dorsal motor nucleus of the vagus and the adjacent nucleus of the tractus solitarius, including its commissural portion (the A2 groups of Dahlström and Fuxe, 1964). This is a complex group that has been shown by enzyme immunohistochemistry to contain adrenaline neurons, noradrenaline neurons, and dopamine neurons

(Hökfelt, unpublished). Similar groups of neurons have been described in primates (DiCarlo *et al.,* 1973; Felten *et al.,* 1974; Garver and Sladek, 1975). Very little is known of the projections of the dorsal tegmental group, and they will not be described in any detail. Lindvall and Björklund (1974*b*) observed axons arising from these cells giving rise to a branch with one collateral ascending in the dorsal periventricular system and another descending into the spinal cord.

The lateral tegmental system appears to have two major components. This is based both on its ontogenetic development (Seiger and Olson, 1973) and on the basis of connections (Lindvall and Björklund, 1974*b,* 1978). Although both the major medullary and pontine lateral tegmental cell groups appear to give rise to ascending and descending projections, each appears to have a major direction of projection. The caudal, medullary cell group appears to provide the majority of the bulbospinal projection, whereas the pontine cell group appears to provide predominantly ascending projections. Within the brain stem itself, it has been very difficult to discern the patterns of projection and to determine the sources of innervation that are evident in brain stem nuclei. In addition, the lateral tegmental projections have been studied in much less detail than the locus coeruleus system. The basis of this is obvious because the locus coeruleus forms a compact, uniform cell group that is technically readily approachable, whereas the lateral tegmental cells are scattered and intermingled among many non-CA neurons. The following text will describe the major projection systems of the lateral tegmental system.

Ascending projections, arising largely from the lateral tegmental group of the pons, but with components from the medullary cell group, ascend in the central tegmental tract, passing through and ventral to the decussation of the superior cerebellar peduncles, and then ascend through the ventral mesencephalic tegmentum into the diencephalon. Some ascend quite ventrally along the course of the ventral tegmental area, whereas others are scattered more dorsal to this (Lindvall and Björklund, 1974*b*). This system, passing through the medial forebrain bundle complex, gives rise to the major innervation of the medial hypothalamus. This includes innervation to the zona interna and subependymal zone of the median eminence and in the arcuate nucleus. Areas of high terminal density are found in the paraventricular, dorsomedial, periventricular, tuberomammillary and anterior hypothalamic nuclei, and in the anterior hypothalamic area and the ventral tuberal hypothalamic area. Although not shown in Fig. 4, it would appear that a significant number of fibers in this system decussate within the supraoptic commissures to terminate on the opposite side in areas that as yet have not been identified. The lateral tegmental noradrenaline compo-

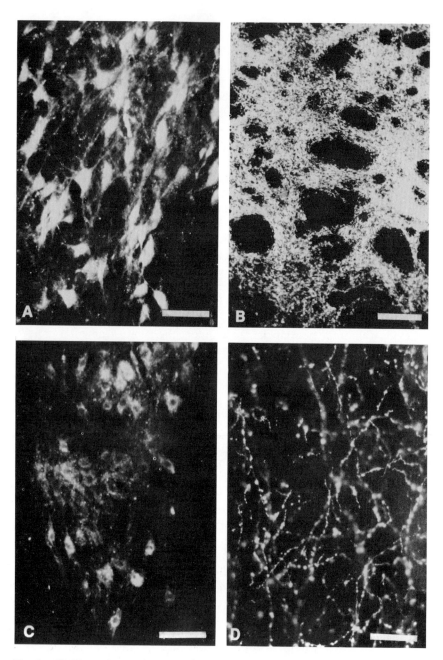

Fig. 5. (A) Photomicrograph of the substantia nigra demonstrating fluorescent cell bodies with dendrites in the pars compacta. Falck–Hillarp method. Marker bar = 50 μm. (B) Caudate–putamen complex demonstrating dense innervation by axons and axon terminals arising from substantia nigra neurons. The open, nonfluorescent spaces are occupied by fibers

nent of the medial forebrain bundle continues rostrally in the lateral hypo-thalamus. Some fibers turn laterally through the ventral amygdaloid bun-dle–ansa peduncularis system to innervate the amygdaloid complex and, to a small extent, the neostriatum. The remaining ascending fibers run in the medial forebrain bundle ventral to the neostriatum. From this position, some turn into the nucleus of the diagonal band and the deep layers of the olfactory tubercle to innervate the interstitial nucleus of the stria terminalis with a very dense plexus and continue into the lateral septal nucleus (see Figs. 6A and C). Whether fibers of this system ascend into the olfactory forebrain or not is unknown at present.

The major descending system is the bulbospinal system. It arises in large part from the cells in the lateral tegmental field of the medulla adjacent to the lateral reticular nucleus, but contains components from the locus coeruleus, the dorsal tegmental cell groups, and probably the pontine lateral tegmental cells. Descending CA axons were identified as a bulbo-spinal noradrenaline system by Carlsson *et al.* (1964) and Dahlström and Fuxe (1965). The organization of the bulbospinal axons was distinguished by Dahlström and Fuxe (1965) into two different systems. The first is a large system of fibers running in the ventral column of the spinal cord and the most ventral part of the lateral column. This terminates in the ventral horn. Another, somewhat smaller, system descends in the lateral funiculus in a somewhat dorsal position and terminates in the dorsal horn and, in the thoracic spinal cord, in the intermediolateral cell column. Within the spinal cord gray, then, there are three areas receiving noradrenaline innervation. The area receiving the densest innervation is the intermediolateral cell column of the thoracic and upper lumbar cord. The majority of the termi-nals appear to be concentrated in the ventral medial portion, where they appear to be in very close approximation to the cell bodies of the pregan-glionic sympathetic neurons. The ventral horn is richly supplied with a noradrenaline terminal plexus. These are most numerous in the ventral two-thirds, and there appear to be both axodendritic and axosomatic arrangements on both motor neurons and on smaller interneurons. The lowest density of innervation is in the dorsal horn, where the axons appear to form a loosely arranged plexus.

---

of the internal capsule traversing the neostriatal complex. Glyoxylic acid method. Marker bar = 80 μm. (C) Locus coeruleus demonstrating cell bodies of a characteristic noradrenaline cell group. Falck–Hillarp method. Marker bar = 80μm. (D) Molecular layer of cortex demonstrat-ing numerous, varicose fibers of locus coeruleus origin terminating in the molecular layer as varicose fibers. Glyoxylic acid method. Marker bar = 50μm.

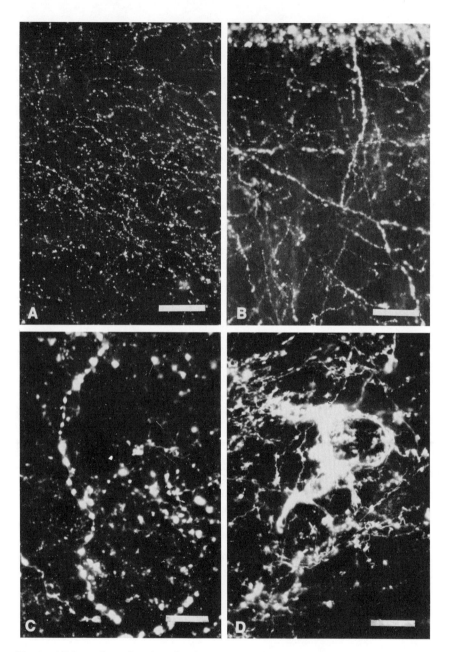

Fig. 6. (A) Lateral septal nucleus showing coarse and fine varicose fibers of the noradrenaline type. Falck–Hillarp method. Marker bar = 80μm. (B) Hippocampal CA1 zone. The intensely fluorescent structures at the top of the figure are autofluorescent pyramidal cells of the CA1 zone. Beneath them are fluorescent axons innervating the hippocampal CA1 stratum radiatum. These arise from locus coeruleus. Falck–Hillarp method. Marker bar = 50μm. (C) Basal

4. Adrenaline System

Adrenaline has been localized within specific regions of the mammalian nervous system by a number of investigators (Vogt, 1954; Gunne, 1962; Koslow and Schlumpf, 1974; Reid *et al.*, 1975; Zivin *et al.*, 1975; Van der Gugten *et al.*, 1976) using a variety of methods including bioassay, spectrofluorometric assay, gas chromatography–mass spectrometry, and radioisotopic–enzymatic assay. In addition, the enzyme that converts noradrenaline to adrenaline, phenylethanolamine-*N*-methyltransferase (PNMT), has been demonstrated to be present in the mammalian CNS (Ciaranello *et al.*, 1969; Pohorecky *et al.*, 1969; Saavedra *et al.*, 1974; Reid *et al.*, 1975, 1976) in a regional distribution. As with the other CA neuron systems, however, assay for the amine itself or for enzymes producing it has given relatively little information concerning the organization of neuron systems utilizing adrenaline as a neurotransmitter. In comparison with noradrenaline and dopamine, though, adrenaline would appear to be a minor CA, since most investigators find it to be present in brain in a range approximating 10% of the noradrenaline content.

The most useful advance in studying adrenaline neuron systems has been the development of an enzyme immunohistochemical method for PNMT (Hökfelt *et al.*, 1973, 1974a). All the PNMT-positive neurons identified by Hökfelt *et al.*, (1973, 1974a) are multipolar neurons of the reticular formation that are organized into two groups. One group, termed the "C1" group, lies among the noradrenaline cells of the lateral reticular formation, whereas the other group, termed "C2," is present in the dorsal medullary cell group. Hökfelt *et al.* (1974a) identified one axon bundle arising from the medullary cell groups. This appears to ascend along with the noradrenaline axons. Terminal axons, as shown by PNMT-positive varicosities, have been identified in a number of areas. These include the dorsal motor nucleus of the vagus, the nucleus of the tractus solitarius, the paraventricular nucleus of the thalamus, the intermediolateral cell column of the spinal cord, the periventricular gray around the fourth ventricle and cerebral aqueduct, the locus coeruleus, the dorsomedial hypothalamic

---

forebrain showing a coarse, intensely fluorescent noradrenaline fiber with numerous, large varicose components. Glyoxylic acid method. Marker bar = 25 μm. (D) Lateral septal nucleus showing numerous dopamine axons forming basket-type synapse around a lateral septal nucleus neuron. The neuron is in the right center of the field. Two dendrites arising from its left border are so heavily innervated as to appear fluorescent. This appearance is due, however, to a confluence of thin dopamine fibers about the proximal dendrites. Glyoxylic acid method. Marker bar = 30 μm.

nucleus, and the perifornical area of the hypothalamus. In addition, a low density of PNMT-positive varicosities is evident in the rhomboid nucleus of the thalamus, the periventricular hypothalamus, the arcuate nucleus of the hypothalamus, the posterior lateral hypothalamus, the medial subthalamus, and the periventricular gray surrounding the central canal of the upper spinal cord. This distribution of terminals demonstrated by immunohisto-chemistry does not conform entirely to the distribution of either PNMT or adrenaline as shown by analytical biochemical methodology. There are two potential interpretations of this. First, the PNMT method has proved a difficult one to work out, and the work thus far carried on may be partially vitiated by a lack of sensitivity of the method. This has been true with most immunohistochemical methods developed to date, and is not meant to be critical of the workers employing these methods. Inevitably, refinements of technique occur and sensitivity increases, demonstrating more substantive evidence for the organization of the neuron system in question. Undoubt-edly, this will occur with the adrenaline neuron system. The second problem is that adrenaline and PNMT themselves present some difficulties in assay, and it is possible that some of the areas that appear to contain either the enzyme or the amine do not. With both the analytical methods and the immunohistochemical method, the problems of analysis and identi-fication are confounded by the low concentrations of adrenaline present in mammalian brain. Nevertheless, the work carried thus far has demon-strated that there are significant adrenaline neuron system projections as well as the better known noradrenaline and dopamine systems.

5. Conclusions

The purpose of this brief review has been to give an overview of the organization of the CA neuron systems in the mammalian brain. These appear to be phylogenetically stable components of the mammalian brain, with only minor variations occurring in species with a wide range of adaptive specializations such as the rat and the primates, including man (cf. Nobin and Björklund, 1973; Olson et al., 1973). Homologies with mamma-lian CA neuron systems can be made throughout the vertebrate line, and although there are major specializations among groups, the similarities are striking (Björklund and Moore, 1978). It should also be noted that the serotonin neuron systems are quite similar to the CA neuron systems in their distribution and phylogenetic stability.

It is beyond the purview of this brief review to go into functional considerations, which will undoubtedly arise elsewhere in this volume. The CA neuron systems have been implicated in many important functions, and undoubtedly participate importantly in neural events that participate in the adaptation of an organization to its environment. There are, in addition, a few anatomical points that should be emphasized. First, the principal CA in the mammalian brain is dopamine. There are two small dopamine neuron systems present in the diencephalon. The first is the tubero–hypophysial system, which innervates the median eminence and the neurointermediate lobe of the pituitary. The second is the incerto–hypothalamic system innervating the dorsal and anterior hypothalamic areas. Both these systems appear topographically organized. In addition, there is a small retinal dopamine neuron system and a periventricular dopamine neuron system that includes, at least in part, the neurons of the dorsal tegmental cell groups in the medulla. Each of these systems is relatively small compared with the major dopamine neuron system, which is composed of a large group of neurons occupying the ventral tegmental area and the pars compacta of the substantia nigra. This system projects as a mesotelencephalic system on the striatum, allocortical basal forebrain structures, and restricted portions of the isocortex. This projection is, at least in large part, topographically organized. Each of the dopamine neuron systems, with the possible exception of the periventricular system, has a relatively restricted projection area. This contrasts the dopamine neuron systems with the noradrenaline neuron systems, which have widespread, diffuse projections. The cell bodies of the noradrenaline neuron systems are found in the brain stem in two major groups, a locus coeruleus group and a lateral tegmental group. The demonstration of the projection of the locus coeruleus group provides one of the most remarkable achievements of recent neuroanatomical investigations. At present, there is substantive evidence that the locus coeruleus projects throughout the neuraxis from the caudal spinal cord, through the brain stem and diencephalon to the telencephalon. With the serotonin neuron projection, it provides the only known direct projection system from brain stem reticular formation to the cerebral cortex. This observation in itself is remarkable, since, until recently, it was believed that all cortical projections arose from neurons no lower than the diencephalon. Another feature of the noradrenaline neuron systems that has not been mentioned in this review is their remarkable plasticity in response to injury (for a review, cf. Moore *et al.,* 1974). Whether the system exhibits such plasticity in response to environmental events is unknown, but the interesting observations of Descarries *et al.* (1977) demonstrating the small number of synaptic contacts made by these neurons in cortex certainly suggests a functional role differing from that of other cortical innervation. Whether this type of innervation holds for other regions receiving projections from the locus coeruleus is unknown. This question and many other questions concerning these fascinating neuron systems remain to be resolved.

Acknowledgments

The preparation of this review and some of the work reported in it was supported by USPHS Grant NS-12080 from the National Institutes of Health. The authors are grateful for the opportunity to contribute to this volume in memory of Harold E. Himwich, who through his own work and the encouragement of others led us for many years in exploring the chemistry of the brain.

6. References

Ajika, K., and Hökfelt, T., 1973, Ultrastructural identification of catecholamine neurones in the hypothalamus periventricular–arcuate nucleus–median eminence complex with special reference to quantitative aspects, Brain Res. 57:97–117.

Ajika, K., and Hökfelt, T., 1975, Projections to the median eminence and the arcuate nucleus with special reference to monoamine systems: Effects of lesions, Cell Tissue Res. 158:15–35.

Andén, N.-E., Carlsson, A., Dahlström, A., Fuxe, K., Hillarp, N.-Å., and Larsson, K., 1964, Demonstration and mapping out of nigro-neostriatal dopamine neurons, Life Sci. 3:523–530.

Andén, N.-E., Dahlström, A., Fuxe, K., and Larsson, K., 1965, Further evidence for the presence of nigro-neostriatal dopamine neurons in the rat, Am. J. Anat. 116:329–334.

Andén, N.-E., Fuxe, K., Hamberger, B., and Hökfelt, T., 1966a, A quantitative study of the nigro-neostriatal dopamine neurons system in the rat, Acta Physiol. Scand. 67:306–312.

Andén, N.-E., Dahlström, A., Fuxe, K., Larsson, K., Olson, L., and Ungerstedt, U., 1966b, Ascending monoamine neurons to the telencephalon and diencephalon, Acta. Physiol. Scand. 67:313–326.

Baumgarten, H. G., Björklund, A., Holstein, A. F., and Nobin, A., 1972, Organization and ultrastructural identification of the catecholamine nerve terminals in the neural lobe and pars intermedia of the rat pituitary, Z. Zellforsch. 126:483–517.

Bedard, P., Larochelle, L., Parent, A., and Poirier, L. J., 1969, The nigrostriatal pathway: A correlative study based on neuroanatomical and neurochemical criteria in the cat and the monkey, Exp. Neurol. 25:365–377.

Berger, B., Thierry, A. M., Tassin, J. P., and Moyre, M. A., 1976, Dopaminergic innervation of the rat prefrontal cortex: A fluorescence histochemical study, Brain Res. 106:133–145.

Bertler, Å., and Rosengren, E., 1959, Occurrence and distribution of catecholamines in brain, Acta Physiol. Scand. 47:350–361.

Björklund, A., and Moore, R. Y., 1978, The Central Adrenergic Neuron, Raven Press, New York, in press.

Björklund, A., and Nobin, A., 1973, Fluorescence histochemical and microspectrofluorometric mapping of dopamine, and noradrenaline cell groups in the rat diencephalon, Brain Res. 51:193–205.

Björklund, A., Falck, B., Hromek, F., Owman, C., and West, K. A., 1970, Identification and terminal distribution of the tubero-hypophyseal monoamine fibre systems in the rat by means of stereotaxic and microspectrofluorimetric techniques, Brain Res. 17:1–23.

Björklund, A., Moore, R. Y., Nobin, A., and Stenevi, U., 1973, The organization of tubero-hypophyseal and reticulo-influndibular catecholamine neuron systems in the rat brain, Brain Res. 51:171–191.

Björklund, A., Lindvall, O., and Nobin, A., 1975, Evidence of an incerto-hypothalamic dopamine neurone system in the rat, *Brain Res. 89*:29–42.

Bloom, F. E., Hoffer, B. J., and Siggins, G. R., 1971, Studies on norepinephrine-containing afferents to Purkinje cells of rat cerebellum. I. Localization of the fibers and their synapses, *Brain Res. 25*:501–521.

Brodal, A., 1969, *Neurological Anatomy,* 2nd Ed., Oxford University Press, New York.

Carlsson, A., Falck, B., and Hillarp, N.-Å., 1962, Cellular localization of brain monoamines, *Acta Physiol. Scand. 56(suppl.*196:1–28.

Carlsson, A., Dahlstrom, A., Fuxe, K., and Hillarp, N.-Å., 1964, Cellular localization of monoamines in the spinal cord, *Acta Physiol. Scand. 60*:112–119.

Carpenter, M. B., and Peter, P., 1972, Nigrostriatal and nigrothalamic fibers in the rhesus monkey, *J. Comp. Neurol. 139*:259–272.

Chu, N.-S., and Bloom, F. E., 1974, The catecholamine-containing neurons in the cat dorsolateral pontine tegmentum: Distribution of the cell bodies and some axonal projections, *Brain Res. 66*:1–21.

Ciaranello, R. D., Barchas, R. E., Byers, G. S., Stemmle, D. W., and Barchas, J. D., 1969, Enzymatic synthesis of adrenaline in mammalian brain, *Nature (London) 221*:368–369.

Corrodi, H., and Jonsson, G., 1967. The formaldehyde fluorescence method for the histochemical demonstration of biogenic monoamines. A review on the methodology, *J. Histochem. Cytochem. 15*:65–78.

Dahlström, A., and Fuxe, K., 1964, Evidence for the existence of monoamine-containing neurons in the central nervous system. I. Demonstration of monoamines in the cell bodies of brain stem neurons, *Acta Physiol. Scand. 62(Suppl. 232)*:1–55.

Dahlström, A., and Fuxe, K., 1965, Evidence for the existence of monoamine neurons in the central nervous system. II. Experimentally induced changes in the intraneuronal amine levels of the bulbospinal neuron systems, *Acta Physiol. Scand. 64(Suppl. 247)*:1–36.

Descarries, L., Beaudet, A., and Watkins, K. C., 1975, Serotonin nerve terminals in adult rat neocortex, *Brain Res. 100*:563–588.

Descarries, L., Watkins, K. C., and Lapierre, Y., 1977, Noradrenergic axon terminals in the cerebral cortex of rat. III. Topometric ultrastructural analysis, *Brain Res.,* in press.

DiCarlo, V., Hubbard, J. E., and Pate, P., 1973, Fluorescence histochemistry of monoamine-containing cell bodies in the brain stem of the squirrel monkey *(Saimuiri sciureus).* IV. An atlas, *J. Comp. Neurol. 152*:347–372.

Dowling, J. E., and Ehinger, B., 1975, Synaptic organization of the amine-containing interplexiform cells of the goldfish and Cebus monkey retinas, *Nature (London) 188*:270–273.

Dupin, J. C., Descarries, L., and de Champlain, J., 1976, Radioautographic visualization of central catecholamine neurons in newborn rat after intravenous administration of tritiated norepinephrine, *Brain Res. 103*:588–596.

Ehinger, B., 1966a, Distribution of adrenergic nerves in the eye and some related structures in the cat, *Acta Physiol. Scand. 66*:123–128.

Ehinger, B., 1966b, Adrenergic nerves to the eyes and to related structures in man and in the cynomolgus monkey *(Macaca irus), Invert. Ophthalmol. 5*:42–52.

Ehinger, B., 1966c, Adrenergic retinal neurons, *Z. Zellforsch. 71*:146–152.

Ehinger, B., and Falck, B., 1969, Adrenergic retinal neurons of some New World monkeys, *Z. Zellforsch. 100*:364–375.

Ehinger, B., Falck, B., and Laties, A. M., 1969, Adrenergic neurons in teleost retina, *Z. Zellforsch. 97*:285–297.

Ehringer, H., and Hornykiewicz, O., 1960, Verteilung von Noradrenalin und Dopamine (3-Hydroxytyramine) in Gehirn des Menschen und ihr Verhalten bei Erkrankungen des extrapiramidalen Systems, *Klin. Wochenschr. 38*:1236–1239.

Falck, B., 1962, Observations on the possibilities of the cellular localization of monoamines by a fluorescence method, *Acta Physiol. Scand. 56(Suppl. 197)*:1–25.

Falck, B., Hillarp, N.-Å., Thieme, G., and Torp, A., 1962, Fluorescence of catecholamines and related compounds condensed with formaldehyde, *J. Histochem. Cytochem. 10*:348–354.

Fallon, J. H., and Moore, R. Y., 1976a, Catecholamine neuron innervation of the rat amygdala, *Anat. Rec. 184*:399.

Fallon, J. H., and Moore, R. Y., 1976b, Dopamine innervation of some basal forebrain areas in the rat, *Neurosci. Abstr., 2(Part 1)*:486.

Felten, D., Laties, A., and Carpenter, M., 1974, Localization of monoamine-containing cell bodies in the squirrel monkey brain, *Am. J. Anat. 138*:153–166.

Ferraro, A., 1928, The connections of the pars suboculomotoria of the substantia nigra, *Arch. Neurol. Psychiatry (Chicago) 19*:177–180.

Freedman, R., Foote, S. L., and Bloom, F. E., 1975, Histochemical characterization of a neocortical projection of the nucleus locus coeruleus in the squirrel monkey, *J. Comp. Neurol. 164*:209–232.

Fuxe, K., 1963, Cellular localization of monoamines in the median eminence and in the infundibular stem of some mammals, *Acta Physiol. Scand. 58*:383–384.

Fuxe, K., 1964, Cellular localization of monamines in the median eminence and in the infundibular stem of some mammals, *Z. Zellforsch. 61*:710–724.

Fuxe, K., 1965a, Evidence for the existence of monoamine-containing neurons in the central nervous system. III. The monoamine nerve terminal, *Z. Zellforsch. 65*:572–596.

Fuxe, K., 1965b, Evidence for the existence of monoamine-containing neurons in the central nervous system. IV. Distribution of monoamine nerve terminals in the central nervous system, *Acta Physiol. Scand. 64(Suppl. 247)*:39–85.

Fuxe, K., and Hökfelt, T., 1966, Further evidence for the existence of tuberoinfundibular dopamine neurons, *Acta Physiol. Scand. 66*:243–244.

Fuxe, K., Hökfelt, T., and Ungerstedt, U., 1970, Morphological and functional aspects of central monoamine neurons, *Int. Rev. Neurobiol. 13*:93–126.

Garver, D. L., and Sladek, J. R., Jr., 1975, Monoamine distribution in primate brain. I. Catecholamine-containing perikarya in the brain stem of *Macaca speciosa, J. Comp. Neurol. 159*:289–304.

Greenfield, J. G., 1963, Paralysis agitans (Parkinson's disease), in: *Greenfield's Neuropathology* (W. Blackwood, A. Meyer, R. M. Norman, W. H. McMenemey, and D. S. Russell, eds.), pp. 582–584, Arnold, London.

Gunne, L.-M., 1962, Relative adrenaline content in brain tissue, *Acta Physiol. Scand. 56*:324–333.

Hartman, B. K., 1973, Immunofluorescence of dopamine-β-hydroxylase. Application of improved methodology to the localization of the peripheral and central noradrenergic nervous system, *J. Histochem. Cytochem. 21*:312–332.

Hattori, T., Fibiger, H. C., McGeer, P. L., and Maler, L., 1973, Analysis of the fine structure of the dopaminergic nigrostriatal projection by electron microscopic autoradiography, *Exp. Neurol. 41*:599–611.

Hillarp, N.-Å., Fuxe, K., and Dahlström, A., 1966, Demonstration and mapping of central neurons containing dopamine, noradrenaline and 5-hydroxytryptamine and their reactions to psychopharmaca, *Pharm. Rev. 18*:727–741.

Hökfelt, T., 1967, Electron microscopic studies on brain slices from regions rich in catecholamine nerve terminals, *Acta, Physiol. Scand. 69*:119–120.

Hökfelt, T., 1968, *In vitro* studies on central and peripheral monoamine neurons at the ultrastructural level, *Z. Zellforsch. 91*:1–74.

Hökfelt, T., and Ljungdahl, Å., 1972, Modification of the Falck–Hillarp formaldehyde fluorescence method using the Vibratome: Simple, rapid and sensitive localization of catecholamines in sections of unfixed or formalin fixed brain tissue, *Histochemie* 29:325–339.

Hökfelt, T., and Ungerstedt, U., 1969, Electron and fluorescence microscopical studies on the nucleus caudatus putamen of the rat after unilateral lesions of nigro-neostriatal dopamine neurons, *Acta Physiol. Scand.* 76:415–426.

Hökfelt, T., Fuxe, K., Goldstein, M., and Johansson, O., 1973, Evidence for adrenaline neurons in the rat brain, *Acta Physiol. Scand.* 89:286–288.

Hökfelt, T., Fuxe, K., Goldstein, M., and Johansson, O., 1974*a*, Immunohistochemical evidence for the existence of adrenaline neurons in the rat brain, *Brain Res.* 66:235–251.

Hökfelt, T., Fuxe, K., Johansson, O., and Ljungdahl, Å., 1974*b*, Pharmacohistochemical evidence of the existence of dopamine nerve terminals in the limbic cortex, *Eur. J. Pharmacol.* 25:108–112.

Hubbard, J. E., and DiCarlo, V., 1973, Fluorescence histochemistry of monoamine-containing cell bodies in the brain stem of the squirrel monkey *(Saimiri sciureus)*. I. The locus coeruleus, *J. Comp. Neurol.* 147:553–565.

Jacobowitz, D. M., and Palkovits, M., 1974, Topographic atlas of catecholamine- and acetylcholinesterase-containing neurons in the rat brain. I. Forebrain (telencephalon, diencephalon), *J. Comp. Neurol.* 157:13–28.

Jones, B. E., and Moore, R. Y., 1974, Catecholamine-containing neurons of the nucleus locus coeruleus in the cat, *J. Comp. Neurol.* 157:43–52.

Jones, B. E., and Moore, R. Y., 1977, Ascending projections of the locus coeruleus in the rat. II. Autoradiographic study, *Brain Res.* 127:23–53.

Jones, B. E., Halaris, A. E., McIlhany, M., and Moore, R. Y., 1977, Ascending projections of the locus coeruleus in the rat. I. Axonal transport in central noradrenaline neurons, *Brain Res.* 127:1–22.

Jonsson, G., Fuxe, K., and Hökfelt, T., 1972, On the catecholamine innervation of the hypothalamus, with special reference to the median eminence, *Brain Res.* 40:271–281.

Koslow, S. H., and Schlumpf, M., 1974, Quantitation of adrenaline in rat brain nuclei and areas by mass fragmentography, *Nature (London)* 251:530–531.

Kromer, L. F., and Moore, R. Y., 1976, Cochlear nucleus innervation by central norepinephrine neurons in the rat, *Brain Res.* 118:531–537.

Kuypers, H. G. J. M., and Maisky, V. A., 1975, Retrograde axonal transport of horseradish peroxidase from spinal cord to brain stem cell groups in the cat, *Neurosci. Lett.* 1:9–14.

Laties, A. M., and Jacobowitz, D., 1966, A comparative study of the autonomic innervation of the eye in monkey, cat, and rabbit, *Anat. Rec.* 156:383–396.

Lindvall, O., 1975, Mesencephalic dopaminergic afferents to the lateral septal nucleus of the rat, *Brain Res.* 87:89–95.

Lindvall, O., and Björklund, A., 1974*a*, The glyoxylic acid fluroescence histochemical method: A detailed account of the methodology for the visualization of central catecholamine neurons, *Histochemie.* 39:97–127.

Lindvall, O., and Björklund, A., 1974*b*, The organization of the ascending catecholamine neuron systems in the rat brain as revealed by the glyoxylic acid fluorescence method, *Acta Physiol. Scand. Suppl.* 412:1–48.

Lindvall, O., and Björklund, A., 1978, Organization of catecholamine neurons in the rat central nervous system, in: *Handbook of Psychopharmacology* (L. Iversen, S. Iverson, and S. H. Snyder, eds.), Vol. 9, Ch. 4, Plenum Press, New York, in press.

Lindvall, O., Björklund, A., Hökfelt, T., and Ljungdahl, A., 1973, Application of the glyoxylic acid method to Vibratome sections for the improved visualization of central catecholamine neurons, *Histochemie* 35:31–38.

Lindvall, O., Björklund, A., Moore, R. Y., and Stenevi, U., 1974a, Mesencephalic dopamine neurons projecting to neocortex, *Brain Res. 81*:325–331.

Lindvall, O., Björklund, A., Nobin, A., and Stenevi, U., 1974b, The adrenergic innervation of the rat thalamus as revealed by the glyoxylic acid fluorescence method, *J. Comp. Neurol. 154*:317–348.

Llamas, A., Reinoso-Suarez, F., and Martinez-Moreno, E., 1975, Projections to the gyrus proreus from the brain stem tegmentum (locus coeruleus, raphe nuclei) in the cat, demonstrated by retrograde transport of horseradish peroxidase, *Brain Res. 89*:331–336.

Lorén, I., Björklund, A., Falck, B., and Lindvall, O., 1976, An improved histofluorescence procedure for freeze–dried paraffin-embedded tissue based on combined formaldehyde–glyoxylic acid perfusion with high magnesium content and acid pH, *Histochemistry 49*:177–192.

Lorente de No', R., 1949, Cerebral cortex: Architecture, intracortical connections, motor projections, in: *Physiology of the Nervous System,* (J. Fulton, ed.), 3rd Ed., pp. 288–312, Oxford University Press, New York.

Maeda, T., and Shimizu, N., 1972, Projections ascendentes du locus coeruleus et e'autres neurones aminergiques pontiques au niveau de prosencephale du rat, *Brain Res. 36*:19–35.

Maler, L., Fibirger, H. C., and McGeer, P. L., 1973, Demonstration of the nigrostriatal projection by silver staining after nigral injections of 6-hydroxydopamine, *Exp. Neurol. 40*:505–515.

Malmfors, T., 1963, Evidence of adrenergic neurons with synaptic terminals in the retina of rats demonstrated with fluorescence and electron microscopy, *Acta Physiol. Scand. 58*:99–100.

Moore, R. Y., 1977, Catecholamine innervation of the basal forebrain. I. The septal area, *J. Comp. Neurol.,* in press.

Moore, R. Y., Bhatnagar, R. K., and Heller, A., 1971, Anatomical and chemical studies of a nigro-neostriatal projection in the cat, *Brain Res. 30*:119–135.

Moore, R. Y., Björklund, A., and Stenevi, U., 1974, Growth and plasticity of adrenergic neurons, in: *The Neurosciences—Third Study Program* (F. O. Schmitt and F. G. Worden, eds.), pp. 961–977, MIT Press, Cambridge.

Mugnaini, E., and Dahl, A.-L., 1975, Mode of distribution of aminergic fibers in the cerebellar cortex of the chicken, *J. Comp. Neurol. 162*:417–432.

Nobin, A., and Björklund, A., 1973, Topography of the monoamine neuron systems in the human brain as revealed in fetuses, *Acta. Physiol. Scand. Suppl. 388*:1–40.

Olson, L., and Fuxe, K., 1971, On the projections from the locus coeruleus noradrenaline neurons: The cerebellar innervation, *Brain Res. 28*:165–171.

Olson, L., Borens, L. O., and Seiger, A., 1973, Histochemical demonstration and mapping of 5-hydroxytryptamine- and catecholamine-containing neuron systems in the human fetal brain, *Z. Anat. Entwicklungsgesch. 139*:259–282.

Palkovits, M., and Jacobowitz, D. M., 1974, Topographic atlas of catecholamine- and acetyl-cholinesterase-containing neurons in the rat brain. II. Hindbrain (mesencephalon, rhombencephalon), *J. Comp. Neurol. 157*:29–42.

Pickel, V. M., Segal, M., and Bloom, F. E., 1974, An radioautographic study of the efferent pathways of the nucleus locus coeruleus, *J. Comp. Neurol. 155*:15–42.

Pohorecky, L. A., Zigmond, M., Karten, H., and Wurtman, R. J., 1969, Enzymatic conversion of norepinephrine to epinephrine by the brain, *J. Pharmacol. Exp. Ther. 165*:190–195.

Reid, J. L., Zivin, J. A., Foppen, F. H., and Kopin, I. J., 1975, Catecholamine neurotransmitters and synthetic enzymes in the spinal cord of the rat, *Life Sci. 16*:975–984.

Reid, J. L., Zivin, J. A., and Kopin, I. J., 1976, The effects of spinal cord transsection and intracisternal 6-hydroxydopamine on phenylethanolamine-*N*-methyl transferase (PNMT) activity in rat brain stem and spinal cord, *J. Neurochem. 26*:629–631.

Russell, G. V., 1955, The nucleus locus coeruleus (dorsal lateralis tegmenti), *Tex. Rep. Biol. Med. 13*:939–988.

Saavedra, J. M., Palkovits, M., Brownstein, M. J., and Axelrod, J., 1974, Localization of phenylethanolamine *N*-methyl transferase in the rat brain nuclei, *Nature (London) 248*:695–696.

Scheibel, M. E., and Scheibel, A. B., 1957, Structural substrates for integrative patterns in the brain stem reticular core, in: *Reticular Formation of the Brain,* (H. H. Jasper, L. D. Proctor, R. S. Knighton, W. C. Moseley, and R. T. Costello eds.), pp. 31–55, Little, Brown and Co., Boston.

Seiger, Å., and Olson, L., 1973, Late prenatal ontogeny of central monoamine neurons in the rat: Fluorescence histochemical observations, *Z. Anat. Entwicklungsgesch. 140*:281–318.

Shimizu, N., and Ohnishi, S., 1973, Demonstration of nigro-neostriatal tract by degeneration silver method, *Exp. Brain Res. 17*:133–138.

Swanson, L. W., 1976, The locus coeruleus: A cytoarchitectonic, Golgi and immunohistochemical study in the albino rat, *Brain Res. 110*:39–56.

Swanson, L. W., and Hartman, B. K., 1975, The central adrenergic system. An immunofluorescence study of the location of cell bodies and their efferent connections in the rat utilizing dopamine-β-hydroxylase as a marker, *J. Comp. Neurol. 163*:467–506.

Thierry, A. M., Blane, G., Sobel, A., Stinus, L., and Glowinski, J., 1973*a,* Dopaminergic terminals in the rat cortex, *Science 182*:499–501.

Thierry, A. M., Stinus, L., Blane, G., and Glowinski, J., 1973*b,* Some evidence for the existence of dopaminergic neurons in the rat cortex, *Brain Res. 50*:230–234.

Ungerstedt, U., 1971, Stereotaxic mapping of the monamine pathways in the rat brain, *Acta. Physiol. Scand. Suppl. 367*:1–48.

Van der Gugten, J., Palkovits, M., Wijen, H. L. J. M., and Versteeg, D. H. G., 1976, Regional distribution of adrenaline in rat brain, *Brain Res. 107*:171–175.

Vogt, M., 1954, The concentration of sympathin in different parts of the central nervous system under normal conditions and after the administration of drugs, *J. Physiol. (London) 123*:451–481.

von Euler, U. S., 1946, A specific sympathomimetic ergone in adrenergic nerve fibers (sympathin) and its relation to adrenaline and noradrenaline, *Acta Physiol. Scand. 12*:73–96.

Zivin, J. A., Reid, J. L., Saavedra, J. M., and Kopin, I. J., 1975, Quantitative localization of biogenic amines in the spinal cord, *Brain Res. 99*:293–301.

Effect of Reserpine on Monoamine Synthesis and on Apparent Dopaminergic Receptor Sensitivity in Rat Brain

Arvid Carlsson and Margit Lindqvist

1. Introduction

There seems to be general agreement that the monoamine-depleting action of reserpine is due to blockade of the uptake mechanisms located in the intracellular storage organelles, generally called "granules" or "synaptic vesicles" (see Carlsson, 1965). Although the monoamine-synthesizing enzymes are not primarily involved, several secondary actions on the activities of these enzymes have been demonstrated or proposed. Dopamine-β-hydroxylase is located in the storage granules, and the blocking action of reserpine on their uptake mechanism may lead to reduced availability of the substrate dopamine (Rutledge and Weiner, 1967). As to the first steps in the synthesis of monoamines, i.e., the hydroxylation of tyrosine and tryptophan, the action of reserpine on the storage mechanism appears to cause rather complex secondary changes in the activity of the enzymes involved. Sustained increases in 5-hydroxyindoleacetic acid (5-HIAA) and homovanillic acid levels in brain after reserpine treatment, outlasting the initial phase of monoamine net release, may indicate increased rates of monoamine synthesis, even though alternative explanations cannot be excluded (Andén *et al.*, 1963, 1964).

Arvid Carlsson and Margit Lindqvist ● Department of Pharmacology, University of Göteborg, Fack S-400 33, Göteborg 33, Sweden

Tozer *et al.* (1966) observed that reserpine retarded the efflux of 5-HIAA from rat brain and pointed out that this alkaloid does not retard 5-HT synthesis. They suggested that the synthesis may even be enhanced.

On the other hand, a reduction of catecholamine synthesis rate lasting for several hours after a single dose of reserpine was observed in mouse vas deferens preparations, in which the tyrosine hydroxylase activity was measured *in vitro* using carboxyl-labeled [^{14}C]L-tyrosine. This reduction was suggested to be due to end-product inhibition by catechols accumulating in the cytoplasmic sap (Weiner *et al.*, 1972). Finally, an induction of tyrosine hydroxylase, slow in onset and lasting for several days, was observed in the adrenals, sympathetic adrenergic neurons, and brains of animals treated with a single dose of reserpine (Mueller *et al.*, 1969; Thoenen *et al.*, 1969). This induction seems to be mediated by neurogenic stimuli.

In the present investigation, we study the effect of reserpine on the hydroxylation of tyrosine and tryptophan in the intact brain *in vivo,* using our method to measure the accumulation of DOPA and 5-hydroxytryptophan (5-HTP) after inhibition of the aromatic L-amino-acid decarboxylase (Carlsson *et al.*, 1972). To investigate whether changes in receptor sensitivity are involved in the actions observed, we also studied the response to the dopamine-receptor agonist apomorphine 4 and 24 hr after reserpine treatment.

2. Methods

Male Sprague–Dawley rats weighing 200–370 g were used.

The following drugs were used: apomorphine HCl· ½H$_2$O (Sandoz, Basel, Switzerland), reserpine (Serpasil®, Ciba-Geigy, Mölndal, Sweden), and the inhibitor of aromatic amino acid decarboxylase NSD 1015 (3-hydroxybenzylhydrazine HCl, synthesized at this department by Dr. Per Martinson). All injections were made intraperitoneally at time and dose schedules given in Section 3. Doses of basic compounds refer to the salts. Control rats always received the same number of injections at corresponding time intervals, isotonic glucose solution replacing reserpine and saline apomorphine.

The rats were killed by decapitation, and the brains were quickly taken out and dissected on an ice-cold glass plate. The following parts of the brain were taken for analyses: (1) corpus striatum; (2) the limbic forebrain, containing *inter alia* the olfactory tubercle, nucleus accumbens (medial part), and nucleus amygdaloideus centralis; and (3) the rest of the hemispheres (referred to as "hemispheres"). For details on the dissection, see Carlsson and Lindqvist (1973).

Immediately after dissection, the brain parts were frozen on dry ice. The parts of 3 brains were pooled and weighed.

The pooled brain parts were homogenized in 10 ml perchloric acid containing 5 mg $Na_2S_2O_5$ and 20 mg EDTA. The extract was purified on a strong cation exchange column (Dowex 50) (Kehr *et al.*, 1972). The following spectrophotofluorimetric analyses were performed: tyrosine (Waalkes and Udenfriend, 1957), DOPA (Kehr *et al.*, 1972), tryptophan (Bédard *et al.*, 1972), and 5-HTP (Atack and Lindqvist, 1973).

Statistics: One-way analysis of variance followed by *t* test (Winer, 1962).

3. Results

3.1. Dose Response

Various doses of reserpine (0.05–5 mg/kg i.p.) were injected 3.5 hr before the inhibitor of aromatic amino acid decarboxylase, NSD 1015, 100 mg/kg i.p. The rats were killed after another 30 min.

Reserpine, 0.2 mg/kg, caused about a 100% increase in DOPA formation both in the striatum and in the limbic forebrain ($p < 0.001$). In the highest doses, i.e., 1 and 5 mg/kg, the increases were about 200 and 125% in striatum and limbic forebrain, respectively ($p < 0.001$ in both cases) (Fig. 1).

In the noradrenaline-predominated hemisphere portion of the brain, the increase in DOPA formation was about 100% after 0.2 mg reserpine/kg ($p < 0.001$), and about 150% after 1 and 5 mg/kg ($p < 0.001$) (Fig. 1).

The formation of 5-HTP was increased in the brain parts studied, but statistical significance was reached only in the striatum after 0.2 and 5 mg reserpine/kg ($p < 0.01$), and in the remaining part of the hemispheres after 0.2 mg/kg ($p < 0.025$) and after 5 mg/kg ($p < 0.01$) (Table I).

The tyrosine levels in the limbic forebrain were significantly decreased after 0.2 and 5 mg reserpine/kg ($p < 0.05$ and $p < 0.01$, respectively). No significant changes in tyrosine levels were observed in the striatum. In the remaining part of the hemispheres, a significant decrease in tyrosine was found after 0.05 mg reserpine/kg ($p < 0.025$) (Table I).

Reserpine did not change the tryptophan levels significantly in any of the brain parts studied (Table I).

Table I. Effect of Various Doses of Reserpine on Tyrosine, Tryptophan, and 5-Hydroxytryptophan in Rat Brain Regions[a]

Dose (mg/kg, i.p.)	Tyrosine (μg/g)			Tryptophan (μg/g)			5-Hydroxytryptophan (ng/g)		
	Limbic	Striatum	Hemispheres	Limbic	Striatum	Hemispheres	Limbic	Striatum	Hemispheres
Control	22.2 ± 0.63 (6)	20.1 ± 0.90 (6)	20.6 ± 1.00 (6)	4.5 ± 0.26 (6)	4.1 ± 0.14 (6)	3.7 ± 0.17 (6)	111 ± 7 (6)	61 ± 5 (6)	58 ± 4 (6)
0.05	20.0 ± 1.25 (2)	18.2 ± 0.05 (2)	15.4 ± 0.20[b] (2)	4.1 ± 0.10 (2)	4.1 ± 0.05 (2)	4.0 ± 0.05 (2)	127 ± 4 (2)	72 ± 1 (2)	78 ± 1 (2)
0.2	17.5 ± 0.80[b] (2)	17.6 ± 0.85 (2)	18.0 ± 0.15 (2)	4.0 ± 0.15 (2)	4.0 ± 0.10 (2)	3.7 ± 0.05 (2)	167 ± 27 (2)	96 ± 7[b] (2)	89 ± 12[b] (2)
1	20.4 ± 0.05 (2)	18.8 ± 0.45 (2)	20.2 ± 1.25 (2)	3.9 ± 0.10 (2)	3.9 ± 0.05 (2)	3.8 ± 0.15 (2)	139 ± 19 (2)	80 ± 13 (2)	82 ± 6 (2)
5	19.5 ± 0.51[c] (5)	17.6 ± 0.67 (5)	19.0 ± 1.04 (5)	4.0 ± 0.21 (5)	3.8 ± 0.27 (5)	3.6 ± 0.18 (5)	151 ± 14 (5)	88 ± 8[c] (5)	87 ± 9[c] (5)

[a]Reserpine was given 4 hr and NSD 1015, 100 mg/kg i.p., 30 min before death. Controls received NSD 1015 alone. Shown are the means ± S.E.M. The figures in parentheses indicate the number of experimental groups, each comprising pooled brain parts of 3 rats.
[b,c] Differs from control: [b] = $p < 0.05$; [c] = $p < 0.01$.

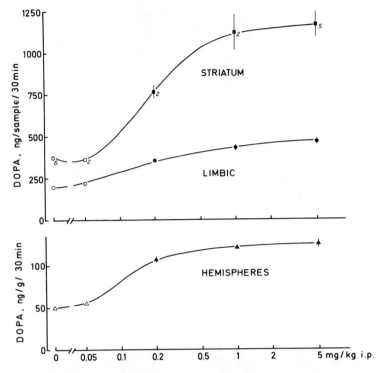

Fig. 1. Effect of various doses of reserpine on DOPA formation in rat brain regions. Reserpine was given 4 hr and NSD 1015 30 min before death. Control animals received NSD 1015 alone. Shown are the means ± S.E.M. The figures on the top curve indicate the numbers of experiments, which were identical for all brain regions. Each experiment comprises pooled brain parts of 3 rats. Solid symbols indicate values significantly different from controls ($p <$ 0.05).

3.2. Time Course

Reserpine, 5 mg/kg i.p., was injected at various time intervals (40 min to 96 hr) before death, followed by NSD 1015, 100 mg/kg i.p., 30 min before death.

At the shortest interval investigated, i.e., 40 min before death, there was a dramatic decrease in DOPA formation by about 90% in the striatum and by about 80% in the limbic forebrain and in the remaining hemisphere part of the brain (Fig. 2). At 20 min later, the synthesis of DOPA had returned to the control level in limbic forebrain and in the hemispheres. In the striatum, the DOPA formation had increased significantly above control ($p <$ 0.05). From 2 hr up to 18 hr, the increase in DOPA formation was

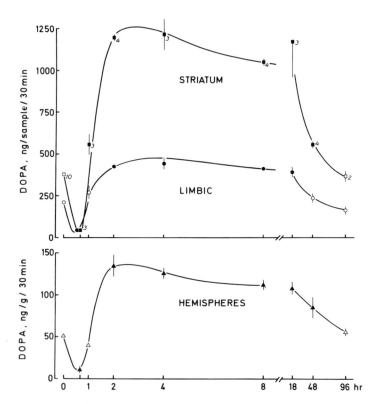

Fig. 2.   Formation of DOPA in rat brain regions after reserpine (5 mg/kg i.p.). All animals received NSD 1015, 100 mg/kg i.p., 30 min before death. For further explanation, see the Fig. 1 caption.

about 200% in the striatum and about 100% in the limbic forebrain. In the remaining part of the hemispheres, the increase was about 150% at 2 and 4 hr and about 115% at 8 and 18 hr. At 48 hr, the increase in DOPA synthesis was much less pronounced, and did not reach significance in the limbic forebrain. At 96 hr, the DOPA formation in all brain parts studied did not differ from the control groups (Fig. 2).

The formation of 5-HTP after reserpine treatment differed markedly from the formation of DOPA. At 40 min, when the DOPA synthesis was considerably decreased, the synthesis of 5-HTP was increased by about 55–65% in all brain parts studied (Fig. 3). At 1 hr, it was further increased, being about 95% in the striatum and 70–75% in the limbic forebrain and in the remaining part of the hemispheres. The increase in 5-HTP was shorter-lasting than the increase in DOPA formation. At 4 hr, 5-HTP formation in

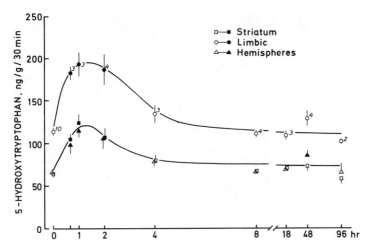

Fig. 3. Formation of 5-HTP in rat brain regions after reserpine (5 mg/kg i.p.). All animals received NSD 1015, 100 mg/kg i.p., 30 min before death. For further explanation, see the Fig. 1 caption.

all brain parts did not differ significantly from the control groups. These levels were maintained in striatum and limbic forebrain throughout the time investigated (up to 96 hr). Also, the formation of 5-HTP in the remaining part of the hemispheres remained at the control level from 4 hr on, except at 48 hr, when a 30% increase was observed ($p < 0.005$) (Fig. 3).

After reserpine administration, there were some moderate and rather complex changes in tryptophan and tyrosine levels (Table II). At 1–2 hr, there was a significant increase in the tryptophan levels in all brain parts studied ($p < 0.025$). At the same time, the tyrosine levels were increased, but significance was reached only in the striatum at 1 hr ($p < 0.01$). At 4–8 hr, both tryptophan and tyrosine levels were decreased. At a longer interval (48 hr), the tryptophan but not the tyrosine levels were significantly increased in all brain parts studied ($p < 0.05$). A decrease in tyrosine was observed in striatum and limbic forebrain at 96 hr ($p < 0.05$).

3.3. Effect of Apomorphine after Pretreatment with Reserpine

Rats were pretreated with reserpine, 5 mg/kg, 4 or 24 hr before death. Apomorphine was injected in doses of 15.6 or 125 μg/kg 37 min and NSD 1015, 100 mg/kg, 30 min before death.

Reserpine stimulated DOPA formation, as compared with NSD 1015 controls, in all brain regions investigated and to the same extent at both time intervals (Fig. 4).

Table II. Tyrosine and Tryptophan Levels in Rat Brain Regions after Reserpine (5 mg/kg i.p.) [a]

Time interval before death	Tyrosine (µg/g)			Tryptophan (µg/g)		
	Limbic	Striatum	Hemispheres	Limbic	Striatum	Hemispheres
Control	22.0 ± 0.42 (10)	20.7 ± 0.49 (10)	20.2 ± 0.71 (10)	4.5 ± 0.15 (10)	4.2 ± 0.10 (10)	3.9 ± 0.11 (10)
40 min	21.2 ± 0.57 (31)	20.6 ± 0.58 (3)	19.3 ± 0.85 (3)	4.5 ± 0.27 (3)	4.5 ± 0.26 (3)	4.3 ± 0.26 (3)
1 hr	25.8 ± 1.71 (3)	24.7 ± 0.73[c] (3)	22.8 ± 1.42 (3)	5.5 ± 0.39[c] (3)	5.3 ± 0.15[d] (3)	4.7 ± 0.56[c] (3)
2 hr	22.9 ± 0.98 (4)	23.0 ± 0.98 (4)	22.0 ± 1.59 (4)	5.2 ± 0.24[b] (4)	5.0 ± 0.06[d] (4)	4.7 ± 0.12[c] (4)
4 hr	18.8 ± 0.21[b] (3)	16.6 ± 0.35[c] (3)	17.5 ± 0.49 (3)	3.8 ± 0.10[b] (3)	3.6 ± 0.06[c] (3)	3.5 ± 0.06 (3)
8 hr	18.7 ± 0.28[c] (4)	18.2 ± 0.69 (4)	17.5 ± 0.48 (4)	3.6 ± 0.18[d] (4)	3.6 ± 0.09[c] (4)	3.2 ± 0.16[c] (4)
18 hr	19.8 ± 1.10 (3)	20.5 ± 1.47 (3)	20.5 ± 1.22 (3)	4.6 ± 0.10 (3)	4.9 ± 0.17[d] (3)	4.2 ± 0.09 (3)
48 hr	21.1 ± 1.98 (4)	22.3 ± 2.26 (4)	21.5 ± 2.58 (4)	5.1 ± 0.18[b] (4)	5.2 ± 0.25[d] (4)	4.8 ± 0.15[d] (4)
96 hr	18.4 ± 1.20[b] (2)	16.9 ± 0.95[b] (2)	17.2 ± 1.30 (2)	4.0 ± 0.10 (2)	4.3 ± 0.25 (2)	3.8 ± 0.25 (2)

[a] All animals received NSD 1015, 100 mg/kg i.p., 30 min before death. Shown are the means ± S.E.M. The figures in parentheses indicate the number of experimental groups, each comprising pooled brain parts of 3 rats.
[b-d] Differs from control: b = $p < 0.05$; c = $p < 0.01$; d = $p < 0.001$.

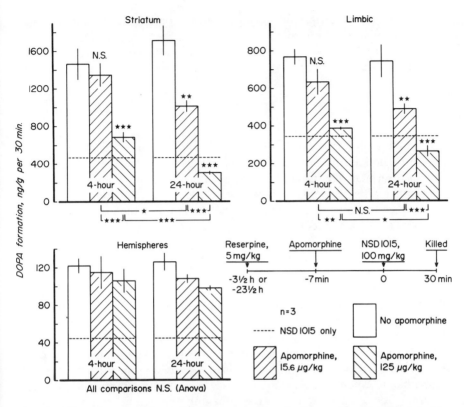

Fig. 4. Effect of apomorphine on DOPA formation in rat brain parts after pretreatment with reserpine 4 or 24 hr previously. All animals were given an intraperitoneal injection of NSD 1015 as indicated, 30 min before death. Injections of reserpine and apomorphine were given intraperitoneally at the time intervals indicated, and the brain parts were analyzed for DOPA. Each experiment comprises pooled brain parts of 3 rats. (*) $p < 0.05$; (**) $p < 0.01$; (***) $p < 0.001$. The asterisks above bars refer to comparison with controls receiving reserpine and NSD 1015, but no apomorphine.

The lower dose of apomorphine (15.6 μg/kg) was inactive when given 4 hr after reserpine, but significantly reduced the reserpine-induced increase in DOPA formation by about 40% in striatum as well as in the dopamine-rich limbic forebrain 24 hr after reserpine. The larger dose of apomorphine (125 μg/kg) reduced the DOPA formation by 50% after 4 hr and by 80% after 24 hr. In the limbic forebrain, as in the striatum, DOPA was reduced by half after 4 hr. At 24 hr, the reduction (65%) was somewhat less pronounced than in the striatum (Fig. 4).

Apomorphine caused no significant effects on DOPA formation in the predominantly noradrenaline-containing hemisphere portion (Fig. 4).

The tyrosine levels were not significantly changed by apomorphine treatment (data not shown).

4. Discussion

Marked retardation of DOPA formation was observed in all three brain regions examined during the period 10–40 min after intraperitoneal injection of reserpine. The most likely explanation of this phenomenon appears to be that after reserpine-induced blockade of the intracellular storage mechanism, catecholamines will accumulate in the cytoplasm in sufficient amounts to cause a direct inhibition of tyrosine hydroxylase (cf. Weiner *et al.*, 1972).

The initial period of inhibition was followed by a prolonged phase of accelerated DOPA formation. This effect reached its maximum a few hours after the administration of reserpine, i.e., at a time when amine depletion and behavioral changes have reached a marked degree. This stimulation of transmitter synthesis may be due to a receptor-mediated feedback response to the declining transmitter concentration in the synaptic cleft. A decrease in receptor sensitivity can be ruled out, in view of the clear-cut response to the receptor agonist apomorphine that appears as soon as 4 hr after reserpine treatment (cf. Kehr *et al.*, 1975). In this respect, reserpine differs clearly from, for example, the phenothiazine and butyrophenone antipsychotics.

The percentage increase in DOPA formation after reserpine treatment was greater in the striatum than in the other dopamine-predominated region, i.e., the limbic portion. A similar difference exists after treatment with phenothiazines and butyrophenones (see Carlsson, 1975), and thus probably reflects a different responsiveness to reduced receptor activation. In the noradrenaline-predominated hemisphere portion, the stimulation of DOPA formation induced by reserpine was about as pronounced as in the limbic portion, suggesting that the receptor-mediated feedback regulation of hemispheric noradrenaline synthesis is quantitatively comparable to that of limbic dopamine synthesis.

The stimulation of DOPA formation appeared to last approximately as long as the gross behavioral signs of reserpine action, i.e., 2 or 3 days. The functional effects of reserpine appear to coincide roughly with the blockade of the intracellular storage mechanism, while the monoamine depletion is known to last much longer (cf. Andén and Henning, 1966). Presumably, an increased receptor sensitivity contributes to the recovery, as indicated, for example, by an increased behavioral response to the dopamine receptor agonist apomorphine, when given one to several days after a single dose of reserpine (Ungerstedt, 1971). This apparent supersensitivity seems to involve also the biochemical feedback response, as indicated by the enhanced effect of apomorphine on DOPA formation observed in the present study 24 hr after reserpine administration. To what extent the receptors involved in this phenomenon are pre- or post-synaptic cannot be determined from the present data.

The 5-HT neurons responded to reserpine in a manner somewhat different from the catecholamine neurons. First, no initial depression of synthesis was observed. This may possibly be related to the fact that tryptophan hydroxylase does not seem to exhibit the phenomenon of end-product inhibition (Jequier *et al.*, 1969). Second, the stimulation of 5-HTP formation was less pronounced and shorter-lasting. This response is possibly receptor-mediated, and thus it appears that this feed-back mechanism is not so strongly developed in the 5-HT as in the catecholamine neurons.

Variations in tryptophan levels (see Section 3) may at most partly explain the fluctuations in 5-HTP formation. As shown in Table I, an increase in 5-HTP formation after reserpine treatment may occur without any concomitant increase in tryptophan levels.

It may be speculated that the short duration of the stimulating action of reserpine on 5-HTP formation is partly due to cessation of the stimulating influence from catecholamine neurons. In favor of such an influence, it was demonstrated that activation of postsynaptic dopamine receptors by apomorphine causes an increase in 5-HT synthesis and metabolism (Grabowska *et al.*, 1973; Carlsson *et al.*, 1976). The α-adrenergic receptor agonist clonidine (Svensson *et al.*, 1975) was shown to inhibit firing and transmitter metabolism of 5-HT neurons, and it was proposed that this action is due to preferential activation of presynaptic receptors, causing inhibition of noradrenaline neurons.

In mice, we reported that reserpine had no influence on the 5-HTP accumulation induced by the decarboxylase inhibitor Ro 4-4602 (Carlsson and Lindqvist, 1972). The measurement was performed about 8 hr after reserpine treatment. At this time interval, there was no effect on 5-HTP in the present study in rats, and thus the question whether reserpine has an influence on 5-HTP formation in mice needs further investigation.

As mentioned in Section 1, Weiner *et al.* (1972) observed a long-lasting inhibition of tyrosine hydroxylase activity in vasa deferentia removed from mice at various intervals after treatment with reserpine. Whether the difference between these and the present results is due to differences in experimental conditions or in the tissues examined cannot be determined at present. The present technique involves blockade by NSD 1015 of the second step of monoamine synthesis, which might be expected to stimulate the first step via feedback. This effect is counteracted, however, by a simultaneous inhibition of monoamine oxidase by NSD 1015, which thus has no marked influence on monoamine levels (Carlsson *et al.,* 1972). We cannot exclude the possibility that the inhibitory action of reserpine on catecholamine synthesis is partially antagonized by NSD 1015, but the opposite effect seems more likely in view of the inhibitory action of this compound on monoamine oxidase, which should enhance the initial accumulation of free amines in the cytoplasm after reserpine treatment.

Even if the actions of reserpine on the first step in the synthesis of catecholamines or 5-HT may be somewhat modified by NSD 1015, the conclusion seems justified that the synthesis of the three major brain monoamines is accelerated by reserpine, apart from an initial inhibitory action on catecholamine synthesis.

In any event, it seems clear that the changes in tyrosine-hydroxylation rates *in vivo* have a time course markedly different from the changes due to induction of the enzyme. Maximum enzyme activities measured *in vitro* have been reported (see Section 1) at a time interval when *in vivo* activities, as observed in the present study, were declining or had already reached pretreatment levels. The stimulation of *in vivo* activities of tyrosine hydroxylase by reserpine thus seems to be due to qualitative changes in the enzyme without any increase in the number of enzyme molecules.

5.   Summary

The effect of reserpine on the synthesis of monoamines in rat brain regions was investigated using an *in vivo* method, in which the accumulation of DOPA and 5-HTP is measured after inhibition of the aromatic L-amino acid decarboxylase by means of 3-hydroxybenzylhydrazine.

Reserpine caused an initial pronounced but short-lasting inhibition of DOPA formation in all brain regions investigated. This effect is suggested to be due to end-product inhibition of tyrosine hydroxylase, caused by catecholamines accumulating in the cytoplasm as a consequence of net release from the synaptic vesicles. This inhibition was followed by a marked stimulation of DOPA formation for more than 24 hr, suggested to be due to receptor-mediated feedback.

The formation of 5-HTP was stimulated by reserpine, but the effect was rather moderate and short-lasting.

The *in vivo* changes in the tyrosine and tryptophan hydroxylases observed after reserpine treatment seem to be poorly correlated to enzyme induction, but rather underline the importance of changes in the activity of preexisting enzyme molecules.

ACKNOWLEDGMENTS

This study was supported by grants from the Swedish Medical Research Council (No. 155) and from Hässle, Mölndal, Sweden. The skillful technical assistance of Miss Birgitta Johansson, Miss Barbro Jörblad, and Miss Gerd Lundgren is gratefully acknowledged. For generous supply of reserpine, we thank Ciba-Geigy, Mölndal, Sweden.

6. References

Andén, N.-E., and Henning, M., 1966, Adrenergic nerve function, noradrenaline level and noradrenaline uptake in cat nictitating membrane after reserpine treatment, *Acta Physiol. Scand.* 67:498.

Andén, N.-E., Roos. B.-E., and Werdinius, B., 1963, 3,4-Dihydroxyphenylacetic acid in rabbit corpus striatum normally and after reserpine treatment, *Life Sci.* 2:319.

Andén, N.-E., Roos, B.-E., and Werdinius, B., 1964, Effects of chlorpromazine, haloperidol and reserpine on the levels of phenolic acids in rabbit corpus striatum, *Life Sci.* 3:149.

Atack, C., and Lindqvist, M., 1973, Conjoint native and orthophthaldialdehyde-condensate assays for the fluorimetric determination of 5-hydroxyindoles in brain, *Naunyn-Schmiedebergs Arch. Pharmakol.* 279:267.

Bédard, P., Carlsson, A., and Lindqvist, M., 1972, Effect of a transverse cerebral hemisection on 5-hydroxytryptamine metabolism in the rat brain, *Naunyn-Schmiedebergs Arch. Pharmakol.* 272:1.

Carlsson, A., 1965, Drugs which block the storage of 5-hydroxytryptamine and related amines, in: *Handbuch der experimentellen Pharmakologie*, Vol. XIX (V. Erspamer, ed.), pp. 529–592, Springer-Verlag, Berlin and Heidelberg.

Carlsson, A., 1975, Receptor-mediated control of dopamine metabolism, in: *Pre- and Postsynaptic Receptors* (E. Usdin and W. E. Bunney, eds.), pp. 49–65, Marcel Dekker, New York.

Carlsson, A., and Lindqvist, M., 1972, The effect of L-tryptophan and some psychotropic drugs on the formation of 5-hydroxytryptophan in the mouse brain *in vivo*, *J. Neural Transm.* 33:23.

Carlsson, A., and Lindqvist, M., 1973, Effect of ethanol on the hydroxylation of tyrosine and tryptophan in rat brain *in vivo*, *J. Pharm. Pharmacol.* 25:437.

Carlsson, A., Davis, J. N., Kehr, W., Lindqvist, M., and Atack, C. V., 1972, Simultaneous measurement of tyrosine and tryptophan hydroxylase activities in brain *in vivo* using an inhibitor of the aromatic amino acid decarboxylase, *Naunyn-Schmiedebergs Arch. Pharmakol.* 275:153.

Carlsson, A., Kehr, W., and Lindqvist, M., 1976, Agonist–antagonist interaction on dopamine receptors in brain, as reflected in the rates of tyrosine and tryptophan hydroxylation, in: *Advances in Parkinsonism: Biochemistry, Physiology, Treatment* (W. Birkmayer and O. Hornykiewicz, eds.), Editiones Roche, Basle, pp. 71–81.

Grabowska, M., Michaluk, J., and Antkiewicz, L., 1973, Possible involvement of brain serotonin in apomorphine-induced hypothermia, *Eur. J. Pharmacol.* 23:82.

Jequier, E., Robinson, D. S., Lovenberg, W., and Sjöerdsma, A., 1969, Further studies on tryptophan hydroxylase in rat brainstem and beef pineal, *Biochem. Pharmacol.* 18:1071.

Kehr, W., Carlsson, A., and Lindqvist, M., 1972, A method for the determination of 3,4-

dihydroxyphenylalanine (DOPA) in brain, *Naunyn-Schmiedebergs Arch. Pharmakol.* *274*:273.

Kehr, W., Carlsson, A., and Lindqvist, M., 1975, Biochemical aspects of dopamine agonists, in: *Advances in Neurology,* Vol. 9 (D. B. Calne, T. N. Chase, and A. Barbeau, eds.), pp. 185–195, Raven Press, New York.

Mueller, R. A., Thoenen, H., and Axelrod, J., 1969, Increase in tyrosine hydroxylase activity after reserpine administration, *J. Pharmacol. Exp. Ther. 169*:74.

Rutledge, C. O., and Weiner, N., 1967, The effect of reserpine on the synthesis of norepinephrine in the isolated rabbit heart, *J. Pharmacol. Exp. Ther. 157*:290.

Svensson, T. H., Bunney, B. S., and Aghajanian, G. K., 1975, Inhibition of both noradrenergic and serotonergic neurons in brain by the α-adrenergic agonist clonidine, *Brain Res. 92*:291.

Thoenen, H., Mueller, R. A., and Axelrod, J., 1969, Trans-synaptic induction of adrenal tyrosine hydroxylase, *J. Pharmacol. Exp. Ther. 169*:249.

Tozer, T. N., Neff, N. H., and Brodie, B. B., 1966, Application of steady state kinetics to the synthesis rate and turnover time of serotonin in the brain of normal and reserpine-treated rats, *J. Pharmacol. Exp. Ther. 153*:177.

Ungerstedt, U., 1971, Postsynaptic supersensitivity after 6-hydroxydopamine induced degeneration of the nigro-striatal dopamine system, *Acta physiol. Scand. Suppl. 367*:69.

Waalkes, T. P., and Udenfriend, S., 1957, A fluorometric method for the estimation of tyrosine in plasma and tissues, *J. Lab. Clin. Med. 50*:733.

Weiner, N., Cloutier, G., Bjur, R., and Pfeffer, R. I., 1972, Modification of norepinephrine synthesis in intact tissue by drugs and during short-term adrenergic nerve stimulation, *Pharmacol. Rev. 24*:203.

Winer, B. J., 1962, *Statistical Principles in Experimental Design,* McGraw-Hill Book Co., New York.

5

The Induction of Tyrosine-3-monooxygenase in Rat Adrenal Medulla: A Model for the Transsynaptic Regulation of Gene Expression

A. Guidotti and E. Costa

1. Introduction

Axelrod and colleagues (Axelrod, 1971; Thoenen, *et al.*, 1969) reported that in rat adrenal medulla, the activity of tyrosine-3-monooxygenase (TH) can be regulated transsynaptically. They found that medullary TH activity increases after the injection of nicotinic receptor agonists or when the activity of cholinergic neurons innervating the medula increases. These changes in TH occur several hours after the stimulus, and depend on RNA transcription (Chuang and Costa, 1976) and protein synthesis (Axelrod, 1971). With the exception of the injection of nicotinic receptor agonists, however, all the other stimuli failed to increase TH activity when applied after adrenal denervation; therefore, this increase of TH was termed "transsynaptic induction." Furthermore, the possibility that the increase in TH was an enzyme induction was corroborated in independent studies carried out in S. Kaufman's (Hoeldtke *et al.*, 1974) and D. Reis's (Joh *et al.*, 1973) laboratories. Using immunotitration experiments, they showed

A. Guidotti and E. Costa ● Laboratory of Preclinical Pharmacology, National Institute of Mental Health, Saint Elizabeths Hospital, Washington, D.C. 20032

that in adrenal, the number of TH molecules increases during transsynaptic induction. These immunotitration experiments do not prove, however, that the transsynaptic induction of TH involves a change in gene expression leading to an increased transcription of the mRNA coding TH synthesis. Since we intended to use the transsynaptic induction of TH as a model to study the transsynaptic regulation of gene expression, we had to show that during the induction, the rate of TH synthesis is increased while the rate of TH degradation remains unaltered. Moreover, it was essential to show that the increase in TH synthesis is preceded by an increase in the rate of synthesis of RNA, which depends on RNA polymerase II.

2.   Measurements of TH Synthesis Rate in Rat Adrenal Medulla

The rates of synthesis and degradation of TH were measured by combining pulse labeling of adrenal protein before and at various times after a stimulus that induces TH transsynaptically (Chuang and Costa, 1974), using immunoaffinity chromatography to assay the incorporation rate of amino acids into TH (Chuang et al., 1975). The rats were killed 90 min after each pulse with [³H]leucine, which was given at various times after an exposure to 2°C for 4 hr. To measure the radioactivity incorporated in medullary TH, the $10^5 g$ supernatant of adrenal medulla homogenate was passed through a Sepharose 4B column conjugated with immunoglobulins directed toward TH. This column, which selectively adsorbs TH, was washed extensively with 20 mM potassium phosphate (pH 7.4), 140 mM KCl, 1 mM $MgCl_2$, and 0.2% Triton X 100. When the radioactivity eluted from the column with this buffer had reached a low background level, the ³H protein adsorbed by the Sepharose anti-TH column was eluted with 6 M guanidine HCl, pH 3.0, and the eluate was immediately neutralized to pH 7 with Tris buffer. This eluate was extensively dialyzed and then lyophilized. The residue was redissolved and subjected to disk gel electrophoresis, using riboflavin as the catalyst. The ³H protein eluted with 6 M guanidine had an electrophoretic mobility identical to that of TH, and contained about 4% of the original ³H protein present in the $1 \times 10^5 g$ supernatant. As shown in Fig. 1, an increase in the ³H incorporation over control was detected from about 10 to 29 hr after the beginning of cold exposure; in contrast, at 48 hr after the stimulus, the incorporation rate of the label was equal in the adrenals of cold-exposed and control rats. The activity of TH was maximally increased at 24 hr, and remained virtually at this maximum for 4 days (Fig. 1).

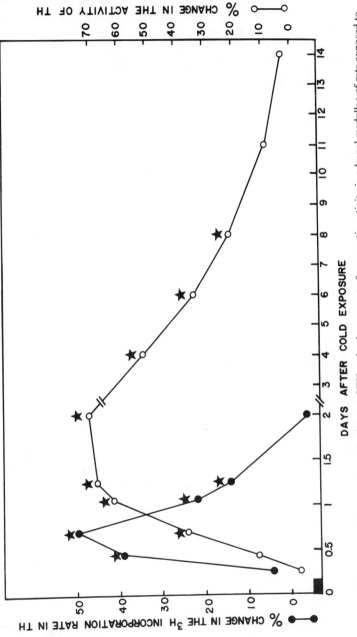

Fig. 1. Time course of increase in synthesis rate of TH and enhancement of enzymatic activity in adrenal medullae of rats exposed to cold. Normal male rats (about 100 g) were kept at 4°C for 4 hr, after which they were returned to 25°C. At various times after stress, and also 90 min prior to death, each rat received 700 μCi [^{3}H]leucine. The incorporation of ^{3}H into TH and the activity of the enzyme were determined as described previously. Each point represents the percentage increase of the mean of 5–7 experiments obtained in stressed rats compared with that obtained in normal rats. (■) Time at 4°C. (★) $P < 0.05$ when the values of stressed rats were compared with those of rats kept at room temperature. Reprinted from Chuang *et al.* (1975) with permission from the publisher.

To measure the degradation rate of adrenal TH in normal and cold-exposed rats, both groups of rats received a pulse of [³H]leucine (Chuang *et al.*, 1975). The rats exposed to cold were pulsed 48 hr after the beginning of cold exposure, because at this time (Fig. 1), the rate of TH synthesis was equal to that of control rats. The decay of radioactivity incorporated into TH was measured during the successive 100 hr. It was found that in both groups of rats, this decay followed first-order kinetics and its $T_{1/2}$ was 68 hr.

With the use of a double-labeling procedure, it was confirmed that the rate of TH degradation is not changed as a result of the transsynaptic induction (Chuang and Costa, 1974). From these results, the rate of TH synthesis was calculated using as a unit the TH activity assayed with saturating concentrations of substrates and cofactors. It was found that in 1 hr, a normal adrenal medulla synthesizes an amount of TH that catalyzes the formation of 58 pmol DOPA/hr^{-1}. In contrast, 20 hr after the beginning of cold exposure, one adrenal medulla synthesizes an amount of TH that catalyzes the formation of 96 pmol DOPA/hr^{-1}. Since in both groups of rats the turnover time of TH is identical, it could be estimated that after the cold exposure, the TH activity will return to normal in about 10 days. The data shown in Fig. 1 entirely support this theoretical calculation, thus confirming that the turnover time of TH is about 100 hr (Chuang *et al.*, 1975).

3. Participation of 3',5'-Adenosine Monophosphate in the Transsynaptic Regulation of Gene Expression in Rat Adrenal Medulla

In 1973, it was proposed that an increase of 3',5'-cyclic adenosine monophosphate (cAMP) content mediates the induction of medullary TH elicited transsynaptically (Guidotti and Costa, 1973). Successive work has supported a crucial role of the increase in the adrenal content of this cyclic nucleotide in mediating the increase in TH synthesis elicited by a prolonged stimulation of nicotinic receptors (Costa and Guidotti, 1973; Costa *et al.*, 1974, 1975a–d; Guidotti *et al.*, 1973a,b, 1974, 1975a; Hanbauer *et al.*, 1975). The evidence supporting this mediation is as follows:

1. All the stimuli that induce TH transsynaptically cause a severalfold increase of cAMP content in medulla. Denervation abolishes the increase in cAMP and the increase of TH induced transsynaptically (Guidotti *et al.*, 1975a,b; Hanbauer *et al.*, 1975).
2. Using cold exposure as the stimulus to induce medullary TH, it was shown that an exposure for 60–90 min is the threshold time of exposure

to induce TH (Guidotti *et al.*, 1973*a,b*). The increase in cAMP elicited by other transsynaptic stimuli that induce TH also lasts from 60 to about 90 min. While the increase in medullary cAMP begins almost simultaneously with the exposure to cold (Guidotti and Costa, 1974*b*), its duration lasts only a maximum of about 90 min, even though the rats are kept in the cold for several hours (Guidotti *et al.*, 1973*a,b*; Costa and Guidotti, 1973; Costa *et al.*, 1974). A plausible explanation is that the duration of the second-messenger response is regulated by the release of an endogenous protein activator of cyclic nucleotide phosphodiesterase that is stored in membranes and chromaffin cells (Uzunov *et al.*, 1975; Gnegy *et al.*, 1976). This protein is bound to synaptic membranes (Gnegy *et al.*, 1977), and its release is promoted by membrane phosphorylation mediated by a cAMP-dependent ATP protein phosphotransferase (protein kinase, PK) (Gnegy *et al.*, 1976).

3. The increase in medullary cAMP and the induction of TH depend on the stimulation of nicotinic receptors (Guidotti *et al.*, 1973*a*; Guidotti and Costa, 1974*a*). In contrast, the stimulation of muscarinic receptors that are also present in adrenal medulla causes a selective increase in the medullary content of $3',5'$-cyclic guanosine monophosphate (cGMP), but not TH induction (Guidotti *et al.*, 1975*a*). Thus, during the development of our thinking, it became convenient to express the second-messenger response elicited by stimuli that cause a transsynaptic induction of TH as the ratio between cAMP and cGMP content of medulla (Guidotti *et al.*, 1973*a*; Costa *et al.*, 1974; Hanbauer *et al.*, 1975). An increase in this ratio that occurs as a first molecular event in the transsynaptic induction of TH estimates how much the nicotinic receptor stimulation prevails over that of muscarinic receptors.

4. Denervation abolishes the cAMP increase and the TH induction elicited by stimuli that increase the release rate of ACh from the nerve terminals that innervate adrenal medulla (Guidotti and Costa, 1973; Costa and Guidotti, 1973; Guidotti *et al.*, 1973*a*). However, a denervation of adrenal medulla performed 5 days before the experiment fails to abolish the increase of cAMP content and the induction of TH elicited by carbamylcholine, a direct stimulant of nicotinic and muscarinic receptors (Guidotti *et al.*, 1973*a*). Interestingly enough, if the denervation is performed 10 days or longer before the experiment, the injection of carbamylcholine progressively loses its capability to increase medullary cAMP content or to induce TH (Hanbauer and Guidotti, 1975).

5. The duration and extent of the increase in cAMP content have a crucial role in eliciting the successive increase in TH. Drugs such as propranolol (Guidotti *et al.*, 1975*a*), dopamine (Costa *et al.*, 1976), and ACTH (Guidotti and Costa, 1974*a*; Guidotti *et al.*, 1974) increase the cAMP

Table I.   Increase of cAMP Content in Adrenal Cortex and Medulla
Elicited by Reserpine: Effect of Dexamethasone[a]

| | cAMP (pmol/mg protein) | |
Treatment	Adrenal medulla	Adrenal cortex
Saline	28 ± 3	10 ± 1.2
Reserpine (16 μmol/ kg i.p.)	75 ± 10^{b}	110 ± 15^{b}
Dexamethasone (0.2 μmol/kg i.p.) + Reserpine (16μmol/kg i.p.)	95 ± 6^{b}	14 ± 2.0

[a]Dexamethasone was injected 120 min before reserpine. The cAMP content was measured in cortex 30 min, and in medulla 60 min, after reserpine.
[b]$P < 0.01$.

content by an extent comparable to that elicited for instance by reserpine, but this increase lasts only 30 min or less, and the TH induction fails to occur. Conversely, a pretreatment with 0.2 μmol dexamethasone/kg delays and considerably reduces the extent of the increase in medullary cAMP/cGMP concentration ratio elicited by reserpine, but it prolongs it from 90 min to several hours, and the induction of TH is slightly delayed but not impaired. It is crucial to keep in mind that this dose of dexamethasone abolishes the increase in cAMP content of adrenal cortex elicited by reserpine (Table I). Moreover, denervation virtually abolishes the increase of cAMP elicited by cold exposure in medulla, but not in adrenal cortex (Guidotti and Costa, 1974a). From these results, we have inferred that the mechanisms that control the second-messenger response are hormonal in cortex and neuronal in adrenal medulla.

4. Protein Kinase Activation and cAMP Content in Rat Adrenal Medulla

It is now widely accepted that some, if not all, of the actions of cAMP in mammalian tissues take place through the interactions of cAMP with the regulatory subunit of cAMP-dependent PK (Krebs, 1972). When the cAMP is bound to the regulatory subunit of PK, the enzyme dissociates into catalytically inactive regulatory subunits that form complexes with cAMP and catalytically active subunits. The content of cAMP in adrenal medulla is in the range of 1.5–2 μmol/kg wet wt., and is increased five- to tenfold by stimuli that induce TH (Guidotti and Costa, 1974*a,b*). When PK is assayed *in vitro,* under conditions of an excess of ligand over enzyme protein, the concentrations of cAMP necessary to activate purified preparations of cAMP-dependent PK half maximally are in the range of 0.2–0.3 μM (Beavo *et al.,* 1974). The apparent dissociation constant for cAMP binding to the regulatory subunit of PK is about 0.2–0.3 μM. However, the concentration of cAMP that causes half-maximum activation (k_A) depends on the concentrations of PK in the tissue and on the concentrations of a heat-stable protein that inhibits PK activity (Ashby and Walsh, 1972, 1973). *In vitro,* when the PK concentration is increased from 9 to 150 nM, the k_A for cAMP activation of PK increases from 0.3 to 1.6 μM (Beavo *et al.,* 1974). Thus, the amount of PK present in a given cell determines the concentration of cAMP that is necessary to express its catalytic activity. Moreover, the concentration of cAMP that causes half-maximum activation (k_A) of PK also depends on the concentrations of the heat-stable protein inhibitor of PK present in the tissue (Beavo *et al.,* 1974). From data published by Beavo *et al.* (1974), one might predict that, for instance, if the inhibitor concentrations present in any given tissue were sufficient to react with 20% of the PK catalytic subunit molecules, only an activation involving more than 20% of the enzyme molecules could be expressed. Changes in the tissue content of the endogenous PK inhibitor may perturb the relationship between increases of cAMP content and PK activation. For instance, when the increase in cAMP content is attenuated but the PK activation can be expressed equally well, one must suspect that changes in the endogenous PK inhibitor content might have occurred. An appreciation of these possibilities suggested to us that it was impossible to rely only on cAMP measurements to estimate a second-messenger response. In fact, during the transsynaptically elicited increase of cAMP, one might surmise that initially the excess of cAMP produced, although bound to PK, cannot promote phosphorylation. Perhaps the PK activity cannot be expressed until the endogenous PK inhibitor has been saturated. Hence, there may be a time period during the cAMP increase when the activation of PK is not expressed. Probably the duration of this silent period is proportional to the extent of the cAMP increase and the amount of endogenous PK inhibitor present. These considerations prompted us to evaluate the cAMP response in terms of its extent and duration, and to consider both parameters of the response as two events functionally interconnected. Only after enough PK is activated to block the function of the endogenous inhibitor of PK with a sufficient number of PK catalytic subunits may one expect a correlation between the increases in cAMP content and the expression of cAMP-independent PK activity. A demonstration that agents can increase the medullary cAMP without modifying the number of free catalytic subunits that can express their activity is shown in Table II. As can be seen, when the cAMP increase lasted only 30 min, the PK activation index at 90 min was not increased, but when the increase of cAMP was prolonged for 60 min, the increase in cAMP caused an increase of the PK activation index for several hours (Kurosawa *et al.*, 1976*a,b*). This index evaluates the percentage of PK activity that can be expressed in the absence of cAMP. In the normal condition, about 18% of the PK activity of medulla can be expressed *in vitro* using histone as P acceptor without addition of cAMP (Table II). This value increases when the PK activity is measured after the medullary cAMP has been elevated for 1 hr (Table II). Since it is technically difficult to establish extent and duration of the increase of cAMP content in medulla, the functional consequences of an increase of cAMP content are now directly estimated by measuring the activation index of PK as indicated in Table II. This index and the PK translocation are, in fact, of great value in establishing the sequence of events initiated by the increase in cAMP content because they express a temporal and spatial amplification of the second-messenger response (Costa *et al.*, 1975*a,d*, 1976; Kurosawa *et al.*, 1976*a,b*,).

Table II. Protein Kinase Activation Index, TH Activity, and Increase of cAMP Content in Rat Adrenal Medulla

Stimulus	cAMP (pmol/mg protein) at 30 min	at 60 min	PK index at 90 min [a]	TH (nmol DOPA/gland per hr^{-1}) at 24 hr
Carbamylcholine (9.2 μmol/kg i.p.)	380 ± 35 [b]	100 ± 9 [b]	0.42 ± 0.05 [b]	11 ± 1 [b]
Reserpine (16 μmol/ kg i.p.)	145 ± 12 [b]	70 ± 10 [b]	0.59 ± 0.03 [b]	10 ± 0.5 [b]
Exposure to 4°C for 2 hr	190 ± 15 [b]	75 ± 20 [b]	0.48 ± 0.04 [b]	8.2 ± 0.8 [b]
ACTH (1 IU/kg i.v.)	225 ± 18 [b]	38 ± 7	0.17 ± 0.005	6 ± 0.4
Dopamine (50 μmol/ kg s.c.)	80 ± 7 [b]	32 ± 7	0.22 ± 0.03	4.8 ± 0.5
Propranolol (40 μmol/ kg i.p.)	100 ± 6 [b]	25 ± 5	0.20 ± 0.01	5.5 ± 0.6
Saline	28 ± 1.1	20 ± 3.2	0.18 ± 0.14	5 ± 0.5

[a] The kinase activation index is the ratio of the activity measured in $2 \times 10^4 g$ supernatant in the absence or in the presence of cAMP (0.7 μM). In all the experiments, the phosphate acceptor was a calf thymus histone mixture (300 μg/ml).

[b] $P < 0.05$ when compared with saline-treated rats. Each value refers to the mean $\pm$ S.E.M. of at least 5 rats.

5. Inconsistency of the Experimental Evidence Supporting a Lack of Correlation Between an Early Increase in cAMP Content and the Delayed Transsynaptic Induction of Medullary TH

Dr. Thoenen's laboratory has published a number of reports showing that the changes in cAMP or in cAMP/cGMP concentration ratios are not an indispensable prerequisite for the subsequent transsynaptic induction of TH (Thoenen *et al.*, 1973, 1975; Thoenen and Otten, 1975). Thus, they have excluded a causal relationship between the two phenomena. Although, as we discussed earlier, there are ample theoretical grounds for apparent discrepancies among extent, rate, duration, and other characteristics of cAMP increase and PK activation, the experiments of Dr. Thoenen's group merely show that only under particular experimental conditions may the neurally mediated TH induction in medulla not be preceded by an increase in cAMP/cGMP concentration ratio that is as prompt or as intense as that reported in ordinary experimental conditions by us and consistently confirmed by Dr. Thoenen's group.

The experiments of Dr. Thoenen's group will be discussed sequentially in chronological order of publication:

5.1. Experiments with Swimming Stress

In 1973, at the IIIrd International Catecholamine Symposium, Dr. Thoenen and his colleagues (Thoenen *et al.*, 1973) reported that they could confirm the good correlation between the early cAMP increase and the delayed TH induction reported by us with cold exposure, carbachol, and reserpine injection. Moreover, they also confirmed the coincidence between the duration of the cAMP increase and the threshold time of cold exposure to elicit TH induction (Guidotti *et al.*, 1973*b*). In their conditions (Thoenen *et al.*, 1973), the exposure to cold causes an increase of cAMP content lasting 90 min, and they could not obtain a delayed induction of TH with 60 min, but 2 hr of cold exposure were sufficient to induce TH (Otten *et al.*, 1973). Interestingly, repeated swimming stress induced medullary TH but caused an exceptionally small increase in cAMP content associated with the stimulus application (Thoenen *et al.*, 1973; Otten *et al.*, 1973). Since the increase in cAMP produced by swimming to exhaustion is much smaller than that during exposure to cold, the validity of the concept that cAMP mediates the transsynaptic induction of TH was questioned (Thoenen *et al.*, 1973). However, when the experimental results were analyzed over a broader time sequence, it was clear that the purported lack of correlation between changes in cAMP and subsequent induction of TH could no longer be maintained (Guidotti and Costa, 1974b).

We report in Fig. 2 (Costa et al., 1975b) a replication of the swimming stress experiments published by Thoenen et al. (1973). The sex, weight, and strain of rats, the water temperature, the number of the swimming stresses, and the time interval between two successive swimming stresses were exactly those reported by Thoenen et al. (1973). However, we measured the body temperature, which, as reported in Fig. 2, falls quite remarkably during this stress. Certainly, as reported by Thoenen et al. (1973), the medullary concentrations of cAMP do not increase during the swimming stress while the rats are severely hypothermic, and of course this is not surprising. As soon as the body temperature returns to basal values, however, 90 min after the termination of the swimming stress, the medullary cAMP content increases, that of cGMP decreases, and the cAMP/cGMP concentration ratio stays elevated for longer than 1 hr (Fig. 2). This ratio, which is normally about 10, becomes 40 at peak effects following the swimming stress. Thus, the swimming stress applied as suggested by Thoenen et al. (1973), but interpreted in the light of basic principles of physiological control in homeothermic rats, confirms and supports our proposal that a second-messenger response always precedes the transsynaptic induction of medullary TH (Guidotti et al., 1973a; Costa et al., 1974).

5.2. Experiments with Reserpine and Propranolol

Thoenen et al. (1975) and Otten et al. (1974a,b) reported that impressive experimental evidence for the dissociation between the rate, extent, and duration of cAMP increase and the subsequent induction of adrenal TH could be obtained by the injection of 40 μmol D,L-propranolol/kg given 30 min before 16 μmol reserpine/kg i.p. They reported that in this condition, reserpine fails to increase medullary cAMP content without impairing TH induction. We (Guidotti et al., 1975b) repeated the experiments exactly as reported by Thoenen et al. (1975) and Otten et al. (1974a,b), but as shown in Fig. 3, a propranolol pretreatment failed to abolish the increase of cAMP content elicited by reserpine. Moreover, propranolol by itself increases cAMP content in medulla for only 30 min, and it fails to activate PK or to induce TH (Fig. 3). In contrast, whether or not reserpine injection is preceded by a propranolol injection, it increases cAMP content, activates PK, and induces TH (Fig. 3). We have on several occasions discussed this discrepancy with Dr. Thoenen, who feels that even though we cannot

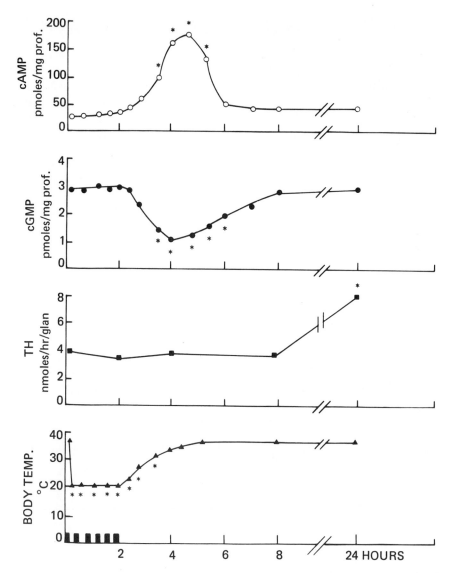

Fig. 2. Body temperature, adrenal medullary cAMP and cGMP concentrations, and TH activity in rats (120 g body wt.) exposed to intermittent swimming stresses in 15°C water. Animals were forced to swim 6 times for a period of 6 min (black bars on abscissa) in 2 hr. In the intervals between swimming trials and after last swimming stress, animals were kept at 25°C. Each value represents the mean of 5 experiments. (*) $P < 0.05$. Reprinted from Costa *et al.* (1975*b*) with permission from the publisher.

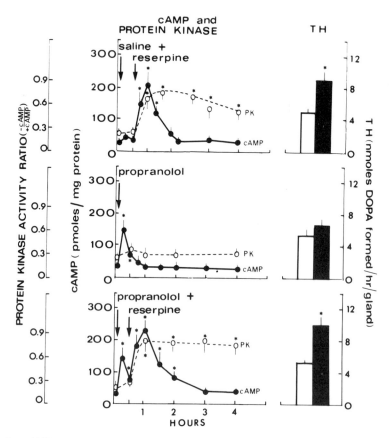

Fig. 3. cAMP concentration and PK and TH activity in adrenal medullae of rat after injection of reserpine, propranolol, and propranolol + reserpine. Reserpine (16 μmol/kg i.p.) was injected 30 min after saline or propranolol (40 μmol/kg i.p.). cAMP concentration and PK activity in the absence or in the presence of 0.7 μM cAMP were measured in the first 4 hr after reserpine administration. TH was measured 48 hr after reserpine or propranolol injection. (*) $P < 0.05$ when compared with control animals. TH: ($\square$) control: ($\blacksquare$) treated. Each value is the mean ± S.E. of at least 10 determinations. Reprinted from Guidotti *et al.* (1975*b*) with permission from the publisher.

repeat his finding, since he could observe the lack of association, the concept of the second-messenger participation in the transsynaptic induction is *ipso facto* open to question. We feel that before the concept is questioned at least another laboratory should be able to reproduce the evidence against the association.

5.3. Experiments with Dexamethasone and Reserpine

As first reported by us (Guidotti *et al.*, 1974; Guidotti and Costa, 1974*a*), high doses of ACTH increase the cAMP content not only of adrenal cortex, but also that of adrenal medulla. Since an increase in pituitary ACTH secretion participates in several stresses used to induce TH, Thoenen and Otten (1975) suggested that the changes in cAMP content in adrenal medulla predominantly reflect the ACTH-mediated increase in this nucleotide content of the adrenal cortex. The experiments reported in Table I clearly show that a dose of dexamethasone (0.2 μmol/kg i.p.) that suppresses the increase in cAMP content of adrenal cortex elicited by reserpine (16 μmol/kg i.p.) fails to abolish the increase in cAMP content of adrenal medulla and the delayed induction of TH (data not shown). The data of Table I show clearly that the increase in cAMP of adrenal medulla elicited by reserpine is independent of a release of ACTH from pituitary. Thus, in adrenal medulla, the increase in cAMP content elicited by reserpine is regulated transsynaptically. These experiments categorically exclude the inference made by Thoenen and Otten (1975) that " . . . there is strong evidence that the changes in cAMP observed in the adrenal medulla mainly reflect the changes occurring in the adrenal cortex which are regulated by the pituitary gland" (p. 281).

5.4. Experiments with Reserpine: A Dose–Response Relationship

Otten and Thoenen (1976) reported that after a dose of 4 μmol reserpine/kg i.p., the increase in cAMP content at 30 min postinjection was smaller than after 16 μmol/kg, and the extent of induction of TH was reduced. We had already published our finding (Guidotti *et al.*, 1975*b*) that is a dose range from 2 to 16 μmol reserpine/kg, the extent of PK activation at 90 min and the induction of TH 24 hr later increase with the dose of reserpine. The increment of both phenomena as a function of dose was quite similar.

Thus, while the data obtained by Otten and Thoenen (1976) and our laboratory (Guidotti *et al.*, 1975*b*) are similar, the emphasis given to these data by Otten and Thoenen is different. We believe that it is inappropriate to exclude on the basis of this data that the increase in cAMP is disocciated from TH induction when we have shown that by using a more precise measurement of the second-messenger response, the association is upheld (Guidotti *et al.*, 1975*b*). We had suggested (Guidotti *et al.*, 1973*a*) that a way to estimate the involvement of the second-messenger response in the induction of TH might be to calculate a ratio between cAMP/cGMP concentration ratio. This ratio was increased every time TH was induced. We also observed that this ratio reached a value of 40 for a number of stimuli we tested. Later (Guidotti et al., 1975b), we realized that a better way to evaluate the second-messenger involvement was to calculate the activation of PK at various times after the stimulus. While Otten and Thoenen (1976) completely confirmed our postulate that the ratio is increased after all the doses of reserpine that induce TH, they argued that with threshold stimuli, an increase is obtained, but it is smaller than that we had originally postulated to be a threshold value for TH induction. We have discussed earlier why one should take into consideration duration and extent of second-messenger responses, and we have explained the theoretical reasons for considering both parameters as concurring factors in the PK activation; therefore, it seems to us unwise to exclude the association of cAMP with TH induction because with small doses of reserpine, the increase is smaller than an arbitrary unit we had chosen to focus our thinking rather than to establish a biological low. In their vain attempts to obtain evidence to dismiss a role of cAMP in the transsynaptic induction of TH, Otten and Thoenen (1976) arbitrarily called our proposal the "ratio theory." Their persistence in this attitude of defining little details as crucial facts rather than trying to develop more consistent measurements of second messenger has merely provided additional evidence in support of the concept that a second-messenger response indicates transsynaptic induction of TH. We must acknowledge that the stubbornness of our opponents has been a healthy stimulus for our research activities and for the consolidation of our concepts.

6. Activation and Translocation of Protein Kinase from Adrenal Medulla Cytosol During Transsynaptic Induction of TH

The kinetic equilibrium of the regulatory and catalytic subunits of cytosol PK was studied by separating the various components of the system chromatographically with Sephadex G200 (Costa et al., 1975a,d; Guidotti et al., 1975b). Two main protein fractions were distinguished: a fraction with high molecular weight the PK activity of which is stimulated by cAMP and corresponds to the whole enzyme, and another protein fraction that includes a PK activity that is cAMP-insensitive, has a low molelcular weight, and possibly corresponds to the free catalytic subunits. Actually, when purified regulatory subunits are added to the latter fraction, its phosphorylating activity becomes dependent on cAMP (Kurosawa et al., 1976a,b; Costa et al., 1976).

Transsynaptic stimuli capable of inducing TH lead to an increase in the number of enzyme molecules present in the part of the chromatographic eluate of medulla supernatant that includes the catalytic subunit of PK (Guidotti *et al.*, 1975*b;* Kurosawa *et al.*, 1976*a*). Hence, in the adrenal medulla supernatant, the activity of PK that retains the capacity to phosphorylate histone in the absence of cAMP is increased 90 min after inducing stimuli. This increase in catalytic subunits of cAMP-dependent PK lasts less than 4 hr. Thus, it does not last long enough to fill the time interval between the application of the transsynaptic stimulus and the increase of TH activity that begins 12–16 hr after the stimulus and is completed at 24 hr (Guidotti *et al.*, 1975*b;* Costa *et al.*, 1975*a,b;* Kurosawa *et al.*, 1976*a,b*). However, the decline in high-molecular-weight cAMP-dependent PK activity of the supernatant lasts up to 18 hr. We became interested in learning more about this temporal correlation because it suggested to us that the termination in the increase in catalytic subunits is not due to the reassociation of these units with regulatory subunits (Kurosawa *et al.*, 1976*a*). In studying the fate of the free catalytic subunits that disappear from cytosol at 4 hr after the stimulus without evidence of reassociating with regulatory subunits, we have found that when the PK activity of the cytosol catalytic subunits is back to normal, the PK activity present in pellets from medulla homogenates is increased. This increase occurred in coincidence with the fractions of the chromatographic eluate that include the catalytic subunits (Costa *et al.*, 1975*a,d*, 1976; Kurosawa *et al.*, 1976*a,b*). The increased activity in the pellet appears to represent an increase in free catalytic subunits, since it is abolished by the addition of purified regulatory subunits (Kurosawa et al., 1976*a*). The affinity for various histones of the catalytic subunits of PK that increase in the pellet at 7 hr after transsynaptic stimuli was studied (Kurosawa *et al.*, 1976*a;* Costa *et al.*, 1976). The histone-substrate specificity of the pellet extracts from animals killed at 7 hr after the stimulus is different from that of the pellets of the control rats, indicating a transfer of a specific category of PK catalytic subunits from cytosol to pellet. A similar transfer of catalytic subunit from cytosol to particulate fraction is mediated by several stimuli that induce TH (Kurosawa *et al.*, 1976*a,b;* Costa *et al.*, 1975*a,d*, 1976).

In other tissues, a similar phenomenon was elicited by hormonal stimulants (Jungmann *et al.*, 1975) and was termed "translocation." By analogy, we have also termed translocation the phenomenon elicited by stimuli that induce TH transsynaptically. At least part of the PK is translocated in nuclei purified from homogenates of adrenal medullae prepared at 7 hr after the application of stimuli that induce TH (Kurosawa *et al.*, 1976*a*). This translocation of PK into the nucleus may be involved in the TH induction by regulating RNA transscription through phosphorylation of

A. Guidotti and E. Costa

Table III. Protein Kinase Translocation and Tyrosine 3-monooxygenase Induction in Intact and Denervated Adrenal Medulla[a]

	Intact			Denervated		
	PK^{32}P incorporated (pmol/mg protein per min)		TH	PK^{32}P incorporated (pmol/mg protein per min)		Th
Stimulus	Cytosol	Pellet extract	(nmol/hr per gland)	Cytosol	Pellet extract	(nmoles/hr per gland)
Saline	163 ± 9	70 ± 11	5 ± 0.5	164 ± 8	63 ± 10	6 ± 0.6
Reserpine (16 μmol/kg i.p.)	100 ± 2[b]	124 ± 4[b]	10 ± 0.5	164 ± 10	52 ± 5	6 ± 0.6
Aminophylline (200 μmol/kg i.p.)	90 ± 8[b]	134 ± 9[b]	12 ± 1.2[b]	150 ± 11	73 ± 9	7 ± 0.4
Carbamylcholine (9.2 μmol/kg i.p.)	120 ± 7[b]	112 ± 5[b]	10 ± 0.5[b]	118 ± 5[b]	110 ± 5[b]	10 ± 0.5[b]
Cold (2 hr at 4° C)	90 ± 8[b]	140 ± 12[b]	9 ± 0.8[b]	157 ± 18	62 ± 6	5 ± 0.5

[a]PK activity was measured at 7 hr after various stimuli in the $1 \times 10^5 g$ supernatant and in the respective pettet extract (for methods, see Kurosawa et al., 1976a). Unilateral denervation was performed 5 days before the experiment. TH activity was measured 24 hr after the stimuli.
[b]$P < 0.02$.

specific nuclear proteins. The significance of translocation as a long-range message in the induction of TH is shown in Table III.

7. Protein Kinase Translocation in Explaining Results Purporting a Lack of Association Between Increase in cAMP and TH Induction

If one adrenal is denervated and the other is left intact, only the intact adrenal shows translocation of PK after reserpine administration (Table III). On the other hand, carbamylcholine injection causes PK translocation and TH induction in both intact and denervated adrenal (Table III). This finding indicates that translocation, like TH induction, is mediated through stimulation of nicotinic receptors. Thus, translocation of PK to particulate fractions including nuclei is a transsynaptically mediated event. Mueller *et al.* (1974) reported that when the adrenal is denervated 4 hr after reserpine injection, the delayed induction of TH is abolished. This finding was confirmed in our laboratory (Kurosawa *et al.*, 1976*b*). Since at 4 hr after reserpine the cAMP content is back to normal, we have selected this experimental protocol to evaluate whether PK translocation is a critical event in the transsynaptic induction of TH. The increase of PK activity in the pellet extract of medullary homogenates from reserpine-treated rats was reversed by denervation, and this decline in pellet PK activity was associated with an increase in the cAMP-dependent PK in cytosol (Table IV). Thus, in the absence of nerve impulses, the PK translocation of catalytic subunits is reversed and reassociation is prompted. This finding supports the view that the translocation of PK into the pellet is a critical

Table IV.   Unilateral Denervation after Reserpine: Effect on Protein Kinase Translocation

Time after Reserpine	Right adrenal gland			Left adrenal gland		
	PK (pmoles/mg protein per min)		TH (nmoles/hr per gland)	PK (pmoles/mg protein per min)		TH (nmoles/hr per gland)
	Cytosol	Pellet		Cytosol	Pellet	
0	143 ± 7	59 ± 4	5.0 ± 0.4	139 ± 8	57 ± 3	5.2 ± 0.4
4[a]	88 ± 12^b	132 ± 9^b		80 ± 8^b	132 ± 9^b	
8	74 ± 12^b	130 ± 20^b		148 ± 26	53 ± 12	
48	143 ± 8	66 ± 8	11 ± 0.9^b	142 ± 10	59 ± 9	5.0 ± 0.6

[a]At 4 hr, the left adrenal nerve was severed.
[b]$P < 0.02$ when compared with respective values at zero time.

step in the chain of events that mediate the transsynaptic control of gene expression leading to the induction of TH. Moreover, it shows that the experiments associating reserpine treatment with adrenal denervation performed 4 hr after reserpine confirm (Kurosawa et al., 1976b) rather than exclude (Mueller et al., 1974) the association between the second-messenger response and the transsynaptic induction of TH.

Hanbauer et al. (1975) and Thoenen et al. (1975) reported that the administration of aminophylline (200 μmol/kg) to adrenal denervated rats causes a more rapid, larger, and more prolonged increase in medullary cAMP of denervated adrenals than did reserpine alone in intact adrenals. Despite this, the delayed TH induction is elicited by reserpine in intact medulla, and is not elicited by aminophylline in denervated medulla. Thoenen and Otten (1975) commented: "Since the induction of TH is not an all or nothing phenomenon but a gradual process it is very difficult to conceive that an arbitrary critical ratio of the two nucleotides should determine whether an induction occurs or not and that ratios very close to each other are followed by no induction or a very marked TH induction" (p. 281). The evidence for the participation of PK activation (Guidotti et al., 1975b) and translocation (Costa et al., 1975a,d; Kurosawa et al., 1976a,b) in the transsynaptic induction of TH elicited by reserpine prompted us to investigate the second-messenger response elicited by aminophylline in denervated medulla in terms of PK activity index of cytosol and translocation of PK to the pellet. In rats with monolateral denervation of adrenal medulla (Costa et al., 1975a), we found (see Table III) that denervation abolishes the translocation of PK and the induction of TH elicited by aminophylline. However, the less marked increase in cAMP content elicited by reserpine is associated with a persistent translocation (Table III). Again, these data also indicate that nerve impulses have a crucial role in maintaining translocation of PK into particulate fraction.

8. Nuclear Phosphorylation and Gene Expression: Role of Protein Kinase Translocation

It is generally accepted now that the PK present in liver nuclei is not stimulated by cAMP (Castagna et al., 1975). Also, in adrenal medulla, the nuclear PK activity is cAMP-independent (Kurosawa et al., 1976a). The PK activity of nuclei at 7 hr after a dose of reserpine that increases TH activity was 144 ± 26 ($N = 3$), while that of saline-treated rats was 65 ± 11, pmol/mg protein per min. Thus, when the synthesis of TH begins to increase (see Fig. 1), the PK activity of nuclei is increased by 100%, and this increase is due to PK translocation (Kurosawa et al., 1976a). This finding raised the question: how can the translocated catalytic subunits of PK that reach the nucleus operate at the molecular level to induce TH? In an attempt to answer this question, we found that the exposure of rats to 4°C for a time period sufficient to induce TH increases the incorporation of [³H]uridine into RNA from 6 to 10 hr later (Chuang and Costa, 1976). During this time, the catalytic subunits of PK are translocated to the nucleus (Kurosawa *et al.*, 1976a). This increased RNA production is not seen in the denervated adrenal medulla of rats exposed to cold (Chuang and Costa, 1976). We also found that this increase in [³H]uridine incorporation occurs primarily in polyA RNA (Chuang and Costa, 1976). Moreover, in nuclei isolated from medullae of rats exposed to 4°C, 8 hr earlier, the increased synthesis of RNA is blocked by α-amanitin (Chuang and Costa, 1974), which inhibits RNA polymerase II (RNAP II) and the mRNA production. We then considered the important question: can phosphorylation of either chromatin or RNAP II lead to such changes in mRNA production?

An *in vitro* transcription system was employed to investigate this question (Chuang *et al.*, 1976). RNAP II from adrenal medullae was incubated in a phosphorylating system containing PK, ATP, and cAMP, and then added to the transcriptional system together with chromatin, also from beef adrenal medulla. Phosphorylation of our preparation of homologous RNAP II did not lead to a significant change in the level of mRNA synthesis. In the converse experiment, chromatin was phosphorylated and then added to a transcriptional system containing RNAP II isolated from either beef adrenal medulla or *Escherichia coli*. Although much of the nonspecific RNA synthesis was seen with the bacterial polymerase, there was only little increase due to chromatin phosphorylation. However, phosphorylation of beef adrenal chromatin led to a large enhancement of mRNA production in the system containing adrenal RNAP II. Thus, it appears that phosphorylation enhances the template activity of the chromatin, presumably by recognition of specific initiation sites for attachment of RNAP II.

9.   Conclusions

The data reported in Fig. 4 show the sequence of molecular events whereby a persistent activation of nicotinic receptors in adrenal medulla causes an increase in the gene expression, including an increase in the synthesis of TH. Stimulation of the nicotinic receptor in the membrane of chromaffin cells leads to a rise in cAMP content and an activation of PK by the release of free catalytic subunits. This increase is not stoichiometrically proportional to the increase in cAMP. The presence of the endogenous

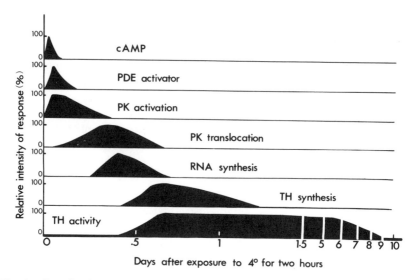

Fig. 4. Cascade of molecular events in adrenal medulla triggered by the increase of cAMP content elicited by cold exposure.

thermostable inhibitor of PK and the relative proportion of ligand and PK molecules determine the extent of PK activation. Moreover, this complex relationship requires that the increase in cAMP persist for a given time. The duration and extent of the cAMP increase play a regulatory role of PK activation within the limits imposed by the number of PK molecules present and the amount of PK endogenous inhibitors. The catalytic sub-units of the PK act on the cell membranes to release the phosphodiesterase activator, and this activator, by interacting in the presence of Ca^{2+} with the high K_m and high V_{max} molecular forms of cyclic nucleotide phosphodies-terase, lowers the K_m of this phosphodiesterase with high catalytic activity and brings to an end the second-messenger response. By this time, how-ever, the message for an effective long-range stimulation of template activity is originated; thus, the activation of PK and the successive nuclear translocation of the PK take place if neuronal activity is preserved. The translocation of catalytic subunits to the nucleus leads to an increased transcription rate of mRNA, which results in an increased synthesis of TH at about 9½ hr after the initiation of the stimulus and an increased number of TH molecules at 12 hr. Several interesting questions are raised by this model: (1) Can this process be generalized to other neuronal cells? (2) How can nerve impulses regulate the time course of PK translocation? (3) What is the molecular mechanism of translocation? (4) How is phosphorylation of selective nuclear protein regulated?

10. References

Ashby, C. D., and Walsh, D., 1972, Characterization of the interaction of a protein inhibitor with adenosine 3′,5′-monophosphate dependent protein kinases. I. Interaction with the catalytic subunit of the protein kinase, *J. Biol. Chem.* 247:6637–6642.

Ashby, C. D., and Walsh, D., 1973, Characterization of the interaction of a protein inhibitor with adenosine 3′,5′-monophosphate dependent protein kinases. II. Mechanism of action with the holoenzyme, *J. Biol. Chem.* 248:1225–1261.

Axelrod, J., 1971, Noradrenaline: Fate and control of its biosynthesis, *Science 173*:598–606.

Beavo, J. A., Bechtel, P. J., and Krebs, E. G., 1974, Activation of protein kinase by physiological concentrations of cyclic AMP, *Proc. Natl. Acad. Sci. U.S.A.* 71:3580–3583.

Castagna, M., Palmer, W., and Walsh, D., 1975, Nuclear protein kinase activity in perfused rat liver stimulated with dibutyryl adenosine cyclic 3′,5′-monophosphate, *Eur. J. Biochem.* 55:193–199.

Chuang, D. M., and Costa, E., 1974, Biosynthesis of tyrosine hydroxylase in rat adrenal medulla after expsure to cold, *Proc. Natl. Acad. Sci. U.S.A.* 71:4570–4574.

Chuang, D. M., and Costa, E., 1976, Trans-synaptic regulation of ribonucleic acid biosynthesis in rat adrenal medulla, *Mol. Pharmacol. 12*:514–518.

Chuang, D. M., Zsilla, G., and Costa, E., 1975, Turnover rate of tyrosine hydroxylase during trans-synaptic induction, *Mol. Pharmacol. 11*:784–794.

Chuang, D. M., Hollenbeck, R., and Costa, E., 1976, Enhancement of template activity in chromatin from adrenal medulla following phosphorylation of chromosomal proteins, *Science 193*:60–62.

Costa, E., and Guidotti, A., 1973, The role of 3′,5′-cyclic adenosine monophosphate in the regulation of adrenal medullary function, in: *New Concepts in Neurotransmitter Regulation* (A. J. Mandel, ed.), pp. 135–152, Plenum Publsihing Co., New York.

Costa, E., Guidotti, A., and Hanbauer, I., 1974, Do cyclic nucleotides promote the trans-synaptic induction of tyrosine hydroxylase?, *Life Sci. 14*:1169–1188.

Costa, E., Chuang, D. M., Guidotti, A., and Uzunov, P., 1975a, Cyclic 3′,5′-adenosine monophosphate dependent molecular mechanisms in the trans-synaptic induction of tyrosine hydroxylase in rat adrenal medulla, in: *Chemical Tools in Catecholamine Research II* (O. Almgren, A. Carlsson, and J. Engel, eds.), pp. 283–292, North-Holland Publishing Co., Amsterdam.

Costa, E., Guidotti, A., and Hanbauer, I., 1975b, Comment on the paper, "Lack of correlation between rate of increase in cAMP and subsequent induction of tyrosine hydroxylase in sympathetic ganglia and adrenal medulla," by T. Thoenen, U. Otten, R. A. Mueller, R. Goodman, and F. Oesch," in: *Neuropsychopharmacology* (J. R. Boissier, H. Hippius, and P. Pichot, eds.), pp. 952–955, Excerpta Medica, Amsterdam.

Costa, E., Guidotti, A., and Hanbauer, I., 1975c, Cyclic nucleotides and trophism of secretory cells: Study of adrenal medulla, in: *Cyclic Nucleotides in Disease* (B. Weiss, ed.), pp. 167–186, University Park Press, Baltimore.

Costa, E., Guidotti, A., and Kurosawa, A., 1975d, Evidence for a role of protein kinase activation and translocation in the trans-synaptic control of tyrosine hydroxylase biosynthesis, in: *Biological Membranes—Neurochemistry*, Vol. 41 (Y. Raoul, ed.), pp. 137–149, North-Holland, Amsterdam.

Costa, E., Kurosawa, A., and Guidotti, A., 1976, Activation and nuclear translocation of histone kinase during the trans-synatpic induction of tyrosine 3-monooxygenase, *Proc. Natl. Acad. Sci. U.S.A., 73*:1058–1062.

Gnegy, M., Costa, E., and Uzunov, P., 1976, The regulation of second messenger responses elicited trans-synaptically: Participation of the endogenous phosphodiesterase activator and protein kinase, *Proc. Natl. Acad. Sci. U.S.A. 73*:352–355.

Gnegy, M., Nathanson, J. A., and Uzunov, P., 1977, Release of the phosphodiesterase activator by cyclic AMP dependent ATP: Protein phosphotransferase from subcellular fractions of rat brain, *Biochim. Biophys. Acta 497*:75–85.

Guidotti, A., and Costa, E., 1973, Involvement of adenosine 3',5'-monophosphate in the activation of tyrosine hydroxylase elicited by drugs, *Science 179*:902–904.

Guidotti, A., and Costa, E., 1974*a,* A role for nicotinic receptors in the regulation of the adenylate cyclase of adrenal medulla, *J. Pharmacol. Exp. Ther. 189*:665–675.

Guidotti, A., and Costa, E., 1974*b,* Association between the increase in cyclic AMP and subsequent induction of tyrosine hydroxylase in rat adrenal medulla: Experiments with swimming stress, *Naunyn-Schmiedebergs Arch. Pharmakol. 282*:217–221.

Guidotti, A., Mao, C., and Costa, E., 1973*a,* Trans-synaptic regulation of tyrosine hydroxylase in adrenal medulla: Possible role of cyclic nucleotides, in: *Frontiers in Catecholamine Research,* (E. Usdin, ed.), pp. 231–236, Pergamon Press, London.

Guidotti, A., Zivkovic, B., Pfeiffer, R., and Costa, E., 1973*b,* Involvement of 3',5'-cyclic adenosine monophosphate in the increase of tyrosine hydroxylase activity elicited by cold exposure, *Naunyn-Schmiedebergs Arch. Pharmakol. 278*:195–206.

Guidotti, A., Mao, C. C., and Costa, E., 1974, Delayed increase of tyrosine hydroxylase activity induced by trans-synaptic stimulation in chromaffin cells: Role of cyclic nucleotides as second messengers, in: *Advances in Cytopharmacology,* Vol. 2 (B. Ceccarelli, F. Clementi, and J. Meldolesi, eds.), pp. 39–46, Raven Press, New York.

Guidotti, A., Hanbauer, I., and Costa, E., 1975*a,* Role of cyclic nucleotides in the induction of tyrosine hydroxylase: A study using the adrenal medulla and the sympathetic ganglion, in: *Advances in Cyclic Nucleotide Research,* Vol. 5 (G. I. Drummond, P. Greengard, and G. A. Robison, eds.), pp. 619–639, Raven Press, New York.

Guidotti, A., Kurosawa, A., Chuang, D., and Costa, E., 1975*b,* Protein kinase activation as an early event in the trans-synaptic induction of tyrosine 3-monooxygenase in adrenal medulla, *Proc. Natl. Acad. Sci. U.S.A. 72*:1152–1156.

Hanbauer, I., and Guidotti, A., 1975, Further evidence for a cAMP dependent regulation of tyrosine 3-monooxygenase induction in adrenal medulla: Effect of denervation, *Naunyn-Schmiedebergs Arch. Pharmakol. 287*:213–217.

Hanbauer, I., Guidotti, A., and Costa, E., 1975, Involvement of cyclic nucleotides in the long term induction of tyrosine hydroxylase, in: *Neuropsychopharmacology* (J. R. Boissier, H. Hippius, and P. Pichot eds.), pp. 932–941, Excerpta Medica, Amsterdam.

Hoeldtke, R., Lloyd, T., and Kaufman, S., 1974, An immunochemical study of the induction of tyrosine hydroxylase in rat adrenal, *Biochem. Biophys. Res. Commun. 57*:1045–1053.

Joh, T. H., Geghman, C., and Reis, D., 1973, Immunochemical demonstration of increased accumulation of tyrosine hydroxylase protein in sympathetic ganglia and adrenal medulla elicited by reserpine, *Proc. Natl. Acad. Sci. U.S.A. 70*:2767–2771.

Jungmann, R. A., Lee, S., and DeAngelo, A. B., 1975, Translocation of cytoplasmic protein kinase and cyclic adenosine monophosphate binding protien to intracellular acceptor sites, *Adv. Cyclic Nucleotide Res. 5*:281–306.

Krebs, E. G., 1972 Protein kinases, in: *Current Topics in Cellular Regulation,* Vol. 5 (Bernard L. Horechker and Earl R. Stadtman, eds.), pp. 99–133, Academic Press, New York.

Kurosawa, A., Guidotti, A., and Costa, E., 1976*a,* Induction of tyrosine 3-monooxygenase elicited by carbamylcholine in intact and denervated adrenal medulla: Role of histone kinase activation and translocation, *Mol. Pharmacol. 12*:420–432.

Kurosawa, A., Guidotti, A., and Costa, E., 1976*b*, Induction of tyrosine 3-monooxygenase in adrenal medulla: Role of protein kinase activation and translocation, *Science 193*:691–693.

Mueller, R. A., Otten, U., and Thoenen, H., 1974, The role of adenosine cyclic 3',5'-monophosphate in reserpine-initiated adrenal medullary tyrosine hydroxylase induction, *Mol. Pharmacol. 10*:855–860.

Otten, U., and Thoenen, H., 1976, Lack of correlation between changes in cyclic nucleotides and subsequent induction of tyrosine hydroxylase in rat adrenal medulla, *Naunyn-Schmiedebergs Arch. Pharmakol. 293*:105–108.

Otten, U., Oesch, F., and Thoenen, H., 1973, Dissociation between changes in cAMP and subsequent induction of TH in the rat superior cervical ganglion and adrenal medulla, *Naunyn-Schmiedebergs Arch. Pharmakol. 280*:129–140.

Otten, U., Mueller, R. A., Oesch, F., and Thoenen, H., 1974*a*, Location of an isoproterenol responsive cyclic AMP pool in adrenergic nerve cell bodies and its relationship to tyrosine 3-monooxygenase induction, *Proc. Natl. Acad. Sci. U.S.A. 71*:2217–2221.

Otten, U., Mueller, R. A., and Thoenen, H., 1974*b*, Evidence against a causal relationship between increase in cAMP and induction of tyrosine hydroxylase in the rat adrenal medulla, *Naunyn-Schmiedebergs Arch. Pharmakol. 285*:233–242.

Thoenen, H., and Otten, U., 1975, Cyclic nucleotides and trans-synaptic enzyme induction: Lack of correlation between initial cAMP increase, changes in cAMP/cGMP ratio and subsequent induction of tyrosine hydroxylase in the adrenal medulla, in: *Chemical Tools in Catecholamine Research II* (Olle Almgren, Arvid Carlsson, and Jorgen Engel, eds.), pp. 275–282, North-Holland Publishing Co., Amsterdam.

Thoenen, H., Mueller, R. A., and Axelrod, J., 1969, Increased tyrosine hydroxylase activity after drug induced alteration of sympathetic transmission, *Nature (London) 221*:1264–1270.

Thoenen, H., Otten, U., and Oesch, F., 1973, Trans-synaptic regulation of tyrosine hydroxylase, in: *Frontiers in Catecholamine Research* (E. Udin and S. Snyder, eds.), pp. 179–186, Pergamon Press, London.

Thoenen, H., Otten, U., Mueller, R. A., Goodman, R., and Oesch, F., 1975, Lack of correlation between rate of increase in cAMP and subsequent induction of tyrosine hydroxylase in sympathetic ganglia and adrenal medulla, in: *Neuropsychopharmacology*, (J. R. Boissier, H. Hippius, and P. Pichot, eds.), pp. 944–951, Excerpta Medica, Amsterdam.

Uzunov, P., Revuelta, A., and Costa, E., 1975, A role for the endogenous activator of 3',5'-nucleotide phosphodiesterase in rat adrenal medulla, *Mol. Pharmacol. 11*:506–510.

6

The Neurophysiological Effects of Diphenylhydantoin and Their Relationship to Anticonvulsant Activity

G. F. Ayala and D. Johnston

1. Introduction

One of the most recent reviews of selected papers on diphenyl-hydantoin (DPH) lists 1712 references (Dreyfus Medical Foundation, 1975). Yet, most of the papers have as an opening remark: "Although DPH is the most widely used anticonvulsant, its mechanism of action is still unknown."

It is by all means not the purpose of this paper to present a unified interpretation of the different data collected so far on DPH. Despite the large amount of data available, such a task seems premature at this time, because of the large number of different preparations used and because in some cases, when key experiments have been repeated in different laboratories, contradictory results have been obtained. The latter occurrence is quite disturbing, especially when the results have been used for extrapolation to a general mechanism of action of DPH.

Two main theories for the activity of DPH are now dominating the field. Both have as a common denominator a decrease of intracellular sodium, but they differ on the specific mechanisms. One theory postulates that DPH increases the activity of the electrogenic, ATPase-dependent,

G. F. Ayala and D. Johnston • Department of Neurology, University of Minnesota, Minneapolis, Minnesota 55455. Dr. Ayala's current affiliation is Department of Neurology, Baylor College of Medicine, Houston, Texas 77030

Na–K active transport system and thereby facilitates the movement of sodium against its electrochemical gradient. The other theory proposes a decrease of the inward sodium flux during the action potential. We will discuss in detail the supporting evidence for each theory in the specific subsections of this chapter. We will also discuss other known effects of DPH on different aspects of membrane and synaptic physiology, and attempt to indicate which ones are consistent with the anticonvulsant and antiarrhythmic properties of the drug. As with most investigations into the mode of action of pharmacologically active substances, a multiplicity of effects are observed. It then becomes necessary to determine which effects are primary or causative with respect to the clinical activity of the drug. Moreover, few but very stimulating data have been reported recently, such as the interference with divalent cation movement across the membrane, which may hold the key for a unified theory of the mechanism of action of DPH. It is becoming apparent, in fact, that the divalent cations may play an important role for several of the membrane and synaptic activities ascribed to DPH.

2.   Active Transport and Electrolyte Balance

2.1.   Biochemical Studies

There is a considerable amount of data concerning the effect of DPH on the active transport of Na^+ and K^+ and on the maintanence of electrolyte balance in excitable tissues. Much of these data, however, are contradictory, and the issue is far from resolved, even after two decades of investigation.

The first report that DPH may stimulate the active extrusion of Na^+ came from the work of Woodbury (1955). He found that the intracellular concentration of Na^+ was decreased in rat brain following the administration of DPH. Since then, a variety of experimental models have been proposed to support or disprove this theory of pump activation. On a biochemical basis, there is much contradictory evidence.

Festoff and Appel (1968) and Escueta and Appel (1971), using synaptosome preparations, showed an increased activity of Na–K–ATPase and an increase in K^+ transport with DPH, but only when the Na/K ratio was abnormally high (30–50:1). They found no effect or a decrease with lower and near-normal ratios of Na/K. These data are extremely interesting, because they suggest an activity of DPH only under abnormal conditions. It is doubtful, however, whether these high Na/K ratios exist *in vivo*.

Escueta *et al.* (1974) found that DPH stimulated potassium uptake in synaptic terminals from epileptogenic freeze lesions and attributed this to two possible mechanisms: an increase in Na–K active transport and an increase in a second K^+-uptake process that is ouabain-insensitive. These data confirmed earlier results of Fertziger *et al.* (1971), who also found an increase in K^+ uptake with DPH using lobster axons, but found no change in K^+ efflux, indicating that DPH stimulates active K^+ influx. More recently, Deupree (1976) presented evidence that DPH does not effect adenosine triphosphates from the brain, even at high Na/K ratios.

Rawson and Pincus (1968) and Pincus and Giarman (1967) found that DPH had no effect, or decreased, the Na–K–ATPase activity in microsomal fractions of rat and guinea pig brain in low to normal ratios of Na^+ to K^+. In other work, Pincus and Rawson (1969) and Pincus *et al.* (1970) also found a decrease in intracellular Na^+ with DPH in lobster nerve, but tentatively concluded that this may be due to a decrease in the passive influx of Na^+ into the neuron. One can imagine how this action of DPH could limit seizure activity, provided the Na^+ equilibrium potential is unaltered and that less sodium enters the cell during excitation. Indeed, Pincus (1972) presented further data on lobster nerves to substantiate his suggestion that DPH has no effect on the Na–K pump, but decreases "downhill" sodium movement. Hasbani *et al.* (1974), also in lobster nerves, found that DPH reduced calcium uptake in stimulated and nonstimulated nerves, with the most dramatic effect observed following stimulation. These and other data concerning the possible interaction between calcium and DPH are discussed more fully in Section 3.1.2.

Experiments using barnacle muscle fibers (Bittar *et al.*, 1973) and frog skeletal muscle fibers (O'Donnell *et al.*, 1975) also failed to show any increase in Na–K active transport. Bittar *et al.* (1973) concluded that DPH inhibits the Na^+ pump, but were unclear as to the significance of their findings in terms of its anticonvulsant and antiarrhythmic properties. O'Donnell *et al.* (1975) found no effect of DPH on active Na^+ or K^+ transport, but did observe a decrease in passive K^+-exchange mechanisms. This latter datum became most significant when they found that DPH reduced the susceptibility to depolarization of fibers bathed in a high-K^+ medium.

2.2. Ouabain Antagonism

There is also a wealth of data that indicates that in several preparations, such as skeletal and cardiac muscles and synaptosomal preparations, DPH interferes with the activity of ouabain. Some authors (Watson and Woodbury, 1973) have interpreted the preventive effect of DPH, on both the arrhythmic and the electrolyte changes of cardiac muscle produced by ouabain, as an indicator of an action of DPH on the active transport of electrolytes across the cell membranes. Baskin *et al.* (1973), however, suggest that the effect of DPH is related to the ability to block ouabain-binding by the cardiac fiber. Other reports (Godfraind *et al.*, 1971), although confirming that DPH reduced the ionic changes induced by oua-bain, indicate that ouabain-binding is not modified by DPH and that the drug acts by stimulating sodium efflux that is not related to a Na–K–ATPase transport system. Moreover, Gibson and Harris (1969) and Spain and Chidsey (1971) showed that DPH is ineffective in reversing the inhibi-tion of ouabain on the cardiac transporting enzyme Na–K–ATPase.

2.3. Frog Skin Preparation

The isolated frog skin also has been used by several groups of investi-gators as a possible model to test, with a less biochemical approach, the hypothesis that DPH alters Na–K active transport. Carroll and Pratley (1970) found that when DPH was applied to the external surface of the skin, the short-circuit current (SCC), which is a measure of active transport in frog skin, was increased. When DPH was applied to the internal surface of the skin, however, the SCC was decreased. Moreover, these results were obtained in zero calcium Ringer. In contrast, Riddle *et al.* (1975) found that DPH increased the SCC, but only with the presence of calcium in the frog Ringer solution. de Sousa and Grosso (1973) and Watson and Woodbury (1972) found a similar increase in the SCC. Although these results tend to substantiate some of the data obtained by more biochemical means, it must be noted, as suggested by Watson and Woodbury (1972), that the frog skin is a rather complex tissue and may not be a suitable model for studying the action of DPH on active transport. Since the frog skin consists of several layers of epithelium, it is difficult to interpret transport data across this tissue in terms of a single neuronal membrane.

2.4. Neurophysiological Studies

There is obviously much conflicting data concerning a mechanism of action of DPH on active transport. Some of this conflict may be attributed to different techniques and different preparations employed for the various studies. What has been singularly unsuccessful, however, is any conclusive demonstration, using electrophysiological techniques, of a DPH stimula-tion of active transport in a normally functioning neuron *in vivo* or *in vitro* (Pincus *et al.*, 1970; Pincus, 1972; Den Hertog, 1972; Ayala *et al.*, 1977*a*). Den Hertog (1972) studied the electrogenic component of the Na$^+$ pump in the rabbit vagus nerve by stimulating, electrically and with a high-K$^+$ medium, posttetanic hyperpolarization (PTH). Both acute and chronic administration of DPH had no effect on the PTH or on the PTH stimulated with high K$^+$. Since the amplitude of the PTH reflects the activity of the electrogenic sodium pump in this preparation, he concluded that DPH does not affect the Na$^+$ pump in the vagus nerve.

In our laboratory, we have studied, using standard electro-physiological techniques, the effects of DPH on the crayfish stretch receptor neuron (SRN) and on certain cells in the abdominal ganglion of *Aplysia* (Ayala *et al.*, 1977*a*). In the crayfish, our efforts were directed toward PTH, which has been shown to be produced by the activation of an electrogenic sodium pump (Nakajima and Takahashi, 1966). PTH was stimulated either with action potentials activated antidromically or by intracellularly applied depolarizing currents, or with the intracellular injection of Na⁺ ions. In all cases, DPH reduced the amplitude of PTH (see Fig. 1). DPH also decreased membrane resistance, but this could not account for the large drop in PTH.

Because of the data of Festoff and Appel (1968) and others who showed that the DPH stimulation of active transport occurred only in conditions of high Na/K ratios, experiments were performed in which the external concentration of K^+ was increased. Even with external K^+ increased 2.5 times above normal, DPH still reduced PTH (Fig. 2). We never observed an increase in PTH and hence an increase in electrogenic Na–K pumping. Lux (1974) measured the increase in extracellular K^+ concentration in mammalian cortex following seizure activity, and did not measure a change greater than 3 times above normal. One would have to conclude, therefore, that if a higher concentration of external K^+ was necessary in our experiments for DPH to stimulate active transport, these conditions would be unphysiological even in epileptic cortex.

An electrogenic sodium pump contributes as much as 50% to the resting membrane potential (RMP) of the giant neuron (R2) in *Aplysia*

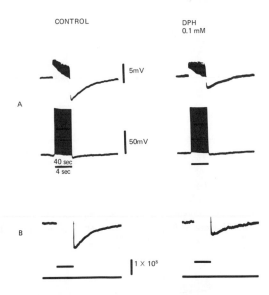

Fig. 1. Effect of 0.1 nM DPH on posttetanic hyperpolarization in the crayfish stretch receptor. In A, the upper and lower traces are different amplifications of the same train of action potentials. In B, only the higher amplification is shown. A train of antidromic action potentials at a rate of 40/sec, with a duration of 4 sec, was elicited in A. In B, the action potentials were obtained by a train of short outward transmembrane currents at the same frequency as A. In all cases, the presence of DPH decreased the amplitude of posttetanic hyperpolarization.

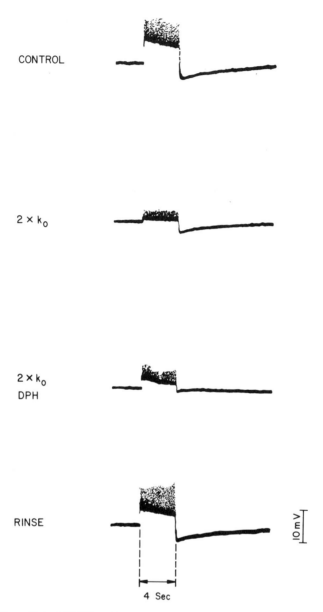

Fig. 2. Effect of 0.1 mM DPH on the membrane resistance and posttetanic hyerpolarization during perfusion with crayfish saline with twice the normal concentration of potassium. The high-potassium solution produced a depolarization of approximately 10 mV. The introduction of DPH decreased the membrane resistance, as well as almost blocking the PTH, which was still present in the saline with $2 \times K_o^+$.

(Carpenter and Alving, 1968). The RMP of this cell is therefore exquisitely sensitive to changes in temperature (2 mV/°C, Carpenter and Alvin, 1968) and to any agents that affect active transport. One would expect that if DPH enhanced active transport mechanisms, it would be easily detectable in these cells. We did these experiments, but were unable to note any significant change in the RMP with DPH.

Other data from our laboratory indicate that DPH does not interfere with the inhibiting effect of ouabain on the electrogenic and electroneutral pump in the crayfish SRN. We have used the same experimental design as outlined above to study PTH. Ouabain abolishes PTH, in agreement with its well-known effect on active transport. DPH fails to reverse or arrest the effect of ouabain on PTH, even when DPH is introduced in the solution before ouabain has completely abolished PTH (Fig. 3). Moreover, DPH does not arrest or reverse the slow depolarization of the neuronal membrane that occurs when the neuron is exposed to ouabain. Both these data

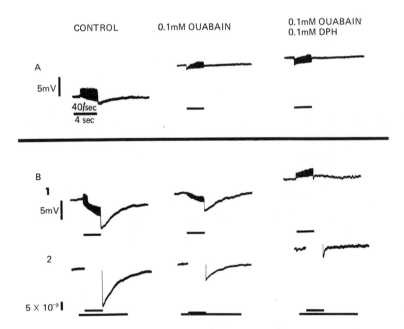

Fig. 3.   Effect of 0.1 mM DPH on the PTH in the SRN pretreated with ouabain (two different experiments). (A) The train of antidromic action potentials was followed by the hyperpolarization, which was abolished by ouabain. DPH failed to reinstate the hyperpolarization. RMP at control − 70 mV. (B) Trains of antidromic action potentials (1) and action potentials triggered by pulses of outward transmembrane current (2). DPH was added to the ouabain solution before the complete disappearance of the PTH. Again, DPH failed to reverse or arrest the effect of ouabain.

indicate that at least in this preparation, DPH does not interfere with the activity of ouabain on the active transport system. These findings are also consistent with the data reported above, i.e., that DPH decreased PTH.

Other evidence indicates, however, that DPH antagonizes the effects of ouabain on certain properties of the neuronal membrane, other than active transport. DPH reverses the increase of input resistance and the "excitability" of the neuron (as tested with pulses of outward transmembrane current) induced by exposure to ouabain. This antagonism of the effects of ouabain is therefore distinct from the activity on active transport.

3. Neurophysiological Studies

3.1. Invertebrate Preparation

3.1.1. Membrane Properties

It is well established that DPH decreases spontaneous firing that occurs in neuronal preparations exposed to low-calcium or high-potassim solutions. However, no changes of RMP have been reported in several neuronal or muscular preparations when exposed to DPH. This observation is quite interesting because in several of the preparations studied, a large part of the RMP is generated by an electrogenic pump. Moreover, no changes of membrane resistance have been reported for skeletal muscles. In our experiments, using both the crayfish stretch receptor and different neurons of the abdominal and buccal ganglion of the *Aplysia,* we have measured a considerable decrease in membrane resistance. Despite the large drop in resistance, however, we have measured very modest or no changes in the RMP. The changes in RMP, if present, were of variable polarity, but never more than a few millivolts. It was our conclusion that the increase in membrane conductance must be primarily for ions with an equilibrium potential close to that of the RMP, i.e., K^+ or Cl^-. We were able to rule out, in most cases, a selective increase of permeability for chloride, because the RMP of the SRN during exposure to DPH was not the same as the equilibrium potential of inhibitory postsynaptic potential (IPSP), which is known, in this preparation, to be chloride-dependent. Very likely all three ions—sodium, potassium, and chloride—are involved, especially in those cases in which a small depolarization occured (Ayala *et al.,* 1977*a*).

The decrease in input resistance produces a dramatic change in the "excitability" of the membrane when tested with pulses of outward current. A pulse of equal amount of current triggers less action potentials during DPH perfusion than in control conditions. Moreover, we have confirmed that DPH blocks spontaneous firing when it occurs in high K_0^+ or during perfusion with ouabain. In this condition, DPH decreases the membrane resistance as observed with normal saline, and does not repolarize the RMP. The latter result is in contrast with the results reported by Su and Feldman (1973) in skeletal muscle membrane. They observed a repolarization of muscle fibers exposed to low K_0^+ when the animal was injected with DPH. The decrease of membrane resistance (and cable properties) may play a very important role because of the resultant decrease in the probability of firing the neuron.

3.1.2. Action Potential

The effect of DPH on the action potential mechanism has received various reports in the literature. Korey (1951) found that DPH had no effect on the normal electrical charateristics of squid axon. However, DPH was found to be extremely effective in reducing the hyperexcitability resulting from a low calcium–magnesium seawater. He also found that DPH rapidly entered the axon. Lipicky *et al.* (1972), using voltage-clamped squid axons, found that DPH reduced the sodium conductance during the action potential, but had little effect on potassium conductance or on the time constant of $_gNa^+$. In contrast, Carnay and Grundfest (1974) found no change in spike amplitude in muscle fibers bathed in DPH. Pincus *et al.* (1970) and Pincus (1972) found a decrease in sodium influx in stimulated lobster nerves with DPH, but Hasbani *et al.* (1974) interpreted this decrease as being secondary to a decrease in calcium uptake.

From experiments in our laboratory (Ayala *et al.*, 1977a), we have found the effect of DPH on the action potential (AP) to be variable, depending on the preparation used for the study. In the crayfish stretch receptor, DPH reduces the overshoot of the AP by an average of 2–3% (Fig. 4a). The negative lobe of the first derivative is also decreased, indicating that the falling phase of the AP is slightly prolonged. In most cells of *Aplysia*, little change in peak amplitude is observed with DPH, although some cells do show a slight decrease in the overshoot. The most prominent effect of DPH on the AP in *Aplysia* neurons, however, is a significant prolongation (Fig. 4b).

Preliminary experiments, in which the ionic currents of the AP were separated and voltage clamping was employed, indicate that DPH is exerting an effect primarily on the potassium conductance mechanisms (Whisler and Johnston, 1975). The AP in *Aplysia* is composed of two inward currents (sodium and calcium) and an outward potassium current. DPH had little effect on the inward sodium or calcium currents during the AP, but

A

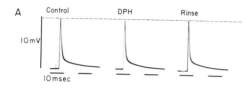

B

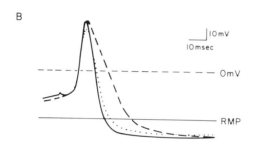

Fig. 4. Changes in shape and amplitude of the APs from the crayfish stretch receptor (A) and from neuron BR$_1$ in the buccal ganglion of *Aplysia* (B). Rinse ($\cdots$), .2mM DPH (---), control (—).

delayed the time to peak of the outward potassium current. Since the inward calcium current was relatively uneffected by DPH, it is doubtful that DPH exerts its effect on the potassium current by limiting calcium influx (Meech and Standen, 1975), but it is possible that DPH could be affecting the internal calcium concentration or the calcium–potassium activation kinetics.

The delay in onset of the potassium conductance may help to explain the almost universal observation that DPH reduces repetitive firing activity. The delay in the potassium conductance results in a prolonged undershoot of the AP and an increased refractory period, which would lead to a decrease in repetitive firing.

3.1.3. Synaptic Transmission

The available data concerning the effects of DPH on synaptic mechanisms are not as inconsistant as in other areas. DPH seems to decrease excitatory postsynaptic potentials (EPSPs) while being quite selective for certain IPSPs. Esplin (1957) found DPH to decrease posttetanic potentiation in the cat spinal cord (see Section 3.2.1 for more complete discussion). Carnay and Grundfest (1974) studied the frog neuromuscular junction and found that DPH, at low concentrations, enhanced the rate of postsynaptic receptor desensitization in low-calcium Ringer and, at higher concentrations, blocked neuromuscular transmission. Pincus and Lee (1973), in keeping with their suggestion that DPH reduces calcium influx, found that with DPH, the stimulus-coupled release of norepinephrine was decreased. Using invertebrate preparations, Barker and Gainer (1973) showed that DPH has a selective action on EPSPs. DPH reduces EPSPs, presumably with a postsynaptic site of action, while exerting no effect on IPSPs. Since the EPSPs in the preparations they studied are Na^+-dependent, and the IPSPs are either Cl^- or K^+-dependent, they concluded that DPH acts selectively on Na^+-dependent synaptic mechanisms without regard to the transmitter involved.

Studies in our laboratory have confirmed some of the results of Barker and Gainer (1973), but we have observed other interesting phenomena that deserve consideration. As shown by Barker and Gainer (1973), DPH decreases Na^+-dependent EPSPs in *Aplysia,* seemingly without regard to transmitter. In *Aplysia,* however, there are many synapses that yield a complex response to stimulation. One such group of synapses is between the interneuron, L_{10}, and the follower cells, L_2–L_6. These cholinergic synapses have a dual response following stimulation of L_{10} (Frazier *et al.,* 1967). With single firings of L_{10}, a simple "short" Cl^--dependent IPSP is elicited. With multiple firings, however, a long K^+-dependent inhibition is obtained that takes many seconds to decay. DPH has little or no effect on the "short" Cl^--dependent IPSP, but does facilitate the long K^+-dependent phase (see Fig. 5). A detailed investigation of this effect has not been completed, but what is immediately obvious is that with DPH, multiple activation of the synapse is not necessary to elicit the long-lasting inhibition. Kehoe (1972) presented data to indicate that there are two separate postsynaptic receptor mechanisms that mediate the short and long responses at this dual synapse. It may be that DPH is selectively enhancing the sensitivity of these receptors for ACh, although other interpretations are also available.

The IPSP in the crayfish stretch receptor has also been studied in our laboratory with quite interesting results. This IPSP is GABA-mediated and Cl^--dependent (Ozawa and Tsuda, 1973), in contrast to the ACh-mediated IPSPs studied in *Aplysia.* DPH dramatically prolongs the IPSP in the crayfish (see Fig. 6A). Iontophoretic injection of GABA to the neurons produced the same prolonged response when DPH was present, suggesting a postsynaptic site of action for this drug (Fig. 6B). Several experiments were performed to try to elucidate the mechanisms involved in the prolongation of this IPSP (Ayala *et al.,* 1977b). Constant current pulses were applied during the IPSP, and the results indicated that DPH prolongs the postsynaptic conductance change. This is also evident by the semilog plot of the falling phase (Fig. 7A). The data in Figs. 6 and 7 also suggest that

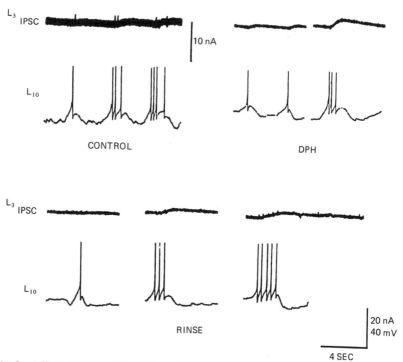

Fig. 5. Effect of DPH on "long" IPSP in *Aplysia*. The follower cell L_3 is voltage-clamped, and the holding potential is near the reversal potential of the short IPSP. It can be seen that multiple firings of the interneuron L_{10} are necessary to elicit the long, potassium-dependent, ACh-mediated IPSP. When Dilantin is added, however, single firings of L_{10} produce a measurable response in L_3. It can also be seen in this figure that the amplitude of the action potential in L_{10} is substantially reduced with Dilantin.

DPH not only prolongs, but also increases, the postsynaptic conductance change. DPH also has a modest effect on the IPSP reversal potential (Fig. 7B), but this change was not always consistent and therefore may not be significant.

    The suggestion made by Pincus and his co-workers that DPH reduces calcium influx to the presynaptic terminal and hence decreases the calcium-activated transmitter release is difficult to reconcile in light of other data. Although DPH reduces EPSPs, the drug is selective for certain inhibitory processes, most notably GABA-mediated IPSPs. Moreover, the effect of DPH seems to be at the postsynaptic membrane and not on the presynaptic release of transmitter. It must be noted, however, that the experiments

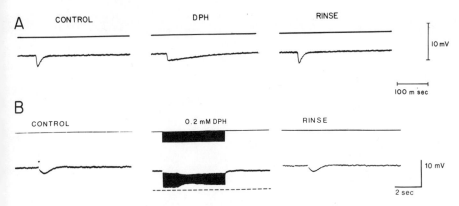

Fig. 6. (A) Effect of 0.1 mM DPH on the IPSP of the crayfish stretch receptor. (B) Effect of DPH on hyperpolarization produced by the iontophoretic application of GABA. A train of brief hyperpolarizing transmembrane currents revealed a continuous changing input conductance at the time of GABA injection. The time course of this change of conductance was much longer than the GABA-induced hyperpolarization as seen in the control.

involved with the iontophoretic injection of transmitter to the postsynaptic neuron (Ayala *et al.*, 1977*b*) do not rule out the possibility that a concomitant change in transmitter release may also be involved. The data with the GABA synapse also suggest that the anticonvulsant properties of DPH could be due to either the prolonged inhibition or the increased synaptic shunting, or both.

3.1.4. Effect of DPH on Bursting Mechanisms

Certain molluscan neurons fire action potentials in rhythmic bursts under normal conditions, the so-called "bursting pacemaker cells" (Frazier *et al.*, 1967). Other neurons, naturally silent, acquire bursting properties when exposed to different convulsant agents (David *et al.*, 1974). The bursting pattern of these neurons consists of alternate periods of membrane-potential depolarization, accompanied by firing of action potentials, which are followed by slow hyperpolarizing waves, the silent period. Essential to the maintenance of this bursting activity is a region of negative slope resistance (NSR) in the current–voltage relationship of these neurons. The NSR represents a region of membrane-voltage instability, and results from a regenerative inward current, probably carried by both sodium and calcium ions (Johnston, 1976), that is responsible for the depolarizing phase of the oscillation. Under voltage-clamp conditions, the NSR can be measured using a series of voltage-step commands from a holding potential near the bottom of the slow oscillation. The hyperpolariz-

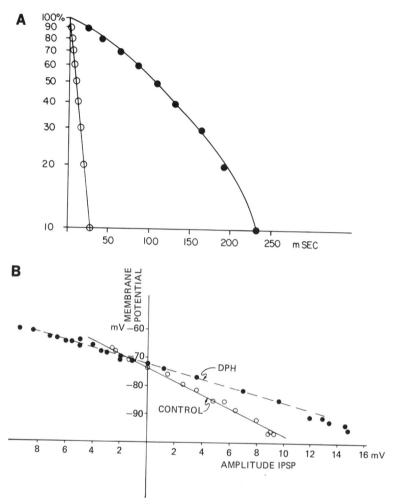

Fig. 7. (A) Semilogarithmic plot of the decay phase of the IPSP. (O) Control; (●) during perfusion with 0.1 mM DPH. The decay is exponential in control condition, but is definitely not exponential with DPH. (B) Amplitude of the IPSP at different levels of membrane potential. Note a very modest change of E_{IPSP} toward a more depolarized level. The slope is decreased during 0.1 mM DPH perfusion, indicating a larger synaptic conductance change.

ing phase is due to a slow increase in potassium conductance that is activated by the influx of calcium during the depolarizing phase (Johnston, 1976).

We have studied in *Aplysia* the effect of DPH on the behavior of spontaneously bursting neurons, and on neurons that were exposed to a convulsant agent.

Two electrodes were inserted into bursting cells L_2–L_6 (Frazier *et al.*, 1967), or into the silent giant cell R2. The cells were routinely voltage-clamped, and the complete current–voltage relationship was obtained before, during, and after administration of DPH. The concentration of DPH ranged from 2×10^{-5} to 2×10^{-4} (5.48–54.8 μg/ml). After about 1–2 hr of DPH perfusion, the characteristic spontaneous bursting activity of these cells was either eliminated or significantly depressed (Figs. 8B and D). No dramatic changes were observed in other electrical properties of the neurons. DPH significantly reduces the NSR (Figs. 8A and C), which is responsible for the reduction in the bursting activity, and also reduces the slow outward potassium current, although to a much lesser extent than the NSR.

Since pentylenetetrazol (PTZ) had been reported to induce bursting activity in normally silent neurons (David *et al.*, 1974) and DPH was found to inhibit this activity, it was of interest to see whether the two drugs might be antagonistic. Figure 9 shows the results of an experiment in which a silent cell R2 was induced to bursting activity with PTZ and then perfused with a combination of PTZ and DPH. The results were quite dramatic. DPH totally suppressed the induced bursting response and the characteristic NSR (Johnston and Ayala, 1975). DPH therefore seems to exert its affect on bursting cells regardless whether it is endogenous to the cell or induced by the convulsant agent PTZ.

The action of DPH in surpressing bursting activity could be interpreted several ways. DPH may be acting by decreasing the sodium influx during the depolarizing phase of the oscillation, or by decreasing the influx of calcium. DPH has been found to have both these effects in various other tissues (Korey, 1951; Lipicky *et al.*, 1972; Hasbani *et al.*, 1974). Unfortunately, no data are presently available to distinguish these two possibilities. The divalent cations, and calcium in particular, have been found to exert a strong regulatory role in bursting pacemaker potentials (Barker and Gainer, 1975; Johnston, 1976).

Sodium conductance seems to be dependent on the external divalent cation concentration, while the movement of calcium regulates the potassium conductance. Whether or not the action on these neurons can be explained on the basis of a primary alteration of the divalent cation control of membrane potential remains to be investigated.

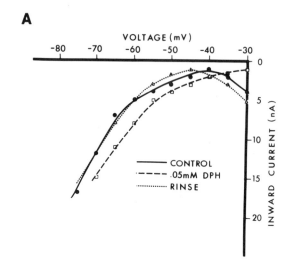

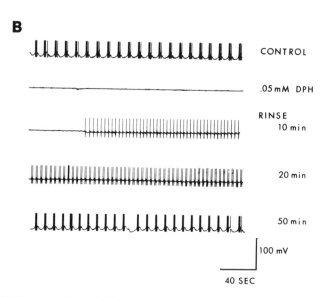

Fig. 8.   (A) Current–voltage (I–V) curves from voltage-clamped bursting cell L_6. Under control conditions, there is a region of negative slope resistance in the I–V curve in the range of the potential oscillation. After 30 min of perfusion with 0.05 mM Dilantin, this NSR has disappeared along with the bursting activity. The region of negative resistance returns with rinse. (B) Effects of Dilantin on bursting pacemaker cell. Cell L_6 is bursting regularly during control. After 30 min of perfusion with 0.05 mM Dilantin, bursting activity has disappeared. The cell slowly returns to control condition after 10, 20, and 50 min of rinse with normal seawater. (The true amplitude of the action potentials cannot be taken from this figure because

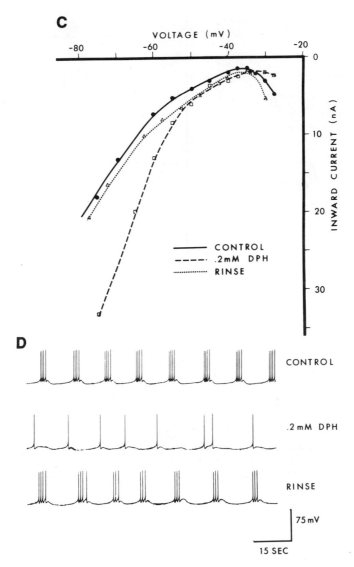

the spikes are being clipped by the pen recorder.) (C) Current–voltage curves from voltage-clamped bursting cell L_6. The bursting decreases but does not fully disappear after more than 60 min of perfusion with 0.2 mM Dilantin. The NRC in the I–V curve decreases but is still present with Dilantin. (D) Dilantin (0.2 mM) is applied to cell L_6 from another ganglion. The bursting pattern is nearly abolished after 60 min of perfusion. The cell, however, is still firing spontaneously but at irregular intervals. Rinsing returns the cell to the control level of activity. Reprinted with permission from Johnston and Ayala (1975) *Science* **189**:1009–1011. Copyright © 1975 by the American Association for the Advancement of Science.

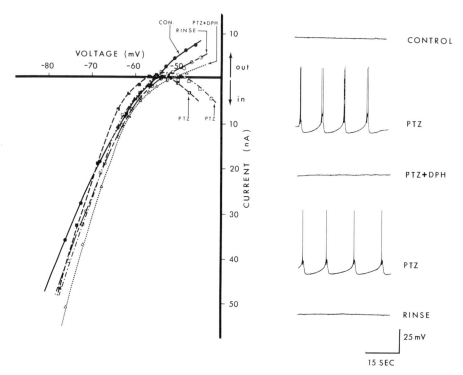

Fig. 9. Antagonism of PTZ and Dilantin. Perfusing the silent giant cell R_2 with 30 mM PTZ produces slow membrane potential oscillations and the characteristic bursting response. Adding 0.1 mM Dilantin to the seawater containing PTZ reverses the action of this convulsant agent, since the bursting activity disappears. Returning to PTZ alone reinstates the bursting, and rinsing with normal seawater returns the cell to its original silent state. Current–voltage curves show a region of negative resistance, which is present during PTZ perfusion but disappears when Dilantin is added. Reprinted with permission from Johnston and Ayala (1975) *Science 189*:1009–1011. Copyright © 1975 by the American Association for the Advancement of Science.

3.2. Mammalian Preparations

3.2.1. Spinal Cord

Experimental studies on the mechanism of action of DPH in mammals have mainly analyzed synaptic transmission in the spinal cord, spontaneous activity of Purkinje cells, inhibitory mechanisms in neocortex, and the behavior of steady potentials and extracellular K.

The most-cited observation is the one of Esplin (1957), who observed the decrease of posttetanic potentiation in the spinal cord. This datum has been further confirmed by several other investigators. The initial interpretation by Esplin was in keeping with the pump theory of Woodbury (1955). DPH enhanced the pump, and "stabilized" the membrane in a less excitable state. Raines and Standaert (1967) further studied this phenomenon, and reported that DPH decreases the hyperpolarization in the dorsal root. Their interpretation was that because the hyperpolarization is due to summation of the positive afterpotentials, which are known to be carried by K^+ currents, DPH should facilitate K^+ outflow during the action potential.

On the other hand, Strittmatter and Somjen (1973) showed in the spinal cord that DPH decreases the steady potential shift that is concomitant with neuronal activity and is now thought to be secondary to the extracellular K^+ accumulation. Heinemann and Lux (1973) showed directly in the neocortex a decrease of K_0^+ accumulation, as well as a more rapid removal of the K_0^+ after injection of DPH. Although both experiments have similar results, Strittmatter and Somjen interpret the data as due to a decreased neuronal activity, while Heinemann and Lux postulate an enhanced pump action for the more rapid removal of K_0^+.

The interpretation of Strittmatter and Somjen is consistent with data concerning the effect of DPH on the AP in *Aplysia* (Whisler and Johnston, 1975) and on repetetive firing of neurons (Ayala *et al.*, 1977a). The data from the former work are also in conflict with the interpretation of Raines and Standaert (1967) on the disappearance of the PTH as recorded from the dorsal root, since they postulate a facilitation of K^+ current.

The problem of the posttetanic potentiation is still open. In some preparations, this phenomenon is sustained by a hyperpolarization of the presynaptic fiber. If this is also the case in the mammalian spinal cord, our data, which show a decrease in PTH during DPH perfusion, can explain the decrease of PTP as reported by Esplin. In other preparations, however, PTP is not related to presynaptic hyperpolarization, but to the accumulation of calcium in the presynaptic terminal, Weinreich (1971). In this case, the data from Pincus (1972) and Lipicky *et al.*, (1972) that DPH decreases the inward Ca^{2+} and Na^+ fluxes may alternatively explain the decrease of PTP.

3.2.2. Cerebellum and Pyramidal Tract Neurons

Other interesting data on the effect of DPH in mammals are those describing the behavior of Purkinje cells. In recent years, the cerebellum has attracted great attention as a possible gaiting mechanism in controlling seizures. The most widely quoted paper is that of Halpern and Julien (1972). They showed in cats that DPH causes a large increase in the rate of firing of the Purkinje cells. This observation fits very well with the gaiting theory. Puro and Woodward (1973), however, using different animals, albino rats, did not observe any change of the rate of spontaneous firing of Purkinje cells after DPH injection, but if the dosage was increased to the point that the animal had signs of drug toxicity, such as cerebellar deficit, the cells stopped firing. A third paper, by Anderson and Raines (1974*a*), shows that at the same dosages as used by Halpern and Julien, there was a change in the rate of neuronal firing, but it was in either direction, without any preferred pattern. However, in those cases in which the rate of firing was increased, it never reached the level reported by Halpern and Julien.

With the available evidence, it seems premature to conclude that DPH increases the Purkinje cell output from the cerebellum, and thus increases any gaiting effect.

Our data from invertebrate preparations that DPH specifically facilitates GABA-mediated inhibition have been confirmed by a study of the recurrent inhibition of the pyramidal tract neurons in the cat. The duration of the recurrent inhibition is prolonged when DPH is injected intravenously (Raabe and Ayala, 1976).

3.2.3. *Receptors*

Another interesting aspect of DPH is the effect on sensory mechanisms, as analyzed by Anderson and Raines in two different preparations: the muscular spindle (Anderson and Raines, 1974*b*) and the cerebellar acoustic evoked response (Anderson and Raines, 1974*a*, 1975). In both cases, they reached the indirect conclusion that DPH alters the ability of the receptor to generate APs. Although our experiments with the crayfish stretch receptor were not specifically designed to investigate the DPH changes on the characteristics of the generator potential, it is reasonable to suspect that the drop of membrane resistance that we have observed would indeed change the amplitude of the generator potential as seen at the trigger zone.

4. *Discussion and Conclusions*

As previously stated, when a chemical agent is studied at the cellular level, a multiplicity of effects are usually uncovered. In the case of DPH, most of the different effects on neuronal activity (from membrane and synaptic properties to more complex behavior of neuronal aggregates) are consistent with the anticonvulsant and antiarrhythmic properties of this drug. In Section 1, we mentioned that several contradictions exist in the literature with regard to some effects of DPH. These contradictions, however, are limited, for the most part, to the problem of accepting from the evidence available the notion that DPH acts to specifically enhance Na–K active transport. We have expressed the opinion that in view of the lack of confirmation of the biochemical data by neurophysiological means, this aspect of DPH activity remains open.

We have reviewed a large body of data concerning the activity of DPH on neuronal systems. One or more of the effects on DPH may indicate in a direct manner the substratum for the clinical manifestation of the drug. These effects are: the selective change in synaptic mechanisms, the decrease in membrane resistance and hence the change in neuronal cable properties, the change in the ionic currents during the action potential, the decrease in repetetive firing, and the suppression of bursting pacemaker activity.

It is intuitive that the effect of DPH on synaptic mechanisms could be of paramount importance in controlling the activity of an epileptic focus. The decrease of the amplitude of the EPSPs and the increase in duration of the IPSPs would compensate the postulated inbalance between excitation and inhibition within the epilepitc focus. The decrease in membrane resistance produced by DPH could also be highly significant for controlling seizure activity. In cortical neurons, excitatory synapses are believed to be located on distal regions of the dendrites, while inhibitory synapses are thought to reside close (both spatially and electrically) to the encoder or trigger zone of the cell. A decreased membrane resistance would decrease the electrotonic length of the dendrites and attenuate synaptic potentials arising from distal regions. This is only a speculative consequence of a decreased membrane resistance, but it could produce a selective decrease in excitation with little or no change in inhibition as seen at the encoder region, without postulating any change in the postsynaptic membrane response. A decrease in repetitive firing would also occur because of a diminished excitatory drive.

The DPH-induced changes in the ionic currents during the AP could be significant from several standpoints. First, a decreased sodium influx would reduce the amplitude of the action potential and thus the amount of Ca^{2+} influx at the presynaptic terminal. One or both of these occurrences might be important for reducing posttetanic potentiation (PTP) at the synapse. The data of Pincus and co-workers showing a direct decrease in Ca^{2+} influx during an AP could also explain the observed decrease in PTP with DPH. Less Ca^{2+} influx might result in less total accumulation of Ca^{2+} and perhaps a decreased PTP. Except for PTP, the bulk of the evidence concerning the effect of DPH on synaptic transmission points to a postsynaptic site of action. If indeed DPH reduces, either directly or indirectly, Ca^{2+} influx to the presynaptic terminal, both excitation and inhibition would presumably be equally affected. This presynaptic action of DPH is probably too small to be observed under normal conditions (i.e., single action potentials), and therefore the postsynaptic action of the drug predominates (decreased excitation and prolonged inhibition). With repetition stimulation like that involved in PTP, however, a decreased Ca^{2+} influx with DPH might play a significant role in reducing PTP.

A second consequence of altered action currents concerns the activity of DPH on potassium efflux. A delayed and prolonged potassium conductance during an action potential would tend to reduce the repetitive firing activity of the neuron. Less activity of the neuron would result in less extracellular accumulation of potassium, less tendency to depolarize, and a further reduction in firing activity. Thus, an alternative explanation for the action of DPH in limiting the spread of a seizure is available.

Finally, the suppression of bursting pacemaker activity by DPH may provide an immediate explanation for the effect of this compound on the ectopic cardiac pacemakers. However, bursting activity may also be significant for epileptogenesis. The idea that neurons within an epileptic focus acquire new qualitative properties has been proposed several times, but no clear demonstration has been presented. There is evidence from invertebrate models that when silent neurons are exposed to convulsant agents and become bursting pacemakers, they acquire a region of unstable membrane potential or negative resistance (David et al., 1974). Spinal motoneurons also seem to acquire a region of unstable membrane potential when exposed to topical penicillin (Kao and Crill, 1972a,b), but no similar phenomenon has been observed in cortical neurons (Ayala et al., 1973). More precisely, these spinal motoneurons do not burst, but exhibit a two-stage equilibrium, one at the normal RMP, the other at a more depolarized level; the "flip-flop phenomenon," in laboratory language, which has some of the properties of bursting, such as a region of negative resistance, without the ability to sustain oscillations. In invertebrate neurons, DPH is specific in suppressing the negative resistance region (and thus bursting activity), regardless whether it is endogenous to the cell or induced by a convulsant agent (Johnston and Ayala, 1975). If DPH is so specific for this kind of behavior, then it is highly suggestive that some of the properties that underlie bursting pacemaker activity may also be involved in epileptogenesis.

The possibility that DPH interferes with the divalent cation control of membrane potential and synaptic transmission is extremely interesting. Divalent cations, and calcium in particular, are intimately involved in every neuronal activity that is affected by DPH. During the AP, Ca^{2+} regulates sodium activation and inactivation, in some neurons carries a substantial portion of the inward current both in the soma and at the presynaptic terminal, and regulates increases in potassium conductance. The amount of transmitter released at the synapse is dependent on the internal calcium concentration, and the postsynaptic response to the mediator may be dependent (although not entirely resolved) on external Ca^{2+}. Internal calcium can regulate the RMP by altering potassium conductance, and many reports are available linking Ca^{2+} with active transport of Na^+ and K^+. Bursting pacemaker activity is also highly dependent on divalent cations, for both the depolarizing and the hyperpolarizing phases of the oscillations.

It may be found that all the effects observed with DPH may be linked to a primary action on the divalent cation control of neuronal activity. This is an exciting area for future research, not only for a better definition of the mechanism of action of DPH, but also for the general problem of epileptogenesis.

5. References

Anderson, R. J., and Raines, A., 1974*a*, Selective diphenylhydantoin suppression of auditory evoked potentials in the cat cerebellar cortex, *Neuropharmacology 13*:749–754.

Anderson, R. J., and Raines, A., 1974*b*, Suppression by diphenylhydantoin of afferent discharges arising in muscle spindles of the triceps surae of the cat, *J. Pharmacol. Exp. Ther. 191*:290–299.

Anderson, R. J., and Raines, A., 1975, Suppression of cerebellar evoked potentials by peripheral action of diphenylhydantoin, *Arch. Int. Pharmacodyn. Ther. 68*:549–554.

Ayala, G. F., Dichter, H., Gumnit, R. J., Matsumoto, H., and Spencer, W. A., 1973, Genesis of epileptic interictal spikes. New knowledge of cortical feedback systems suggests a neurophysiological explanation of brief paroxysms, *Brain Res. 52*:1–18.

Ayala, G. F., Lin, S., and Johnston, D., 1977*a*, The mechanism of action of diphenylhydantoin on invertebrate neurons. I. Effects on basic membrane properties, *Brain Res. 121*:245–258.

Ayala, G. F., Johnston, D., Lin, S., and Dichter, H. N., 1977*b*, The mechanism of action of diphenylhydantoin on invertebrate neurons. II. Effects on synaptic mechanisms, *Brain Res. 121*:259–270.

Barker, J. L., and Gainer, H., 1973, Pentobarbital: Selective depression of excitatory synaptic potentials, *Science 182*: 720–722.

Barker, J. L., and Gainer, H., 1975, Studies on bursting pacemaker potential activity in molluscan neurons. II. Regulation by divalent cations, *Brain Res. 84*:479–500.

Baskin, S. I., Dutta, S., and Marks, B. H., 1973, The effects of diphenylhydantoin and potassium on the biological activity of ouabain in the guinea-pig heart, *Br. J. Pharmacol. 47*:85–96.

Bittar, E. E., Chen, S. S., Danielson, B. A., and Tong, E. Y., 1973, An investigation of the action of diphenylhydantoin on sodium efflux in barnacle muscle fibres, *Acta Physiol. Scand. 89*:30–38.

Carnay, L., and Grundfest, S., 1974, Excitable membrane stabilization by diphenylhydantoin and calcium, *Neuropharmacology 13*:1097–1108.

Carpenter, D. O., and Alvin, B. O., 1968, A contribution of an electrogenic Na^+ pump to membrane potential in *Aplysia* neurons, *J. Gen. Physiol. 52*:1–21.

Carroll, P. T., and Pratley, J. N., 1970, The effects of diphenylhydantoin on sodium transport in frog skin, *Com. Gen. Pharmacol. 1*:365.

David, R. J., Wilson, W. A., and Escueta, A. V., 1974, Voltage clamp analysis of pentylenetetrazol effects on *Aplysia* neurons, *Brain Res. 67*:549–554.

Den Hertog, A., 1972, The effect of diphenylhydantoin on the electrogenic component of the sodium pump in mammalian nonmyelinated nerve fibres, *Eur. J. Pharmacol. 19*:94–97.

de Sousa, R. C., and Grosso, A., 1973, Interaction of diphenylhydantoin with norepinephrine, theophilline and cyclic AMP in frog skin, *Experientia 29*:748–749.

Deupree, J. D., 1976, Evidence that diphenylhydantoin does not affect adenosine triphosphatases from brain, *Neuropharmacology 15*:187–195.

Dreyfus Medical Foundation, 1975, *DPH.*

Escueta, A. V., and Appel, S. H., 1971, Diphenylhydantoin and potassium transport in isolated nerve terminals, *J. Clin. Invest. 150*:9–15.

Escueta, A. V., Davidson, D., Hartwing, G., and Reilly, E., 1974, The freezing lesion. III. The effects of diphenylhydantoin on potassium transport within nerve terminals from the primary foci, *Brain Res. 86*:85–96.

Esplin, D., 1957, Effect of diphenylhydantoin on synaptic transmission in the cat spinal cord and stellate ganglion, *J. Pharmacol. Exp. Ther. 120*:301–323.

Fertziger, A. P., Liuzzi, S. E., and Dunham, P. B., 1971 Diphenylhydantoin (Dilantin): Stimulation of potassium influx in lobster axons, *Brain Res. 33*:592–596.

Festoff, B. W., and Appel, S. H., 1968, Effect of diphenylhydantoin on synaptosome sodium potassium ATPase, *J. Clin. Invest. 47*:2752–2758.

Frazier, W. T., Kandel, E. R., Kupfermann, I., Waziri, R., and Coggeshall, R. E., 1967, Morphological and functional properties of identified neurons in the abdominal ganglion of *Aplysia california, J. Neurophysiol. 30*:1288–1351.

Gibson, K., and Harris, P., 1969, Diphenylhydantoin and human myocardial microsomal (Na^+, K^+)–ATPase, *Biochem. Biophys. Res. Commun. 35*:75–78.

Godfraind, T., Lesne, M., and Pousti, A., 1971, The action of diphenylhydantoin upon drug binding ionic effects and inotropic action of ouabain, *Arch. Int. Pharmacodyn. Ther. 191*:66–73.

Halpern, L. M., and Julien, R. M., 1972, Augmentation of cerebellar Purkinje cell discharge rate after diphenylhydantoin, *Epilepsia 13*:377–385.

Hasbani, M., Pincus, J., and Lee, S. H., 1974, Diphenylhydantoin and calcium movement in lobster nerves, *Arch. Neurol. 31*:250–254.

Heinemann, V., and Lux, H. D., 1973, Effects of diphenylhydantoin on extracellular (K^+) in cat cortex, *Electroencephalogr. Clin. Neurophysiol. 34*:735.

Johnston, D., 1976, Voltage clamp reveals basis for calcium regulation of bursting pacemaker cells in *Aplysia, Brain Res. 107*:418–423.

Johnston, D., and Ayala, G. F., 1975, Diphenylhydantoin: The action of a common anticonvulsant on bursting pacemaker cells in *Aplysia, Science 189*:1009–1011.

Kao, L. J., and Crill, W. E., 1972a, Penicillin induced segmental myoclonus. I. Motor responses and intracellular recording from motor neurons, *Arch. Neurol. 26*:150–161.

Kao, L. J., and Crill, W. E., 1972b, Penicillin induced segmental myoclonus. II. Membrane properties of cat spinal motoneurons, *Arch. Neurol. 26*:162–168.

Kehoe, J. A., 1972, Ionic mechanisms of a two component cholinergic inhibition in *Aplysia* neurons, *J. Physiol. 225*:85–114.

Korey, S. R., 1951, Effect of Dilantin and Mesatoin on the giant axon of the squid, *Proc. Soc. Exp. Biol. Med. 79*:297–299.

Lipicky, R. J., Gilbert, D. L., and Stillman, I. M., 1972, Diphenylhydantoin inhibition of sodium conductance in squid giant axon, *Proc. Natl. Acad. Sci. U.S.A. 69*:1758–1760.

Lux, M. D., 1974, The kinetics of extracellular potassium: Relation to epileptogenesis, *Epilepsia 15*:375–394.

Meech, R. W., and Standen, N. B., 1975, Potassium activation in *Helix aspersa* neurones under voltage clamp: A component mediated by calcium influx, *J. Physiol. 249*:211–239.

Nakajima, S., and Takahashi, K., 1966, Post-tetanic hyperpolarization and electrogenic Na pump in stretch receptor neurone of crayfish, *J. Physiol. 187*:105–127.

O'Donnell, J. J., Tikovacs, B., and Szabo, S., 1975, Influence of membrane stabilizer diphenylhydantoin on potassium and sodium movements in skeletal muscle, *Pfluegers Arch. 358*:275–288.

Ozawa, S., and Tsuda, K., 1973, Membrane permeability change during inhibitory transmitter action in crayfish stretch receptor cell, *J. Neurophysiol. 36*:805–816.

Pincus, J. H., 1972, Diphenylhydantoin and ion flux in lobster nerves, *Arch. Neurol. 26*:4–10.

Pincus, J. H., and Giarman, N. H., 1967, The effect of diphenylhydantoin on sodium, potassium, and magnesium stimulated adenosine triphosphatase activity of rat brain, *Biochem. Pharmacol. 16*:600–603.

Pincus, J. H., and Lee, S. H., 1973, Diphenylhydantoin and calcium, *Arch. Neurol. 29*:239–244.

Pincus, J. H., and Rawson, M. D., 1969, Diphenylhydantoin and intracellular sodium concentration, *Neurology 19*:419–422.

Pincus, J. H., Grove, I., Marino, B. B., and Glasser, G. E., 1970, Studies on the mechanism of action of diphenylhydantoin, *Arch. Neurol. 22*:566–571.

Puro, D. G., and Woodward, D. J., 1973, Effects of diphenylhydantoin on activity of rat cerebellar Purkinje cells, *Neuropharmacology 12*:433–440.

Raabe, W., and Ayala, G. F., 1976, Diphenylhydantoin increases cortical postsynaptic inhibition, *Brain Res. 105*:597–601.

Raines, A., and Standaert F. G., 1967, An effect of diphenylhydantoin on post-tetanic hyperpolarization of intramedullary nerve terminals, *J. Pharmacol. Exp. Ther. 156*:591–597.

Rawson, M. D., and Pincus, J. H., 1968, The effect of diphenylhydantoin on sodium, potassium, magnesium-activated adenosine triphosphate in microsomal fractions of rat and guinea-pig brain and on whole homogenates of human brain, *Biochem. Pharmacol. 17*:573–579.

Riddle, T. R., Mandel, L. J., and Goldner, M. M., 1975, Dilantin–calcium interaction and active Na transport in frog skin, *Eur. J. Pharmacol. 33*:49–192.

Spain, R., and Chidsey, B. A., 1971, Myocardial Na/K adenosine triphosphatase activity during reversal of ouabain toxicity with diphenylhydantoin, *J. Pharmacol. Exp. Ther. 179*:594–598.

Strittmatter, W. J., and Somjen, G. G., 1973, Depression of sustained evoked potential and glial depolarization in spinal cord by barbiturates and by diphenylhydantoin, *Brain Res. 55*:333–342.

Su, P. C., and Feldman, D. S., 1973, Motor nerve terminal and muscle membrane stabilization by diphenylhydantoin administration, *Arch. Neurol. 28*:376–779.

Watson, E. L., and Woodbury, D. M., 1972, Effects of diphenylhydantoin on active sodium transport in frog skin, *J. Pharmacol. Exp. Ther. 180*:767–782.

Watson, E. L., and Woodbury, D. M., 1973, The effect of diphenylhydantoin and ouabain, alone and in combination, in the electrocardiogram and on cellular electrolytes of guinea-pig heart and skeletal muscle, *Arch. Int. Pharmacodyn. Ther. 201*:389–399.

Weinreich, D., 1971, Ionic mechanism of post-tetanic potentiation at the neuromuscular junction of the frog, *J. Physiol. 212*:431–446.

Whisler, J. W., and Johnston, D., 1975, Diphenylhydantoin and calcium on *Aplysia* neurons, 5th Annual Meeting of the Society of Neuroscience, Toronto, abstract 1106.

Woodbury, D. M. 1955, Effect of diphenylhydantoin on electrolytes and radiosodium turnover in brain and other tissues of normal, hyponatremic and postictal rats, *J. Pharmacol. Exp. Ther. 115*:74–95.

7

Some Molecular Aspects of Neural Mechanisms

J. R. Smythies

1. Introduction

This contribution to the volume of scientific papers in memory of my old teacher Harold Himwich will review seven years' work in a field that might variously be regarded as structural molecular biology or else as neuroanatomy at the molecular level. The strategy that I have used to guide my approach to these problems has been based on my training as a neuroanatomist. The majority of workers currently in molecular neurobiology have reached it via biochemistry or biophysics, and hence functional relationships have been to the fore in their work, whereas structural aspects of molecular neural mechanisms, as the ultimate basis of all behavior, are equally important.

The work to be described is based on the following strategies:

(1) *The search for complementarity.* Biological molecules, in general, interact by virtue of their mutual complementarity. For example, when a small molecule such as a transmitter or a hormone binds to a specific receptor site on a macromolecule, it does so because it fits into a cavity specifically adapted for it. That is, the three-dimensional shape of the ligand together with the distribution in three-dimensional space of charged groups, lipophilic areas, and hydrogen-bonding moieties will bear a "key–lock"

J. R. Smythies • Department of Psychiatry and the Neurosciences Program, University of Alabama in Birmingham, Birmingham, Alabama 35294

relationship to the three-dimensional complementary cavity with its array in three-dimensional space of complementary charged groups, lipophilic areas, and hydrogen-bonding moieties. The same will be true when two macromolecules interact (e.g., histone and DNA in chromatin), except that the key–lock simile should be replaced by another, e.g., scaffolding and building. The most famous discovery of such complementarity in nature was of course the relationship of guanine to cytosine and of adenine to thymine that gave the clue to the structure of DNA. Thus, if we study the molecular structure of a number of different chemical agents that act either as agonists or antagonists at one common receptor, it may be possible to envisage the shadowy outlines of a unique complementary protein struc-ture, and, by the use of Corey–Pauling–Kaltun (CPK) molecular models, to build these in the form of tentative hypothetical structures.

(2) *The use of speculative hypotheses.* The comparative neglect in recent times in neurobiology of the powerful scientific tool of the specula-tive hypothesis was recently discussed by Eccles (1970). An essential ingredient in a developed science is a hypothesis that does not merely codify the data, but that goes *beyond* the data. It says: "Let us imagine that X is the case—if so, what follows from it? What predictions does it lead to that can be tested by experiment?" Or, alternatively, if the problem is the molecular structure of, for example, the sodium channel, we can ask: "What *possible* ways are there of constructing a tube through a membrane that could conduct ions? In such tubes, how could we construct gates to turn the ion flow on and off?" A hypothesis should be evaluated, not on the basis of its degree of speculation ("too speculative") but on the basis of (a) whether it "explains the data" and (b) whether it can be rigorously tested by experiment, i.e., subjected to a crucial experiment or series of experiments.

2. Molecular Structure of Receptors for Transmitters

Our work in this area has been based on the ideas of three previous workers:

(1) In 1962, two Russian pharmacologists, Kusnetsov and Ghokov (1962) suggested, on the basis of structure–activity relationship studies on neuromuscular blockers, that the molecular basis of receptors might be two parallel β-pleated protein chains linked by their complementary opposed amino acids (Fig. 1). We have called this structure a "Kusnetsov–Ghokov grid." There is a whole family of possible grids, depending on the amino acids involved, but the ones we will be concerned with here are those based

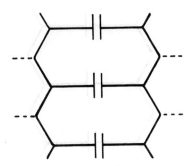

Fig. 1. A Kusnetsov–Ghokov grid.

mainly on the double resonating ionic bonds between Arg and Glu and on hydrogen bonds between Gln and Gln. The stereochemical relationship of these two links is shown in Fig. 2. Note the directional feature of the former bond, unlike an ordinary ionic bond, which has no directional properties. Note also the capacity for additional hydrogen bonding provided by the unused protons and spare electron pairs shown in the figure.

(2) The second hypothesis was formulated by Gill (1965): that the most likely conformational change in the receptor protein engineered by highly charged transmitters such as ACh, GABA, glutamate, glycine, and others interacting with their specific receptors would depend on the disruption of an ionic bond, i.e., between a basic amino acid (Lys, Arg) and an acidic one (Glu, Asp, phosphoser).

(3) Barlow (1964) suggested that the ACh receptor at the neuromuscular junction contains an anionic grid with negatively charged groups some 14 Å apart—to explain the neuromuscular blocking action of polydecamethioniums (where $n \approx 37$). A β-pleated chain of protein in which every other amino acid is Glu, Asp, or phosphoser will generate such a grid.

A Kusnetsov–Ghokov grid by itself, however, is not enough. No particular complementarity can be demonstrated between such grids and transmitters, their agonists and antagonists. What is needed is not a receptor grid, but a receptor cup. How, then, to construct such a cup on the basis

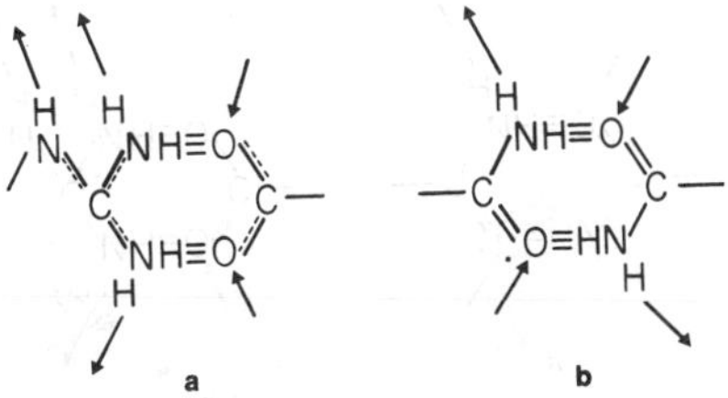

Fig. 2. Stereochemical features of Arg-Glu ionically bonded (a) and Gln–Gln hydrogen-bonded (b). The arrows mark spare protons and spare electron pairs and bond angles.

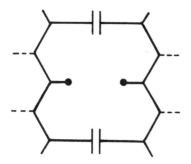

Fig. 3. A Kusnetsov–Ghokov grid based on Gln-Gln cross-links to form the basis of a receptor cup.

of the grid? The simplest answer is to turn each β-pleated chain into a β-pleated sheet by adding two more peptide chains (secondary chains, one to each side). Take, for example, a grid in which the primary chains are cross-linked by three Gln–Gln bonds. In this case, a cup can be generated if amino acids Nos. 1 and 5 of each secondary chain are Gln and the middle opposed amino acid (i.e., No. 3) is small (Fig. 3). The molecular models indicate that if we have a Gln–Gln double hydrogen bond between two primary chains, and if we superimpose a second Gln–Gln link between the two secondary chains, then we can obtain two more hydrogen bonds between the Gln's of each chain, as illustrated in Fig. 4. If the cross-linked amino acids on the primary chains are lipophilic (e.g., Met–Met), then two lipophilic amino acids of the same length at the overlying loci will form one wall of the cup. If the primary link is between Arg and Glu, then there is no pair of amino acids with the necessary complementarity to form the super-imposed secondary link. We can run the secondary peptide chain itself across, however, if we put a right-angled bend (?Pro) at locus 1. The peptide chain itself, through its CO and NH groups, has the requisite complementarity to the spare proton and spare electron pair of an Arg–Glu ionic bond (Smythies, 1975a). Clearly, there are a large number of possible receptor cups of this kind based on Kusnetsov–Ghokov grids, depending on the particular amino acid sequences involved and the number of rungs on the grid.

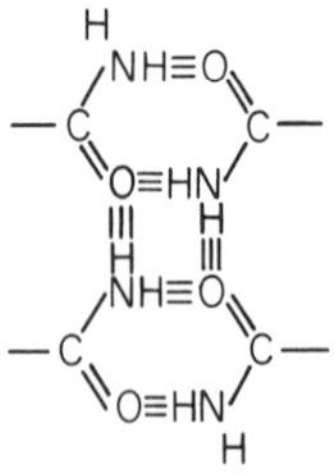

Fig. 4. Further development of a receptor cup based on a Kusnetsov–Ghokov grid (see the text).

There are two possible actions of a transmitter or a hormone acting at such a site. The inactivated state of the receptor grid (R) may be with the complementary amino acids bound to each other, and the action of the transmitter may be to disrupt one or more links, leading to disruption of the grid (R_1). Alternatively, the inactivated state of the receptor may be with these cross-links unmade (R_1), and the action of the transmitter may be to promote the formation of the grid (R). In each case, this primary conformational change may trigger others in the receptor protein in such a way that as that adjacent ionic channel is opened, an enzymatic site is activated, bound calcium is released, or some other phenomenon occurs.

On this basis, we have constructed hypotheses concerning the possible molecular structure of receptor sites for a number of transmitters: ACh and catecholamines (Smythies, 1975*a*), GABA and glycine (Smythies, 1974), prostaglandins (Smythies *et al.*, 1975*a*), and enkephaline (the "opiate" receptor) (Smythies, 1975*b*, 1977). These hypotheses "explain the data," and have led to a number of predictions, some of which are currently being tested by experiment (Collins *et al.*, 1975; Dray, 1975; Curtis and Johnston, 1974). In the case of the nicotinic ACh receptor in the neuromuscular junction, we have further been able to suggest how the mechanism linking activation of the receptor to opening of an adjacent ion-conducting channel may operate (Smythies *et al.*, 1975*b*). This hypothesis specifies a particular conformation for the snake neurotoxins (such as cobrotoxin and α-bungarotoxin) that act at this site. The hypothesis can therefore be tested by determining the X-ray structure of these toxins. In the case of the glycine receptor, the specification that we have made is actually for the "strychnine receptor," since the model receptor was constructed from a consideration of the molecular structure of known glycine antagonists such as strychnine, thebaine, lordanosine, and others. The glycine receptor may be a part of the larger strychnine receptor, in whole or in part, or the relationship between the two may be allosteric. The same considerations may apply to other receptors, e.g., the GABA receptor, on the basis of these structural relationships. A prediction that tetramethylenedisulfotetramine (TETS) and cunaniol (as well as the related molecule of cicutoxin) are GABA antagonists has been tested. Cunaniol has been found to be a GABA antagonist with no action at glycine receptors, and TETS has been found to antagonize both GABA and glycine. It is of course easier to predict that a molecule is too large to fit a certain receptor (as in the case of cicutoxin and the "glycine" receptor) than to predict whether a small glycine receptor occupant may not also find a way of filling a part of the larger GABA receptor.

This analysis depends on the widely held hypothesis that receptors are made largely if not entirely of protein. Protein is found mainly in three conformations: α-helix, β-sheet, and random coil. We have investigated how receptor "cups" could be constructed on the basis of the α-helix, but the stereochemistry comes out all wrong. In the case of a random coil conformation, we cannot, of course, exclude the possibility that some receptors may be based on this conformation that approaches a β-sheet conformation in its molecular structure. In other words, our β-sheet hypothesis may be in part an oversimplification. The value of a hypothesis is, however, in its usefulness more than in its absolute "truth." The various hypotheses that we have constructed have led to a number of specific predictions that may be rigorously tested by experiment. A previous hypothesis concerning the molecular structure of the opiate receptor (Smythies *et al.*, 1971) was refuted by experiment (Smythies, 1975*b*), and so an entirely new hypothesis was constructed that again leads to a new set of predictions that are in turn testable by experiment (Smythies, 1977).

3. Molecular Structure of the Sodium Channel

The sodium channel in the excitable membrane of nerve and muscle is activated by a change in the potential difference across the membrane, rather than by a chemical transmitter. It contains an external recognition site for the hydrated sodium ion and an internal gate or gates that control the flow of sodium ions through the channel. Fortunately, there are two sets of toxins of complex molecular structure that act on elements of this system. Tetrodotoxin (TTX) and saxitoxin (STX) block the external orifice of the channel, probably by interacting with the ion-recognition mechanism. The "h" gate, which cuts off the ion flow, is prevented from closing by the action of batrachotoxin (BTX), aconitine, and veratridine, which all act on one site, and by scorpion neurotoxins, which act at a second site (Catterall, 1975). A study of all the possible ways of forming a tube or channel across a membrane out of a protein molecule(s) equipped with an electrogenic gate controlling the ion flow, together with an examination of the molecular structures of BTX, aconitine, and veratridine, suggested a simple protein structure capable of acting as the required mechanism. A protein molecule, or molecules, could form a tube across a membrane on the basis of α-helices, β-sheets, random coils, or various admixtures of these conformations (Smythies,1975*c*). One of these possible structures consists of a variant of a Kusnetsov–Ghokov grid, i.e., two five-(or more)-tiered antiparallel β-sheets, each of the sequence –Gln–X–Gln–. The two sheets face each other in parallel, and bind to each other by two Gln–Gln double hydrogen bonds at each tier. This structure forms a tube inside the protein molecule as a whole. The tube is open if each opposed Gln–Gln pair binds in addition to its two *vertical* neighbors (one above, one below) using

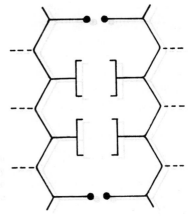

Fig. 5. Model of a Gln–Gln "shutter" inside a Met:Met "tube." The Met:Met structure is merely one example of how the "sides" of the tube may be completed. Other protein or even lipid structures are possible.

the binding pattern shown in Fig. 4. The tube may be closed by breaking these vertical hydrogen bonds, rotating the Gln side chains through 90° at the α-β carbon–carbon bond, and reforming the Gln–Gln accessory hydrogen bonds, this time with the *horizontal* neighbor. This mechanism acts like a venetian blind (Fig. 5).

Although the molecular structure of BTX, aconitine, and veratridine are very different from each other (Fig. 6), they are nevertheless all

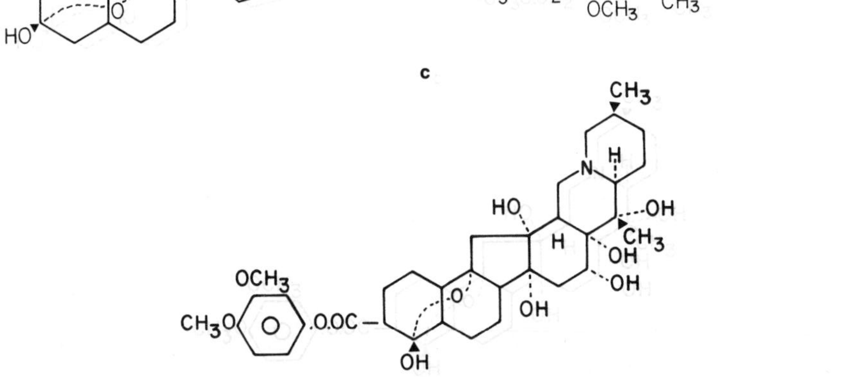

Fig. 6. Structures of batrachotoxin (a), aconitine (c), and veratridine (c).

complementary in different ways to the simple Gln–Gln "shutter" described here. They can all bind to it to prevent the "h" gate from being closed as shown in diagrammatic form in Fig. 7. We have further been able to suggest the detailed tertiary conformation for all three scorpion neurotoxins of known amino acid sequence that probably act at the inner orifice of the channel. We postulate that all three (of materially different sequence) have a doughnut shape and bind to the internal orifice of the "h" gate (–X–Gln–X–Gln–X–) (×2) structure described above) in such a manner as to prevent the Gln–Gln "venetian blind" mechanism from closing, and to further allow the Na^+ ions to escape through the central hole of the doughnut-shaped molecule. This hypothesis may be rigorously tested by determining the X-ray structure of the three scorpion neurotoxins, which the hypothesis predicts in some detail (Smythies *et al.*, 1977).

On the basis of determining which organic cations will, and which will not, pass through the Na^+ channel, Hille (1971) suggested that the external orifice of the channel consists of a quasirectangular orifice some 3×5 Å in size, lined with six oxygen atoms and bearing one formal negative charge. From a consideration of the molecular structures of TTX and STX, which block this orifice, we have suggested that the simplest way of constructing such a mechanism from protein is by the sequence –Asp–Pro–Gln–Pro–Gln–Pro–Gln–Pro–Asn–Pro–Gln–, forming a ring. The Asp and Asn go "down" and bind to each other, forming one wall of the 3×5 Å orifice. The four Gln's go "up" and form a hydrogen-bonding structure complementary to $Na^+ \cdot 6(H_2O)$ [and to the TTX molecule, which to a certain degree mimics $Na^+ \cdot 6(H_2O)$]. This mechanism could recognize and bind $Na^+ \cdot 6(H_2O)$ and remove four or five molecules of the water of hydration, transmitting $Na^+ \cdot (H_2O)$ or $Na^+ \cdot (2H_2O)$ through the 3×5 Å hole (any

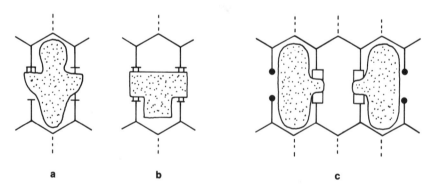

     a   **b**   **c**

Fig. 7. Model of interaction of specific toxins with Gln-Gln shutter mechanism: (a) BTX; (b) aconitine; (c) veratridine. Hydrogen bonds marked as—.

larger number of water molecules of hydration remaining render the molecular complex too large to pass through the 3×5 Å aperture).

4. Molecular Structure of Nucleohistone

The long DNA molecule must be tightly wound up to fit inside the confined space in the chromosome. Recent evidence from a number of sources indicates that chromatin (nucleohistone) has a "bead-and-string" structure (Olins and Olins, 1974; Kolata, 1975; Crick and Klug, 1975). In each bead, some 140–200 base pairs of DNA are tightly complexed with two molecules of each of the histones except histone I. Each bead, or v body, forms a spheroid structure some 100 Å in diameter. The beads are separated by short segments of DNA ("string"). Histone I, it is thought, binds in a 1:1 ratio mainly to the string portion. Crick and Klug (1975) recently suggested that the basis for the mechanism for winding the DNA molecule into these spheroid beads is the "kinky helix," i.e., segments of DNA double helix of length $10 \times n$ base pairs separated by kinks of approximately 90° produced by a simple rotation at the C_4^1–C_5^1 bonds into the minor groove. Owing to the detailed stereochemistry involved, such a system will generate a "kinky" helix the form of which will depend on (1) the number assigned to n for each section and (2) the value of α—the kink angle. Crick and Klug (1975) suggest a simple helix in which $n = 2$ for all segments and $\alpha \approx 98°$. Figure 8 shows how such a helix would look. If $\alpha = 90°$, the opposite segments will be parallel. If $\alpha = 98°$, there will be some rotation in the system. Weintraub *et al.* (1976) presented an alternative model in which the DNA forms a nonkinked coil around a central core of histone (Fig. 9). The internal diameter of the coil is approximately 80 Å, and the external diameter approximately 120 Å. The interior of the coil is packed by two identical paired tetramers of the four histones.

There is direct evidence to suggest that the DNA is wound around the outside of a central histone core. One might imagine that the mechanical support needed to maintain the system could be supplied by histone molecules of the form suggested in Figs. 9 or 10, or variations on this theme. There is also evidence that the basic portions of each histone

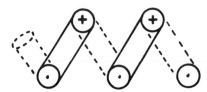

Fig. 8. Diagram of a $(20)_{10}$ Crick–Klug kinky helix: arrow convention.

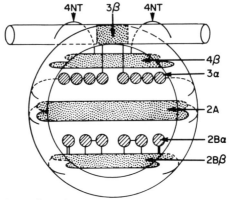

Fig. 9. Diagram of the Weintraub model with my postulated detail of histone structure superadded. (NT) N-terminal. The locations for 2A and 2B may be reversed, or the two may be intertwined.

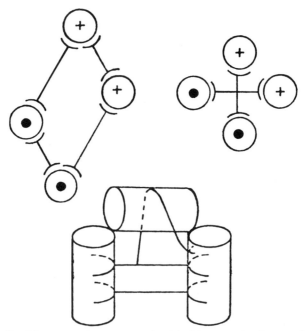

Fig. 10. Possible structural supports rendered by histone molecules to a Crick–Klug kinky helix. In a Weintraub coil, the topology is the same.

(mainly *N*-terminal) bind to DNA (presumably in part to phosphate), and that histone–histone interactions are based on lipophilic interaction between α-helices in the non-basic parts of the molecule.

Since it seems that each ν body contains pairs of each of the major histones, one might expect to see some twofold symmetry in the structure to provide identical or nearly identical binding sites in pairs for these four histones. Careful examination of a simple wire model of the (20)7 original Crick–Klug kinky helix for various values of α failed to reveal any such symmetry. We have found, however, that a simple modification of this helix provides a possible answer. We have approached this problem from a consideration of how each individual histone could bind to so specified a target as a DNA double helix (Smythies *et al.*, 1972, 1974 *a,b*), using the "rules" published by Fasman *et al.* (1976) for predicting secondary protein structure (α-helix, β-sheet, β-turn) from the amino acid sequence. These rules by themselves, of course, do not permit the prediction of tertiary structure, for this "matching-to-target" and the satisfaction of simple engineering principles are necessary, together with extensive model-building using CPK molecular models.

We supposed that a protein molecule, to bind strongly to a DNA double helix, should bind ionically to the phosphate groups via Lys or Arg ("roof"), and also to the grooves via hydrogen-bonding, and lipophilic and multiple Van der Waals' interactions ("packing"). Histones must also have portions that bind to DNA double helix and other portions that cross between DNA double helices.

4.1. Histone H_4

The amino acid sequence of this histone is given in Fig. 11 (Delange *et al.*, 1969). Application of the Chou and Fasman rules (Fasman *et al.*, 1976) suggests the following secondary structure:

α-helix (1) 15–22 (u = unstable)
(2) 31–39 (u)
(3) 57–67 [3 A: (s = stable 63–67)]
β-sheet (1) 26–30
(2) 46–51
(3) 69–73
(4) 80–90
(5) 96–100

β-Turns 2–5, 4–7, 7–10, 11–14, 22–25, 39–42, 53–56, 76–79, 92–95
Possible $\alpha \rightarrow \beta$ change 57–63 (3 A)

ser	gly	arg	gly	lys	gly	gly	lys	gly	leu	10
gly	lys	gly	gly	ala	lys	arg	his	arg	lys	20
val	leu	arg	asp	asn	ile	gln	gly	ile	thr	30
lys	pro	ala	ile	arg	arg	leu	ala	arg	arg	40
gly	gly	val	lys	arg	ile	ser	gly	leu	ile	50
tyr	glu	glu	thr	arg	gly	val	leu	lys	val	60
phe	leu	glu	asn	val	ile	arg	asp	ala	val	70
thr	tyr	thr	glu	his	ala	lys	arg	lys	thr	80
val	thr	ala	met	asp	val	val	tyr	ala	leu	90
lys	arg	gln	gly	arg	thr	leu	tyr	gly	phe	100
gly	gly									

Fig. 11.   Amino acid sequence of histone H_4.

The long β-sheet chain (4) is closely related to the shorter β-chains on each side (3) and (5). The length of (3) + (5) $\approx$ 4. If they form one β-sheet, as depicted in Fig. 12, this locates two short loops at each end, each with three basic amino acids, suggesting that this section of H_4 forms a strut joining two DNA double helices with their centers some 70 Å apart. The end of this β-pleated sheet is only one residue away from the short stable helix 3 A (63–67). This helix leads directly into a further probable recurrent β-pleated sheet (62–46), which is eight residues long including the apical β-turn (56–53) (Fig. 12). This may also form part of the strut. If the two H_4 molecules are closely associated with each other in chromatin, such a strut could have $(1\frac{1}{2} + 1\frac{1}{2}) = 3 \beta$ strands of approximately equal length.

The rest of H_4 is adapted to run along a major groove of DNA binding by lipophilic and Van der Waals' interactions (in the groove) and ionic bonds to phosphate as follows (Fig. 13): α2 (39–31) has the required groove-binding form for an α-helix –B–L–L–L–B–B–L–L–B–B– (L = lipophilic, B = basic amino acid) in which the lipophilic groups are all on the (down) side and the basic groups on the (up) side; this is followed by a "packing" segment (30–21) packed in the floor of the groove, then a

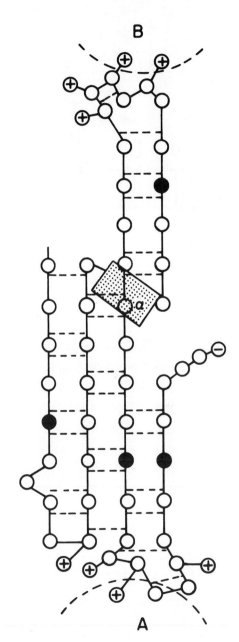

Fig. 12. Postulated β structure for histone H₄ C-terminal.

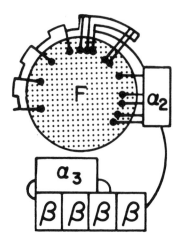

Fig. 13. Postulated mode of binding of *N*-terminal of H₄ to DNA.

recurrent "roof" segment of the form −B−B−B−B−B− running back over this packing segment, and finally a multiple β-turn segment with "packing" amino acids (Leu, Ala, Gly, Ser) interspersed with basic amino acids opposite DNA phosphates. This DNA "groove-binding" segment is located over the middle of the "strut" described earlier, which suggests binding under a kinked or nonkinked DNA arch (Fig. 13).

4.2. Histone H₃

Fasman *et al.* (1976) suggest the following secondary structure for this histone (sequence from DeLange *et al.,* 1972) (Fig. 14):

$$\alpha\text{-helix (1)} \quad 16\text{--}27 \text{ (u)}$$
$$\text{(2)} \quad 45\text{--}53 \text{ (s, 45--50)}$$
$$\text{(3)} \quad 58\text{--}65 \text{ (s)}$$
$$\text{(4)} \quad 67\text{--}79 \text{ (u)}$$
$$\text{(5)} \quad 88\text{--}98 \text{ (s, 88--95)}$$
$$\beta\text{-sheet (1)} \quad 99\text{--}104$$
$$\text{(2) } 109\text{--}113$$
$$\text{(3) } 117\text{--}120$$
$$\text{(4) } 124\text{--}128$$

β-Turns 10–13, 31–34, 37–40, 42–45, 55–58, 84–87, 106–109, 121–124
Possible $\alpha \rightarrow \beta$ change 45–48 and 67–71

This arrangement suggests a recurrent antiparallel β-sheet between (1) β₁ and β₂ apexed by β-turn (106–109) and (2) β₃ and β₄ apexed by β-turn (121–124). Molecular models indicate that these two β-sheets can form a single

ala	arg	thr	lys	gln	thr	ala	arg	lys	ser	10
thr	gly	gly	lys	ala	pro	arg	lys	gln	leu	20
ala	thr	lys	ala	ala	arg	lys	ser	ala	pro	30
ala	thr	gly	gly	val	lys	lys	pro	his	arg	40
tyr	arg	pro	gly	thr	val	ala	leu	arg	glu	50
ile	arg	arg	tyr	glu	lys	ser	thr	glu	leu	60
leu	ile	arg	lys	leu	pro	phe	gln	arg	leu	70
val	arg	glu	ile	ala	gln	asp	phe	lys	thr	80
asp	leu	arg	phe	gln	ser	ser	ala	val	met	90
ala	leu	gln	glu	ala	ser	glu	ala	tyr	leu	100
val	gly	leu	phe	glu	asp	thr	asn	leu	cys	110
ala	ile	his	ala	lys	arg	val	thr	ile	met	120
pro	lys	asp	ile	gln	leu	ala	arg	arg	ile	130
arg	gly	glu	arg	ala						

Fig. 14. Amino acid sequence of histone H_3.

parallel four-tiered β-pleated sheet, of which one side is wholly lipophilic and contains the single Cys (110) (Fig. 15). Moreover, the two sides of two H_3 molecules are complementary, if opposed so as to form a disulfide bond, by means of interlocked lipophilic amino acids. This results in a compact rectangular structure with four basic amino acids at each end (Fig. 16), suitable for binding two DNA helices together with their centers some 40 Å apart. This sheet continues directly with a series of four α-helices separated by eight, two, and four residues. Each α-helix is largely amphoteric, with one lipophilic side and one charged side. The N-terminal segment (1–42) is suitable for packing a DNA major groove with alternative "roof" and "packing" segments.

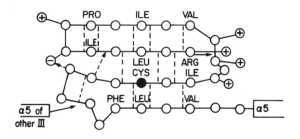

Fig. 15.   Suggested quadruple β-sheet for the *N*-terminal of H₃.

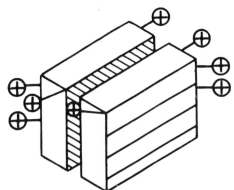

Fig. 16.   Diagram of two postulated H₃ *N*-terminal quadruple β-sheets.

4.3.   Histone H₂B

The analysis by Fasman *et al.* (1976) indicates the following probable structure (sequence from Yeoman *et al.,* 1972) (Fig. 17):

$$
\begin{array}{ll}
\alpha\text{-helix (1)} & 15\text{--}24 \text{ (u)} \\
\quad\quad\quad(2) & 69\text{--}82 \text{ (s, 76--82)} \\
\quad\quad\quad(3) & 93\text{--}102 \text{ (s)} \\
\quad\quad\quad(4) & 105\text{--}113 \text{ (s)} \\
\beta\text{-sheet (1)} & 39\text{--}48 \\
\quad\quad\quad(2) & 61\text{--}66 \\
\quad\quad\quad(3) & 88\text{--}90 \\
\quad\quad\quad(4) & 117\text{--}122
\end{array}
$$

β-Turns 10–13, 24–27, 35–38, 49–52, 66–69, 84–87, 102–105, 122–125
Possible $\alpha \rightarrow \beta$ transition 93–102

pro	gln	pro	ala	lys	ser	ala	pro	ala	pro	10
lys	lys	gly	ser	lys	ala	val	thr	lys	lys	20
ala	gln	lys	lys	asp	gly	lys	lys	arg	lys	30
arg	ser	arg	lys	glu	ser	tyr	ser	val	tyr	40
val	tyr	lys	val	leu	lys	gln	val	his	pro	50
asp	thr	gly	ile	ser	ser	lys	ala	met	gly	60
ile	met	asn	ser	phe	val	asn	asp	ile	phe	70
glu	arg	ile	ala	gly	glu	ala	ser	arg	leu	80
ala	his	tyr	asn	lys	arg	ser	thr	ile	thr	90
ser	arg	glu	ile	gln	thr	ala	val	arg	leu	100
leu	leu	pro	gly	glu	leu	ala	lys	his	ala	110
val	ser	glu	gly	thr	lys	ala	val	thr	lys	120
tyr	thr	ser	ser	lys						

Fig. 17. Amino acid sequence of histone H$_2$B.

This contains one long β-segment (39–48) with a β-turn at each end, giving a possible 10 to 14-residue β-pleated sheet. There are two further β-segments (2) and (4) of six residues each, so that the three can form one β-pleated sheet of approximately 12 residues. There are also three stable α-helices predicted: α-2 is contiguous via a β-turn with β2, and α3 and α4 are separated by only two residues from each other.

4.4. Histone H_2A

The analysis of probable secondary structure is as follows (sequence from Iwai *et al.,* 1970) (Fig. 18):

α-helix (1)   9–15 (u)
         (2)   47–66 (s)
         (3)   81–88 (s)
         (4)   91–97 (s)
         (5) 118–127 (u)
β-sheet (1)   23–27
          (2)   30–34
          (3)   76–79
          (4) 100–104
          (5) 111–116

β-Turns 2–5, 5–8, 16–19, 27–30, 35–38, 44–47, 66–69, 71–74, 73–76, 88–91, 108–111

Possible $\alpha \rightarrow \beta$ transformations 49–55, 57–63, 83–87

ser	gly	arg	gly	lys	gln	gly	gly	lys	ala	10
arg	ala	lys	ala	lys	thr	arg	ser	ser	arg	20
ala	gly	leu	gln	phe	pro	val	gly	arg	val	30
his	arg	leu	leu	arg	lys	gly	asn	tyr	ala	40
glu	arg	val	gly	ala	gly	ala	pro	val	tyr	50
leu	ala	ala	val	leu	glu	tyr	leu	thr	ala	60
glu	ile	leu	glu	leu	ala	gly	asn	ala	ala	70
arg	asp	asn	lys	lys	thr	arg	ile	ile	pro	80
arg	his	leu	gln	leu	ala	ile	arg	asn	asp	90
glu	glu	leu	asn	lys	leu	leu	gly	lys	val	100
thr	ile	ala	gln	gly	gly	val	leu	pro	asn	110
ile	gln	ala	val	leu	leu	pro	lys	lys	thr	120
glu	ser	his	his	lys	ala	lys	gly	lys		

Fig. 18.   Amino acid sequence of histone H_2A.

β-Sheet segments (1) and (2) are connected by the β-turn 27–30, and they are therefore likely to form an antiparallel sheet. Unlike the previous examples, this histone reveals a certain symmetry, i.e., (helix)–sheet–sheet–long helix–sheet–two short helices–sheet–sheet–(helix). The under surfaces of all three stable α-helices are extensively lipophilic.

5. Possible Structures for the Nucleosome

If we now compare these predicted secondary structures with various Crick–Klug kinky helices and with the Weintraub model, the following may be suggested:

In the Weintraub model, the only possible binding site for the postulated quadruple β-sheet of III is where the incoming and exiting parts of the DNA loop cross at the "stalk" of the loop. In this case, the major β-sheets of the two H_4 molecules would act as a strut between the DNA some little way down the loop, as shown in Fig. 9. Presumably, the α-helices of H_3 would reinforce this major strut, since H_3 and H_4 bind closely together *in vitro* to form a tetramer. The β-sheet of the two H_2B molecules could form a strut in the equivalent lower part of the loop, and the two H_2A molecules could form an equatorial strut, or vice versa, as diagrammed in Fig. 9. The basic N-termini of all four histones would bind to the adjacent DNA double helix to anchor the struts.

In the original Crick–Klug model in which there are seven to nine kinks with an interkink DNA length of 20 base pairs, there is no locus for the postulated quadruple β-sheet of H_3, since there are no two parallel or quasiparallel DNA strands approximately 40 Å apart. However, a minor modification of this helix (base pair interkink numbers X (A), 20 (B), 20 (C), 20 (D), 10 (E), 20 (F), 20 (H), X (I), in which X is the lead into the adjacent "string" portion, could be 5, 10, or 15 or some other number) allows this. If we number the components of this kinky helix A–I as above, then a locus to bind the quadruple β-sheet of H_3 is the 40 Å gap (as measured between the centers of the DNA double helices involved) between D and F (Fig. 19). One H_4 strut now runs between B and D with the N-terminal loop over C, and the other H_4 strut runs between F and H with N-terminal loop over G.

Each $H_4\beta$ strut would be reinforced by a criss-crossing pattern of attached H_3 α-helices as before. The N-terminal of one H_3 would wind down the major groove of B and that of the other down H. The main portion of one H_2B could then act as a strut between B and F and of the other between D and H. The two H_2A molecules could act as a strut between B and H, with various interactions between the α-helices of H_2B and H_2A. The middle β-sheet of H_2A could interact with the C-terminal β-

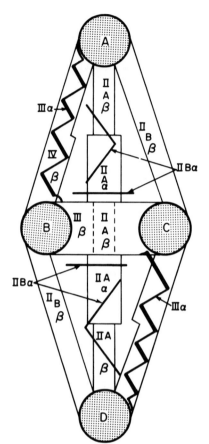

Fig. 19. Possible mode of binding of histones to one form of the Crick–Klug kinky helix.

sheet of H_3, and the two terminal β-sheets of H_2A could likewise interact with the β-sheet of H_4.

Cross-linking experiments should eliminate one of these models, since the propinquity of the different histones is very different in each of them; e.g., in my version of the Weintraub model, the two H_4 molecules are widely contiguous, whereas in my version of the Crick–Klug model, they do not touch at all.

6. References

Barlow, R. B., 1964, *Introduction to Chemical Pharmacology,* Methuen, London.
Catterall, W. A., 1975, Activation of the action potential Na$^+$ ionophore of cultured neuroblastoma cells by veratridine and batrachotoxin, *J. Biol. Chem. 250*:4053.

Collins, J. F., Hill, R. G., and Roberts, F., 1975, A study of tetramethylenedisulphotetramine (TETS) and related compounds as antagonists of presynaptic inhibition and microiontophoretically applied γ-aminobutyric acid (GABA) and glycine in the rat cuneate nucleus, *Br. J. Pharmacol. 54*:239P.

Crick, F. H. C., and Klug, A., 1975, Kinky helix, *Nature (London) 255*:530.

Curtis, D. R., and Johnston, G. A. R., 1974, Convulsant alkaloids, in: *Neuropoisons,* Vol. 2 (L. L. Simpson and D. R. Curtis, eds.), pp. 207–248, Plenum, New York.

DeLange, R. J., Famborough, D. M., Smith, E. L., and Bonner, J., 1969, Calf and pea histone IV. III. Complete amino acid sequence of pea seedling histone IV; comparison with the homologous calf thymus histone, *J. Biol. Chem. 244*:5669.

DeLange, R. J., Hooper, J. A., and Smith, E. L., 1972, Complete amino acid sequence of calf thymus histone III, *Proc. Natl. Acad. Sci. U.S.A. 69*:882.

Dray, A., 1975, Tetramethylenedisulphotetramine and amino acid inhibition in the rat brain, *Neuropharmacology 14*:703.

Eccles, J. R., 1970, *Facing Reality,* Springer-Verlag, New York.

Fasman, G., Chou, P. Y., and Adler, A. J., 1976, Prediction of the conformation of the histones, *Biophys. J. 16*:1201.

Gill, E. W., 1965, Drug receptor interactions, *Prog. Med. Chem. 4*:39.

Hille, G., 1971, The permeability of the sodium channel to organic cations in myelinated nerve, *J. Gen. Physiol. 58*:599.

Iwai, K., Ishikawa, K., and Hayashi, H., 1970, Amino acid sequence of slightly lysine rich histone, *Nature (London) 226*:1056.

Kolata, G. B., 1975, Chromatin structure: The supercoil is superseded, *Science 188*:1097.

Kusnetsov, S. G., and Ghokov, S. N., 1962, *Synthetic Atropine-like Substances,* State Publishing House of Medical Literature, Leningrad.

Olins, D. E., and Olins, A. L., 1974, Spheroid chromatin units (v bodies), *Science 183*:330.

Smythies, J. R., 1974, Relationships between chemical structure and biological activity of convulsants, *Annu. Rev. Pharmacol. 14*:9.

Smythies, J. R., 1975*a,* The molecular structure of acetylcholine and adrenergic receptors: An all protein model, *Int. Rev. Neurobiol. 17*:131.

Smythies, J. R., 1975*b,* Possible molecular forms of the opiate receptor, *Life Sci. 16*:1819.

Smythies, J. R., 1975*c,* The molecular structure of the sodium channel, in: *Molecular and Quantum Chemistry* (E. Bergmann and B. Pullman, eds)., pp. 573–581, Reidel, Boston.

Smythies, J. R., 1977, On the molecular structure of the opiate receptor, *Psychoneuroendocrinology 2*:71.

Smythies, J. R., Antun, F., Yank, G. O., and York, C., 1971, Molecular mechanisms of storage of transmitters in synaptic terminals, *Nature (London) 231*:185.

Smythies, J. R., Benington, F., and Morin, R. D., 1972, A mechanism for the interaction of a histone and DNA, *J. Theor. Biol. 37*:151.

Smythies, J. R., Benington, F., Bradley, R. J., Morin, R. D., and Romine, W. O., Jr., 1974*a,* On the mechanism of interaction between histone I and DNA and histone III and DNA, *J. Theor. Biol. 47*:309.

Smythies, J. R., Benington, F., Bradley, R. J., Morin, R. D., and Romine, W. O., Jr., 1974*b,* On the mechanism of interaction between histone IIB₁ and DNA and histone IIB₂ and DNA, *J. Theor. Biol. 47*:383.

Smythies, J. R., Benington, F., and Morin, R. D., 1975*a,* On the molecular structure of receptors for co-carcinogens and some anti-cancer drugs, *Psychoneuroendocrinology 1*:20.

Smythies, J. R., Benington, F., Bridgers, W. F., Bradley, R. J., Morin, R. D., and Romine, W. O., Jr., 1975*b,* The molecular structure of the receptor–ionophore complex at the neuromuscular junction, *J. Theor. Biol. 51*:111.

Smythies, J. R., Benington, F., Bradley, R. J., and Morin, R. D., 1977, A molecular mechanism of action of scorpion neurotoxins, *Ala. J. Med. Sci. 14*:68.

Weintraub, H., Worcel, A., and Alberts, B., 1976, A model for chromatin based on two symmetrically paired half-nucleosomes, *Cell 9*:409.

Yeoman, L. C., Olson, M. O., Sugano, N., Jordan, J. J., Taylor, C. W., Starbuck, W. C., and Busch, H., 1972, Amino acid sequence of the center of the arginine-lysine-rich histone from calf thymus: The total sequence, *J. Biol. Chem. 247*:6018.

8

Seven Neurons of Psychopharmacology: Adaptive Regulation in Biogenic Amine Neurons

Arnold J. Mandell

1. Introduction

The mind of the medical clinician, no less than that of the researcher, travels often to models of physiological function. Although he knows such cartoonlike, mechanistic scenarios to be less than perfect, they serve to organize his observations. Vague discomfort arises when one must make such models explicit, for we know there is evidence missing for many steps in their pictorial development and the false steps we must knowingly take to ensure their continuity. Likewise, I didn't enjoy the news that the mathematical models used to predict the tides for the next ten years had nothing to do with the mechanisms of tide formation, or the fact that Wall Street chartists often don't know anything about the companies the stock prices of which they predict. Chloral hydrate does not decompose to chloroform in the body, even though a century ago this explanatory model predicted much of its clinical pharmacology: latency, duration, interactions with other drugs, and effects of overdose. The bromides are not antiepileptic because they reduce the frequency of masturbation, although that was the reason given for their first use.

Arnold J. Mandell, M.D. • School of Medicine, University of California at San Diego, La Jolla, California 92093

Models of central nervous system function that relate biological processes to behavior have been the most imaginative, and the most desperate, that doctors have had to face. The brain's remoteness as calvarial prisoner, its heterogeneity and unique interactional complexity, and the innate difficulties in describing and quantifying its input and output functions have led researchers and clinicians alike to reach everywhere from the value systems of their childhood to the newest finding in molecular biology for help in constructing their personal images of its reality. The neurologist's telephone switchboard, the under-pressure gland bag of the psychoanalyst, the pediatric psychiatrists's developmental freeze, the psycholinguist's grammar-generating machine, the gestaltist's holography, the experimental psychologist's forest of S–R trees, the self-help group's power greater than the conscious self, the internist's liver between the ears, and the Buddha's experiential moment of now—all can be useful models of brain function.

The sources of psychopharmacological data over the past twenty years have been relatively remote from the living brain of man and of enormous variety as to technique. Enzymatic and metabolic studies of animal brain, histofluorescence microscopy of chemically specifiable brain systems, microelectrode and microiontophoretic studies of single brain cells, scalp and depth electrode recordings, human cerebrospinal fluid metabolite determinations, measurement of psychotropic drug effects on normal behavior and clinical syndromes, auditory and visual evoked potential recordings in man, urinary amine metabolite assessments, enzymatic studies of biopsied muscle—all are examples of the breadth of the accruing data base. This diffuseness requires modeling for a sense of comprehension and intelligibly integrated discourse, even for the courage to go on! The situation is somewhat reminiscent of the state of the art in nephrology before the era of micropuncture, electron microscopy, renal biopsy, and the new radiological techniques. Models predicting the behavior of nephrons, derived from such data as differential renal clearances, membrane function in artificial systems, stop-flow analyses, and metabolically distant body fluids were constructed diagrammatically—always including the escape clauses of brain stem, pulmonary, and cardiovascular physiology. Inferences were made from these varied sources and summarized as model nephrons in the journals and textbooks. The practitioners of research and clinical care operated with those pictures as their current reality, revising them as new findings emerged.

Since its birth in the mid-1950's there has been much model-building in psychopharmacology to represent our concepts of how the new agents work on the brain and, implicitly, how the brain itself works. The form of each model is cast in the conceptual matrix of the dominant research

1i.tt

techniques of its time. During the earliest days, when the EEG machine, oscilloscope, and primitive computer supplied the machinery for drug studies, the nervous system was pictured as an organization of conduction and relay systems. Conversations with the brain were in terms such as *drug-in* and *electricity-out*. Orientation, attention, arousal, hyperarousal, sleep, and coma were the experimental and clinical behaviors of interest. The "reticular formation" and the "limbic system" were used as biobehavioral as well as neuroanatomical concepts. We thought we had accounted for the psychopharmacology of the states of consciousness and sleep—an organization arranged along a unitary dimension and driven by the cells of the brain stem's reticular core. Sedatives moved the brain toward slow waves, sleep, and the coma of delta waves; stimulants, toward fast waves and alertness. Low-voltage "awake" waves were soon found to occur in deep (dreaming) sleep, the just-introduced phenothiazines made fast and spiky waves although animals and man became somnolent from them, and the model was in trouble. Was the difficulty inherent in the transliteration of the research language of drug-to-electricity-to-behavior?

2. Seven Model Neurons

During the twenty years that have followed, the neural representations of psychopharmacology have become predominantly chemical, with electrophysiological data relegated until recently to the status of confirmatory epiphenomena. *Chemical-in* and *chemical-out* characterize the new conversational tone. In addition, the pictures have shrunk to a more manageable size, to a set of model neurons, seven of which I will present below. Each of these models was derived from a set of basic and clinical research findings and conveys a group of insights that are potentially valuable in the management of patients, but suffers as do all such oversimplifications from unaccounted for or inconsistent data. We must introduce important indeterminacies from the beginning. For example, the chemical identity of the biogenic amine neurotransmitter will seldom be specified; the chemical coding for neural or behavioral action is far from coherent in the literature and too seductive should we pretend to know. Is dopamine a modulator of motor movement, repetitious thought and action, rage, territoriality? Does too little or too much brain norepinephrine represent endogneous depression? Is serotonin an inhibitory transmitter, a modulator, or not a neurotransmitter in the usual sense at all? It pays us now to speak more generally of psychopharmacological neurons, treating expectantly the need for closure that substitution of substance for symbol that the future will supply.

2.1. Model Neuron 1

The first ideas about biogenic amine transmitters and drug action are represented in Fig. 1. Transmitters after synthesis are stored in vesicles that are synthesized in the cell body, transported along the axons to nerve endings, and, under the influence of cellular activation, gather together at the nerve-ending membrane, adhere to it, and release their informational content into the synapse. After impingement on receptors, neurotransmitter molecules can be inactivated metabolically, washed away to be inactivated by another cell, or returned into the nerve ending via an active reuptake mechanism. Pictured also (Fig. 1) is a three-way cytoplasmic equilibrium among the functions of synthesis, storage, and degradation. This model, on the basis of over two decades of research on animal brains, some corroborating shadows gathered from the spinal fluid and urine of man, and a resonance with the intuitive, psychiatrically promulgated concept of brain as a closed energy system without adaptive capacity (and subject therefore to being depleted, dammed up, or exhausted) has been used to explain the actions on behavior of most psychotropic drugs (von Euler, 1958; Axelrod, 1959; Trendelenburg, 1959; Kirshner, 1962; Kopin, 1964; Carlsson *et al.,* 1966). Monoamine oxidase inhibitors increase psychic energy by increasing the stores of transmitter; reserpine's sedation comes from impairing vesicu-

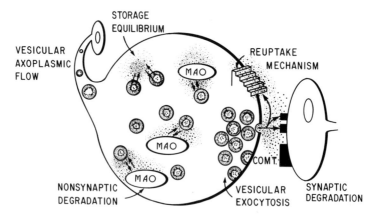

Fig. 1. Model neuron illustrating regulation of neurotransmission by transmitter storage, release, and reuptake, a concept of the brain as a closed energy system without adaptive capacities. Monoamine oxidase (MAO) and catechol-O-methyltransferase (COMT) are the enzymes involved in, respectively, pre- or nonsynaptic and synaptic degradation of biogenic amine neurotransmitters.

lar stores, which leads to depletion; tricyclic antidepressants increase functional levels by lengthening the synaptic half-life of transmitter as they impair the reuptake process; antipsychotic drugs impede the access of transmitters to receptors by preventing their release or blocking the receptor function, or both; amphetamine facilitates release and impedes reuptake; lithium impedes release; cocaine releases; and opiates block receptors. The model has become a psychopharmacological cosmology, explaining almost everything. Recited like a novena before critical clinical decisions, it brings reassurance.

There are, however, troubling implications with this essentially hydrodynamic model, which have led to further work and other models. Whereas this model predicts that drugs lead to almost instantaneous changes in cellular chemical function, the associated behavioral changes in man may require several days, weeks, or months to become manifest. Lithium's prophylactic action against recurrent depression may take years to express itself fully. Why do tricyclic antidepressants take three to six weeks to be effective if they block reuptake as soon as a therapeutic blood level is achieved, usually within a week or so? Why do antipsychotic drugs, immediately sedating and motor-retardant, take days to weeks to alter features in a patient's pathology of thought? In addition to the absence of temporal factors in this most-used of the model neurons, we must deal with the disturbing premise that the brain is passive: done to, it stays done to. All of us know better. Seldom does one encounter an organ more resistant to direct manipulation. Evidence for the brain's intrinsic negativity can be gathered from sources as varied as the phenomena of rebound to experience and drugs (postecstasy ennui; the progressive augmentation of fear that follows the regular invocation of alcohol's courage) to the poor rate of compliance with authoritarian cardiovascular management programs.

The brain responds in its own ways to perturbation. Reserpine's depletion of neurotransmitter is associated with increased neurotransmitter synthesis, as is the blockade of receptor function by antipsychotic drugs. The levels of catecholamine metabolites in human cerebrospinal fluid are reduced by chronic treatment with the tricyclic antidepressant drugs, although catecholamine transmission is said to be facilitated. Lithium treatment, though it initially increases the turnover of serotonin, results eventually in a decrease in animal brain tryptophan hydroxylase and indoleamine metabolites in human cerebrospinal fluid. The complexities involved in the brain's development of a new, drug-treated steady state require conceptualization of a number of model neurons, each encompassing a family of phenomena, all seen as operating at the same time, although we are unable to say which are prepotent.

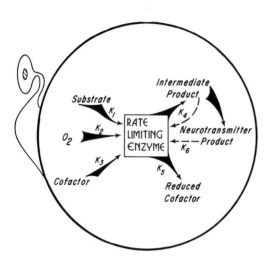

Fig. 2. Model neuron illustrating regulation of neurotransmitter biosynthesis by kinetic factors such as concentrations of substrates and their interactions with intermediate and final reaction products.

2.2. Model Neuron 2

The earliest studies of metabolic events following acute drug effects suggested that there were adaptive changes involving the kinetic parameters in the biosynthesis of biogenic amine neurotransmitters. The coordination of amino acid substrate, pterin cofactor, and oxygen on the active site of the rate-limiting, mixed-function oxidase can be seen as influencable by the concentrations of the substituents and products (Fig. 2) (Alousi and Weiner, 1966; Ikeda *et al.,* 1966; Udenfriend, 1966; Neff and Costa, 1968; Weiner and Rabadjija, 1968). There is evidence in catecholamine systems that too much amino acid substrate, perhaps by disrupting an orderly sequence of binding on the active site, can reduce the rate of the biosynthetic process. The rate-relevant concentrations of substrates as well as the interaction of intermediate and final products (DOPA and 5-hydroxytryptophan as K_4; dopamine and norepinephrine as K_6) with the substituents in the enzymatic reaction (K_1 to K_3) can be regulatory. Pharmacological studies of peripheral autonomic structures, showing that an activated system made preferential use of newly synthesized transmitter over that stored in vesicles, helped focus attention on the factors that regulate transmitter synthesis in contrast to the previous emphasis on those that regulate subcellular mobility. Studies of these influences have shown that substrate, breed of cofactor, and concentrations of products can play important roles. The most commonly invoked kinetic explanation for adaptive changes in intact systems is that the change in the cytoplasmic concentrations of amines (K_6) regulates the rate of their biosynthesis as the amine product competes for the cofactor site. Amphetamine, releasing and blocking the reuptake of dopamine, frees tyrosine hydroxylase from the tonic inhibitory effect of intraneuronal dopamine, which has been competing with the pterin cofactor for its site on the enzyme (K_3 process vs. K_6). Cocaine and the tricyclic antidepressants also increase relative rates of synthesis in some systems, which is explained by a similar reduction in cytoplasmic level of amine and the level of tonic inhibition of the enzyme. The monoamine oxidase inhibitors, increasing the intraneuronal concentration of the amines, reduce the biosynthetic rate, and this is explained by the converse of the situation described above. Product-feedback inhibition can be demonstrated unambiguously in the catecholamine biosynthetic systems. For those involving serotonin, the test-tube demonstration of competitive inhibition at reasonable product or intermediate-metabolite concentrations has been more ambiguous and dependent on the structure of the pteridine cofactor used.

2.3.   Model Neuron 3

Pharmacological alterations in the concentration and subcellular mobility of neurotransmitter (see Fig. 1) and the resulting kinetic adjustments in their biosynthetic rates (see Fig. 2) are short in latency and quick to stop after the drug influence is gone. In Fig. 3 are illustrated a group of adaptive phenomena resulting in alterations in the activity state of the rate-limiting biosynthetic enzymes that, once triggered, have half-lives of minutes to several hours, often lasting significantly beyond the peak effect of a

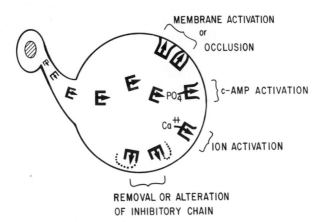

Fig. 3.   Model neuron illustrating regulation of neurotransmitter biosynthesis by alterations in enzyme conformation. Such changes are intermediate in latency and duration between kinetic determinants and changes in amount of enzyme.

drug. These conformationally influenced changes in enzymatic rates are not as quick as the kinetic dance of metabolic intermediates, not as slow or long-lasting as increments or decrements in enzyme protein would be. Evidence has accumulated that the shape or accessibility, or both, of the enzyme's active site, reducing or increasing the thermodynamic barrier to biosynthetic fit of the reaction's participants, can be influenced by the impingement of drugs on intact neural systems (Kuczenski and Mandell, 1972; Fisher and Kaufman, 1973; Costa *et al.*, 1974; Lloyd and Kaufman, 1974; Knapp *et al.*, 1975; Abita *et al.*, 1976; Raese *et al.*, 1976). Whether the intermediate steps involve changes in cellular discharge rates or indicate a new kind of drug–neuron interaction remains to be explored and settled. Enzyme activation, represented in Fig. 3 by the splayed arms of the E's, can be mediated by polyanionic membrane component effectors such as the sulfated mucopolysaccharides, lysolecithin, and phosphatidyl serine. Neural activation and associated changes in the swimming pattern of the subcellular citizens may move the biosynthetic machinery into membraneous walls (vesicular, reticular, or nerve-ending), which work allosteric acrobatics on the protein and change the affinity for its cosubstrates. Other mechanisms to explain the induction of postural change and readiness for enzyme productivity include a cAMP-mediated phosphorylation of the enzyme or increment in polyanionic phosphates, interaction with divalent cations such as calcium, and the flip-flop, curtain-raising, or proteolytic digestion of an enzyme's regulatory chain, the role of which at the active site can be gatekeeping.

Do antipsychotics, blocking dopamine receptors, lead to immediate and sustained increases in dopamine synthesis in the corpus striatum via an alternation in the activity state of the enzyme in addition to the kinetic possibilities? Is this change mediated by phosphorylation? Membrane binding? Activation by calcium? Amphetamine, a releaser of amines into the synapse and thus an indirect provocateur of a kinetically mediated increase in synthesis, also reduces enzyme activity for several hours after the behavioral activating effect of the drug is gone. Is this mediated by a family of influences on conformation? Clinically, could it account for lethargy after a period of behavioral activation in response to the drug? Awareness of these neurobiological adaptations that outlast the primary drug effect may sensitize clinicians to observe the "off" periods in their patients' psychopharmacological treatment. After-drug reactions, though subtle, are often more pervasive than the primary and anticipated effects, especially of acutely acting drugs. How much more depressed or fearful in attitude is the neurotic patient treated long-term with stimulants, sedatives, or sedative (minor) tranquilizers—not in the language of overt symptoms of anxiety but in terms of a deep dread in the self?

2.4.   Model Neuron 4

In a fourth model neuron (Fig. 4), consider adaptive changes in the amount of enzyme protein *per se,* mechanisms that, in contrast to temporary alterations in the physical state of existing enzyme molecules (see Fig. 3), are longer-lasting codifications of accommodation (Mueller *et al.,* 1969; Dahlstrom, 1971; Segal, D.S., *et al.,* 1971; Joh *et al.,* 1973; Mandell, 1975). Reserpine, that tried-and-true disturber of amine system homeostasis, which temporarily increases cytoplasmic concentrations of amines for competition with the cofactor but in the long run reduces this competition by depleting stores of transmitter, leads over the still longer run (hours, days, or weeks) to a compensatory increase in the amount of enzyme protein for use in the sustained augmentation in synthesis of neurotransmitter. Such increases or decreases in enzyme protein first appear in cell-body regions, are carried by energized waves of microtubular protein down axonal sluices, to remain at a new level in the nerve ending for days or weeks. The rate of axonal transport may vary. The decrease in biosynthetic enzymes induced by regular treatment with tricyclics may take days to reach the biogenic amine nerve endings in the miniheaded rat. Does it take weeks to reach man's more peninsular forebrain from the brain stem's

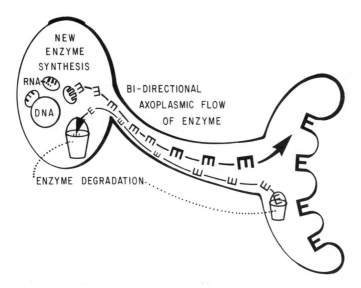

Fig. 4.   Model neuron illustrating regulation of neurotransmitter biosynthesis by alterations in the level of enzyme protein. Experimentally induced shifts in amount of enzyme appear first in cell-body regions and, after various lengths of time for axonal transport, are measurable in regions rich in nerve terminals.

protein workshops? Does the time required for changes in the manufacturing policy and delivery of enzyme protein account for the long latency to effect of the antidepressant drugs? The anorectic fenfluramine can induce a reduction in tryptophan hydroxylase in the serotonergic system that may last three or four weeks after a single drug administration. Should these possibilities not sensitize the physician to look weeks later for the effect of today's change in drug dose? Should we not withhold for several days or weeks the decision that the tricyclics, antipsychotics, or lithium aren't working, since all these drugs lead to changes of this sort in enzyme protein, holding the patient in treatment through charm and guile during the drug's early peripheral and irrelevant central side effects until the full symphony of drug effect and echoing cascades of metabolic events can be realized?

2.5. Model Neuron 5

The model depicted in Fig. 5 will likely soon be of interest to practicing physicians. There remain a few years of testing the influence of amino acid loads on the mind. It is said that tryptophan, the serotonin precursor, will soon be introduced as an over-the-counter sleep-inducing preparation. The work leading to this model makes us aware of the potential relationship

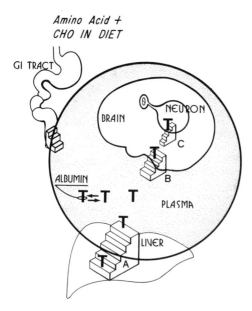

Fig. 5. Model neuron illustrating regulation of neurotransmitter biosynthesis by substrate supply. In this case, T represents the serotonin precursor tryptophan; stairways A–C represent active transport mechanisms at which other amino acids and psychotropic drugs can exert influence, ultimately affecting serotonin synthesis by affecting the substrate supply.

between nutritional status, central nervous system state, and neural responsivity to psychotropic drugs. It also teaches us more about the regulation of neurotransmitter biosynthesis (Moir and Eccleston, 1968; Olendorf, 1971; Knapp and Mandell, 1975; Paoletti *et al.*, 1975; Cohen and Wurtman, 1976). The substrate requirements, dictated by kinetic constants, when combined with the levels of aromatic amino acids as determined in animal brains, have suggested that although the tyrosine hydroxylase of dopamine and norepinephrine synthesis is saturated and more precursor would not lead to more product, the tryptophan hydroxylase of serotonin synthesis is not. More tryptophan in the diet can lead to more serotonin in the brains of animals and more indole acids in the cerebrospinal fluid of man. (Likewise, recent work has shown that more choline in the diet increases brain concentrations of acetylcholine.) In rats, *chronic* dietary tryptophan deprivation lowered brain tryptophan and serotonin, whereas, acutely, intake of a tryptophan-free, high-carbohydrate meal resulted in increased brain tryptophan and serotonin. Recent speculation has suggested that brain tryptophan and serotonin levels may determine protein hunger. Memories are invoked of the rigid refusals of meat seen commonly in the psychotically ill. Psychotropic drugs alter the hepatic metabolism of protein such that plasma levels of tryptophan are altered, sometimes for hours or days.

Tryptophan exists in the plasma in two forms: free and bound to albumin, a binding that has relevance to clinical pharmacology. Substances such as free fatty acids, salicylates, and clofibrate compete for tryptophan's binding site, changing the fraction that is free and the associated dynamics of blood–brain transport. As can be visualized from Fig. 5 (stairways A–C), there are at least three energy-dependent, somewhat stereospecific, amino-acid-uptake processes between the gastrointestinal hepatic treatment of protein and the transport of tryptophan into the neuron. There is competition for the common stairs among the neutral amino acids such that even alphatic ones like leucine and isoleucine can take the place of aromatic tryptophan. Psychotropic drugs can interact with these transport systems. For example, lithium stimulates the high-affinity uptake of tryptophan into the neuron, leading first to an increase in serotonin synthesis by the cells containing tryptophan hydroxylase, which can be seen in animal brains and is reflected in temporary increments of indole acids in human spinal fluid. With longer treatment and compensatory changes in enzyme protein (cf. Fig. 4), there is a decrease in rat brain enzyme and human spinal fluid metabolites. Cocaine blocks this neuronal tryptophan-transport system and reduces brain serotonin. Clinical case reports suggest that the lithiumized individual will not respond to cocaine. Is this an example of a drug–drug interaction on stairway C (Fig. 5) or an antagonism in the neurotransmitter-release function (see Fig. 1)?

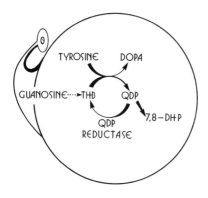

Fig. 6. Model neuron illustrating potentially regulatory dynamics in the concentration and disposition of reduced pterins, which are essential cofactors for the hydroxylation of monoamine precursors.

2.6. Model Neuron 6

There is a possibility that amine biosynthesis can also be regulated through changes in the rate of synthesis or disposition, or both, of the nonfolate pterins in brain (Fig. 6). These compounds, long known to be the cofactor catalysts of tyrosine and tryptophan hydroxylation, more or less efficient depending on structure, have recently been seen to have dynamic properties (Kaufman, 1967; Musacchio *et al.*, 1971; Buff and Dairman, 1975; Bullard *et al.*, 1976). Reserpine raises and amphetamine lowers pterin concentration, which is correlated with changes in nerve-ending amine biosynthesis. Guanosine seems to be the precursor of the most active of the known cofactors, tetrahydrobiopterin, which is oxidized to the quinoid 7,8-dihydro form during the hydroxylation of the amino acid and is regenerated by a quinoid dihydropterin reductase that is much in excess. If the quinoid form is isomerized to the nonquinoid form, however, the reduction cannot be effected. As study continues on these compounds, the determinants of functional levels of nonfolate pterins with regulatory potential will become more clear. Is it possible that the dramatic mood changes associated with the chemotherapy of cancer are related to interference with the biosynthesis or disposition of these biogenic-amine-related pterins? New structures for psychotropic and blood-pressure medication are also suggested by the implications of these studies.

2.7. Model Neuron 7

The models in Figs. 2–4 can be construed as representing the brain's armaments of control, maintaining the *status quo*. Kinetic "feedback" effects, changes in the physical state of the biosynthetic enzymes, and alterations in the amount of enzyme protein, tuned to move biogenic-amine production in a direction opposite to the acute effect of the drug, all help keep the aminergic system from running off. These mechanisms exhibit a redundancy of biochemical inhibitory control reminiscent of that first brought to prominence in the nervous systems modeled by Sherrington and Jackson in neurophysiology at the turn of the century. Although neurophysiology had been relegated to the prehistory of psychopharmacology, recent studies of the single units of aminergic systems in brain during response to drugs have returned neurophysiology to the frontier of psychopharmacology and suggested another set of inhibitory controls, at least four interneuronal feedback loops (Fig. 7): (1) an autoreceptor loop, perhaps dendritic processes metabolically equipped like axonal endings so they can inform the cell body directly what its downstream terminals are up to; (2) a postsynaptic feedback loop that ends on a presynaptic nerve ending; (3) a postsynaptic feedback loop that ends on the presynaptic cell body; and (4) a postsynaptic feedback loop that ends on an interneuron, which in turn passes the information to the presynaptic cell (Aghajanian *et al.,* 1972; Segal, M., and Bloom, 1974; Gallager and Aghajanian, 1975; Groves *et al.,* 1975). Drugs like LSD, with its indole conformation, which can easily be imagined to take the place of serotonin as an agonist or antagonist on the postsynaptic cell, have been shown to influence serotonergic cells directly. Thinking about *alpha* and *beta* receptors, long denied in the brain, has come to life with the advent of new *alpha* and *beta* agonists that act centrally. Propanolol, depressing and sedating to patients, appears to be one. Discoveries of more exquisitely specifiable receptors in brain are being made at an accelerating rate.

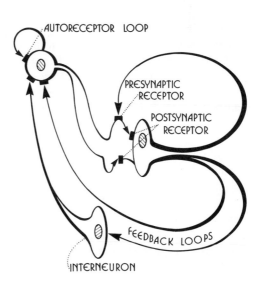

Fig. 7. Model neuron illustrating potential regulatory feedback loop suggested by recent neurophysiological studies of single-unit phenomena.

3. Discussion and Speculation

The primary effects of psychotropic drugs, taken with the compensatory mechanisms, explain something about the processes that might be involved in the prophylactic action achieved by the chronic treatment of psychiatric patients with such agents as lithium, the tricyclic antidepressants, and the antipsychotic drugs. All have been convincingly shown to reduce the incidence of recurrence of symptoms. Such a drug-induced steady state appears to accomplish for the brain increased stability against disturbance. The brain's range of response to disease-activating traumata may be reduced by this buffering action. Chronic treatment with psychotropic drugs, by moving such adaptive mechanisms to the ends of their ranges, may create a circumstance in which the system is no longer as responsive to input, yet is fixed within a zone between the maintained primary drug effect and the biological limit of the adaptive mechanisms (Mandell and Knapp, 1976). Perhaps the psychoses, like the illnesses in general medicine that have been most elusive (collagen, neoplastic, glandular), result from deregulated attempts at physiological adaptation to disrupting stimuli; if so, not only psychotropic drug mechanisms but those of some psychiatric diseases may be found in the models illustrated in Figs. 2–7.

It appears that there would be a message for the clinician in the imagined functioning of these seven model neurons: *the importance of time in psychopharmacology*. Taught by our personal systems of psychological causality to look only at the immediate temporal environment for the evoker of our feelings; brought up in a medical practice dominated by central nervous system drugs like sedatives, minor tranquilizers, and stimulants, which act *now;* learning a psychiatry that related the symptomatology of today to an etiology of the first five years of life, we lack brain shelves for the determinant events in the intermediate past. This blindness for intermediate periods of causality is not new to mankind.

Even today, aboriginal tribes in central and northern Australia do not comprehend the relationship between fornication and childbirth. They have had little experience with the kinds of studies such proofs would require (a longitudinal crossover design with difficult-to-control control groups; the immunoassay of urinary hormones), and their intuitions do not reach far enough. The same can be said for many practicing physicians and the psychotropic drugs. The full neurochemical effects of psychotropic drug action (and perhaps of life events as well) take longer to manifest themselves in subjective state and behavior than is generally appreciated. The brain's reverberating adaptive mechanisms, each with a different time constant, require varying periods to reveal their final statements about what has happened to them.

ACKNOWLEDGMENT

The author's research is supported by Grant No. DA-00265-05 from the National Institute on Drug Abuse, United States Public Health Service. This article was written while Dr. Mandell was the recipient, Johananoff International Fellowship for Advanced Biomedical Studies at the Mario Negri Institute for Pharmacological Research in Milan, Italy, 1976–1977.

4. References

Abita, J., Milstien, S., Chang, N., and Kaufman, S., 1976, *In vitro* activation of rat liver phenylalanine hydroxylation by phosphorylation, *J. Biol. Chem. 251*:5310.

Aghajanian, G. K., Haigler, H. J., and Bloom, F. E., 1972, Lysergic acid diethylamide and serotonin: Direct actions on serotonin containing neurons in rat brain, *Life Sci. 11*:615.

Alousi, A., and Weiner, N., 1966, The regulation of norepinephrine synthesis in sympathetic nerves: Effect of nerve stimulation, cocaine, and catecholamine-releasing agents, *Proc. Natl. Acad. Sci. U.S.A. 56*:1491.

Axelrod, J., 1959, Metabolism of epinephrine and other sympathomimetic amines, *Physiol. Rev. 39*:751.

Buff, K., and Dairman, W., 1975, Biosynthesis of biopterin by two clones of mouse neuroblastoma, *Mol. Pharmacol. 11*:87.

Bullard, W. P., Mandell, A. J., and Russo, P. V., 1976, Dyanamics and disposition of reduced pterins in the rat brain (abstract), Society for Neuroscience.

Carlsson, A., Fuxe, K., Hamberger, B., and Lindqvist, M., 1966, Biochemical and histochemical studies on the effects of imipramine-like drugs and (+)-amphetamine on central and peripheral catecholamine neurons, *Acta Physiol. Scand. 67*:481.

Cohen, E. L., and Wurtman, R. L., 1976, Brain acetylcholine: Control by dietary choline, *Science 191*:561.

Costa, E., Guidotti, A., and Zivkovic, B., 1974, Short- and long-term regulation of tyrosine hydroxylase, in: *Neuropsychopharmacology of Monoamines and Their Regulatory Enzymes* (E. Usdin, ed.) pp. 161–175, Raven Press, New York.

Dahlstrom, A., 1971, Axoplasmic transport (with particular respect to adrenergic neurons), *Philos. Trans. R. Soc. London 261*:325.

von Euler, U.S., 1958, The presence of the adrenergic neurotransmitter in intraaxonal structures, *Acta Physiol. Scand. 43*:155.

Fisher, D. B., and Kaufman, S., 1973, The stimulation of rat liver phenylalanine hydroxylase by lysolecithin and α-chymotrypsin, *J. Biol. Chem. 248*:4345.

Gallager, D. W., and Aghajanian, G. K., 1975, Effects of chlorimipramine and lysergic acid diethylamide on efflux of precursor-formed ^{3}H-serotonin: Correlations with serotonergic impulse flow, *J. Pharmacol. Exp. Ther. 193*:785.

Groves, P. M., Wilson, C. J., Young, S. J., and Rebec, G. V., 1975, Self-inhibition by dopaminergic neurons, *Science 190*:522.

Ikeda, M., Fahien, L. A., and Udenfriend, S., 1966, A kinetic study of bovine adrenal tyrosine hydroxylase, *J. Biol. Chem. 241*:4452.

Joh, T. H., Geghman, C., and Reis, D. J., 1973, Immunochemical demonstration of increased tyrosine hydroxylase protein in sympathetic ganglia and adrenal medulla elicited by reserpine, *Proc. Natl. Acad. Sci. U.S.A. 70*:2767.

Kaufman, S., 1967, Pteridine cofactors, *Annu. Rev. Biochem. 36*:171.

Kirshner, N., 1962, Uptake of catecholamines by a particulate fraction of the adrenal medulla, *J. Biol. Chem. 237*:2311.

Knapp, S., and Mandell, A. J., 1975, Effect of lithium chloride on parameters of biosynthetic capacity for 5-hydroxytryptamine in rat brain, *J. Pharmacol. Exp. Ther. 193*:812.

Knapp. S., Mandell, A. J., and Bullard, W. P., 1975, Calcium activation of brain tryptophan hydroxylase, *Life Sci. 16*:1583.

Kopin, I. J., 1964, Storage and metabolism of catecholamines: The role of monamine oxidase, *Pharmacol. Rev. 16*:179.

Kuczenski, R. T., and Mandell, A. J., 1972, Regulatory properties of soluble and particulate rat brain tyrosine hydroxylase, *J. Biol. Chem. 247*:3114.

Lloyd, T., and Kaufman, S., 1974, The stimulation of partially purified bovine caudate tyrosine hydroxylase by phosphatidyl-L-serine, *Biochem. Biophys. Res. Commun. 59*:1262.

Mandell, A. J. (ed.), 1975, Neurobiological mechanisms of presynaptic metabolic adaptation and their organization: Implications for a pathophysiology of the affective disorders, in: *Neurobiological Mechanisms of Adaptation and Behavior,* pp. 1–32, Raven Press, New York.

Mandell, A. J., and Knapp, S., 1976, A neurobiological model for the symmetrical prophylactic action of lithium in bipolar affective disorder, *Pharmakopsychiatr./Neuro-Psychopharmakol. (Stuttgart) 9*:116.

Moir, A. T. B., and Eccleston, D., 1968, The effects of precursor loading in the cerebral metabolism of 5-hydroxyindoles, *J. Neurochem. 15*:1093.

Mueller, R. A., Thoenen, H., and Axelrod, J., 1969, Inhibition of transsynaptically increased tyrosine hydroxylase activity by cycloheximide and actinomycin D, *Mol. Pharmacol. 5*:463.

Musacchio, J., D'Angelo, G. L., and McQueen, C. A., 1971, Dihydropteridine reductase: Implication on the regulation of catecholamine biosynthesis, *Proc. Natl. Acad. Sci. U.S.A. 68*:2087.

Neff, N. H., and Costa, E., 1968, Application of steady-state kinetics to the study of catecholamine turnover after monoamine oxidase inhibition or reserpine administration, *J. Pharmacol. Exp. Ther. 160*:40.

Oldendorf, W. H., 1971, Brain uptake of radiolabeled amino acids, amines, and hexoses after arterial injection, *Am. J. Physiol. 221*:1629.

Paoletti, R., Sirtori, C., and Spano, P. F., 1975, Clinical relevance of drugs affecting tryptophan transport, *Annu. Rev. Pharmacol.15*:73.

Raese, J., Patrick, R. L., and Barchas, J. D., 1976, Phospholipid-induced activation of tyrosine hydroxylase from rat brain striatal synaptosomes, *Biochem. Pharmacol. 25*:2245.

Segal, D. S., Sullivan, J. L., Kuczenski, R. T., and Mandell, A. J., 1971, Effects of long term reserpine treatment on brain tyrosine hydroxylase and behavioral activity, *Science 173*:847.

Segal, M., and Bloom, F. E., 1974, The action of norepinephrine in the rat hippocampus *Brain Res. 72*:79.

Trendelenburg, U., 1959, The supersensitivity caused by cocaine, *J. Pharmacol. Exp. Ther. 125*:55.

Udenfriend, S., 1966, Tyrosine hydroxylase, *Pharmacol. Rev. 18*:43.

Weiner, N., and Rabadjija, M., 1968, The regulation of norepinephrine synthesis. Effect of puromycin on the accelerated synthesis of norepinephrine associated with nerve stimulation, *J. Pharmacol. Exp. Ther. 164*:103.

Wurtman, R. J., and Fernstrom, J. D., 1974, Effects of diet on brain neurotransmitters, *Nutr. Rev. 32*:193.

Epilogue

Seymour Kety

Harold Himwich was a neuroscientist long before that word was coined, and before a coherent body of knowledge had developed to justify the existence of a new discipline. His career spanned six decades and as many disciplines: biochemistry, embryology, physiology, and pharmacology, and all of these coupled with clinical investigations in medicine and psychiatry. His fertile mind blazed a logical path through and among these fields, tying them together in a way that helped to develop the concept of neuroscience and the dependence of an understanding of normal and abnormal behavior upon all of them.

On a foundation of excellent biochemical training with Meyerhoff, he proceeded to examine the processes of energy metabolism in muscle and a number of other tissues. His demonstration of a respiratory quotient of unity for the brain *in vivo* and *in vitro* emphasized a remarkable dependence of the brain on glucose as its major energy-yielding substrate, which holds as true today as it did in 1929 for physiological conditions. Only in severe starvation is the brain known to turn to other substrates. So closely is the uptake of glucose in the brain coupled with its functional activity that it is now possible to employ that uptake, quantified and visualized by means of ^{14}C-labeled deoxyglucose, as a means of delineating regions of high functional activity in the brain.

Himwich's studies on the neonatal brain, among the earliest in what would now be called developmental neurochemistry, rapidly became classics. They demonstrated with undisputed clarity the remarkable resistance of the neonatal brain to anoxia, an adaptation the biochemical basis of which we are only now beginning to appreciate. Developmental neuro-chemistry, in which he pioneered, is an arena of considerable ferment at the present time, in which advances in molecular biology have been brought to bear upon the process of gene expression in the developing brain. Although progress has been rapid, the processes undoubtedly involved in the miracle of embryology are so numerous and complex, and so intimately inter-woven, that it will be many years before this field will become prosaic.

Himwich was primarily a physiologist in the original sense of that broad discipline of which biochemistry, biophysics, pharmacology, endo-crinology, and neurobiology were all a part. His identification with physiol-ogy touched upon all of these fields. The respiratory quotient and the importance of glucose metabolism to the brain's economy led him and Williamina, his wife and collaborator, to examine both the anaerobic and the oxidative metabolism of that substance, as well as the utilization of oxygen by the brain in a number of clinical states, notably mental retardation and anesthesia. It was his identification with physiology that permitted him to explore the electrical activity of the brain and the effects of a variety of classical neurotropic drugs. It was that which prepared him, when the psychoactive neuroleptic agents became available, to be among the first to examine their physiology and pharmacology by means of electrophysiologi-cal recording.

His interest in glucose metabolism brought him naturally to a confron-tation with the major clinical disorder of glucose metabolism that is seen in diabetes mellitus. During that period of time insulin hypoglycemia was widely used in the treatment of schizophrenia. It is not difficult to see how a curious and thoughtful mind would be challenged by this perplexing disor-der and how it might become a major theme in the research he was to conduct later on.

It was his interest in schizophrenia, undoubtedly, that led him to develop the Thudicum Psychiatric Research Laboratories at Galesburg, where he spent the last 25 years of his career. There he was able to bring into convergence the sciences in which he had pioneered. He brought to this problem not only his previous competence but also his eagerness to keep abreast of new developments, so that the biogenic amines, transmeth-ylation, the neuroendocrine system, became important fields of exploration for him and his colleagues.

This volume, representing as it does contributions by a substantial number of outstanding investigators who were trained or influenced by him in all the disciplines that he encompassed, is an appropriate tribute to Harold Himwich, to the wide range of his interests, and to his productive career in the service of science and humanity.

Bibliography of Harold E. Himwich

1920 Rhabdomyoma of the ovary, *J. Cancer Res.* 5:227.

1921 Terotomas and their relation to age, *J. Cancer Res.* 6:261.

1923 Studies in the physiology of muscular exercise. I. Changes in acid–base equilibrium following short periods of vigorous muscular exercise, *J. Biol. Chem.* 55:495 (with D. P. Barr and R. P. Green).

1923 Studies in the physiology of muscular exercise. II. Comparison of arterial and venous blood following short periods of vigorous muscular exercise, *J. Biol. Chem.* 55:525 (with D. P. Barr and R. P. Green).

1923 Studies in the physiology of muscular exercise. V. Oxygen relationships in the arterial blood, *J. Biol. Chem.* 57:363 (with D. P. Barr).

1924 Studies of the effect of exercise in diabetes. I. Changes in acid–base equilibrium and their relation to the accumulation of lactic acid and acetone, *J. Biol. Chem.* 59:265 (with R. O. Loebel and D. P. Barr).

1924 Studies of the effect of exercise in diabetes. II. Lactic acid formation in phlorhizin diabetes, *J. Biol. Chem.* 61:9 (with R. O. Loebel, D. P. Barr, and E. Tolstoi).

1924 Beitrag zum Kohlehydratsoffwechsel des Warmblutermuskels, insbesondere nach einseitiger Fetternährung, *Pflugeers Arch. gesamte Physiol. Menschen Tiere* 205:415 (with O. Meyerhof).

1924 Über die Milchsäurebildung bei Muskelcontracturen, *Klin. Wochenschr.* 3:392 (with O. Meyerhof).

1926 The respiratory quotient of resting muscle, *Am. J. Physiol.* 76:188 (with W. B. Castle).

1926 The respiratory quotient of exercising muscle, *Proc. Soc. Exp. Biol. (N.Y.)* 23:169 (with M. I. Rose).

1926 Changes in the respiratory quotient produced by subcutaneous injection of dioxyacetone and glucose, *Proc. Soc. Exp. Biol. (N.Y.)* 24:238 (with M. I. Rose and M. R. Malev).

1927 Studies in the metabolism of muscle. I. The respiratory quotient of resting muscle, *Am. J. Physiol.* 83:92 (with W. B. Castle).

1927 Formation of lactic acid in excised organs, *Proc. Soc. Exp. Biol. (N.Y.)* 25:53 (with S. A. Jacobson).

1927 The oxygen saturation of hemoglobin in the arterial blood of exercising patients, *J. Clin. Invest.* 5:113 (with R. O. Loebel).

1928 Changes in lactic acid and glucose in the blood on passage through organs, *Proc. Soc. Exp. Biol. (N.Y.)* 25:347 (with Y. D. Koskoff and L. H. Nahum).

1929 Respiratory quotient of the brain, *Proc. Soc. Exp. Biol. (N.Y.)* 26:496 (with L. H. Nahum).

1929   Utilization of fat by resting and exercising muscles of diabetic dogs, *Proc. Soc. Exp. Biol. (N.Y.) 27*:193 (with H. Friedman, E. Berry, and W. H. Chambers).

1929   Studies in the metabolism of muscle. II. The respiratory quotient of exercising muscle, *Am. J. Physiol. 88*:663 (with M. I. Rose).

1929   The respiratory quotient of testicle, *Am. J. Physiol. 88*:680 (with L. H. Nahum).

1929   Studies in glandular metabolism. I. The source of the lactic acid produced on incubation of the testicle and the submaxillary gland, *Am. J. Physiol. 91*:172 (with M. A. Adams).

1930   Effect of adrenalin on blood fat, *Proc. Soc. Exp. Biol. (N.Y.) 27*:814 (with M. L. Petermann).

1930   Effect of pituitary extract on basal metabolic rate, *Proc. Soc. Exp. Biol. (N.Y.) 27*:815 (with F. W. Haynes).

1930   Effects of posterior pituitary extracts on the lactic acid of blood, *Proc. Soc. Exp. Biol. (N.Y.) 28*:331 (with J. F. Fazekas).

1930   Effects of posterior pituitary extract on plasma concentration and fat content and on blood sugar, *Proc. Soc. Exp. Biol. (N.Y.) 28*:332 (with F. W. Haynes and M. A. Spiers).

1930   Effect of ephedrine on blood glucose and lactic acid and plasma fat, *Proc. Soc. Exp. Biol. (N.Y.) 28*:333 (with H. Henstell and J. F. Fazekas).

1930   Effect of stimulation of hypothalamus on blood sugar, *Am. J. Physiol. 93*:658 (with A. D. Keller).

1930   Regulation of the respiration in nephritis with nitrogen retention, *Am. J. Physiol. 93*:667 (with R. O. Loebel and D. P. Barr).

1930   Studies in carbohydrate metabolism. I. A glucose lactic acid cycle involving muscle and liver, *J. Biol. Chem. 85*:571 (with Y. D. Koskoff and L. H. Nahum).

1930   Studies in carbohydrate metabolism. II. Glucose lactic acid cycle in diabetes, *J. Biol. Chem. 90*:417 (with W. H. Chambers, Y. D. Koskoff, and L. H. Nahum).

1930   Studies in glandular metabolism. II. Carbohydrates of resting and secreting submaxillary glands, *J. Biol. Chem. 93*:568 (with Y. D. Koskoff and L. H. Nahum).

1931   The vitamin B complex in relation to food intake during hyperthyroidism, *Proc. Soc. Exp. Biol. (N.Y.) 28*:646 (with W. Goldfarb and G. R. Cowgill).

1931   Effects of adrenalin on the glucose and lactic acid exchange of the brain, *Proc. Soc. Exp. Biol. (N.Y.) 29*:72 (with L. H. Nahum).

1931   Effects of posterior pituitary extracts on oxygen consumption of excised tissue, *Proc. Soc. Exp. Biol. (N.Y.) 29*:233 (with R. Finkelstein and K. E. Humphreys).

1931   The effects of acetylcholine injections on blood fat and glucose, *Proc. Soc. Exp. Biol. (N.Y.) 20*:234 (with M. J. Bruhn).

1931   The degree of saturation of blood fats mobilized during diabetes, *Proc. Soc. Exp. Biol. (N.Y.) 29*:235 (with M. A. Spiers).

1931   Effect of noxius stimulation on blood fat, *Proc. Soc. Exp. Biol. (N.Y.) 29*:236 (with J. F. Fazekas and M. A. Spiers).

1931   Organs capable of producing acetone substances, *Science 74*:606.

1931   A modification of the method of Stewart and White for the determination of blood-fat, with observations on several species in postabsorptive conditions, *Biochem. J. 25*:1839 (with H. Friedman and M. A. Spiers).

1931   Effects of posterior pituitary extracts on basal metabolism, *Am. J. Physiol. 96*:640 (with F. W. Haynes).

1931   The effect of emotional stress on blood fat, *Am. J. Physiol 97*:533 (with F. Fulton).

1931   The effects of adrenalin, ephedrine and insulin on blood fat, *Am. J. Physiol. 97*:648 (with M. A. Spiers).

1931   The effect of various organs on the acetone content of the blood in phlorhizin and pancreatic diabetes, *J. Biol. Chem. 93*:337 (with W. Goldfarb and A. Weller).

1932 Note on the determination of blood fat, *Proc. Soc. Exp. Biol. (N.Y.) 29*:777.
1932 Respiratory quotient of various parts of the brain, *Proc. Soc. Exp. Biol. (N.Y.) 30*:366 (with J. F. Fazekas).
1932 The physiological action of alcohol, in: *Alcohol and Man* (H. Emerson, ed.), pp. 1–23, MacMillan, New York.
1932 The role of lactic acid in the living organism, *Yale J. Biol. Med. 4*:259.
1932 Changes in blood fat produced by fasting, phlorhizin and pancreatectomy, *Am. J. Physiol. 99*:619 (with W. H. Chambers, A. L. Hunter, and M. A. Spiers).
1932 Studies in the physiology of vitamins. XVII. The effect of thyroid administration upon the anorexia characteristic of lack of undifferentiated vitamin B, *Am. J. Physiol. 99*:689 (with W. Goldfarb and G. R. Cowgill).
1932 Effects of alcohol on metabolism, *Am. J. Physiol. 101*:57 (with L. H. Nahum, N. Rakieten, J. F. Fazekas, and D. DuBois).
1932 The respiratory quotient of the brain, *Am. J. Physiol. 101*:446 (with L. H. Nahum).
1932 Effect of posterior pituitary extracts on the constituents of the blood, *Am. J. Physiol. 101*:711 (with F. W. Haynes and J. F. Fazekas).
1932 Studies on subcutaneous absorption, *Am. J. Physiol. 102*:365 (with G. S. Goldman and M. Y. Krosnick).
1932 Insulin and appetite. I. A method for increasing weight in thin patients, *Am. J. Med. Sci. 183*:608 (with L. H. Nahum).
1933 Effects of alcohol on metabolism, *Arch. Sci. Biol. (Bologna) 18*:179.
1933 Ketone substance production and destruction in certain tissues of diabetic dogs, *J. Biol. Chem. 101*:441 (with W. Goldfarb).
1933 Respiratory quotient of cerbral cortex in B_1 avitaminosis, *Proc. Soc. Exp. Biol. (N.Y.) 30*:903 (with J. F. Fazekas, N. Rakieten, and R. Sanders).
1933 Effect of methylene blue and cyanide on respiration of cerbral cortex, testicle, liver and kidney, *Proc. Soc. Exp. Biol. (N.Y.) 30*:904 (with J. F. Fazekas and M. H. Hurlburt).
1933 Effects of methylene blue on respiratory metabolism of the rat, *Proc. Soc. Exp. Biol. (N.Y.) 30*:906 (with W. Goldfarb).
1933 Effect of methylene blue on the respiratory quotient of the brain *in situ, Proc. Soc. Exp. Biol. (N.Y.) 30*:907 (with N. Rakieten, L. H. Nahum, D. DuBois, and R. Sanders).
1933 The ketogenic–antiketogenic ratio, *Am. J. Physiol. 105*:50 (with W. Goldfarb).
1933 The metabolism of alcohol, *J. Am. Med. Assoc. 100*:651 (with L. H. Nahum, N. Rakieten, J. F. Fazekas, D. DuBois, and E. F. Gildea).
1934 The influence of glycine on creatinuria in peripheral neuritis, *Am. J. Med. Sci. 188*:560 (with M. J. C. Allinson and H. H. Henstell).
1934 Changes of the carbohydrate metabolism of the heart following coronary occlusion, *Am. J. Physiol. 109*:403 (with W. Goldfarb and L. H. Nahum).
1934 Diabetic hyperpyrexia, *Am. J. Physiol. 110*:19 (with J. F. Fazekas, L. H. Nahum, D. DuBois, L. Greenburg, and A. Gilman).
1934 A study of subcutaneous absorption in the adrenalectomized rat, *Am. J. Physiol. 110*:153 (with S. B. Barker and J. F. Fazekas).
1934 The metabolism of tissues excised from adrenalectomized rats, *Am. J. Physiol. 110*:348 (with J. F. Fazekas, S. B. Barker, and M. H. Hurlburt).
1934 The lipid components of the lymph of the thoracic duct of the dog, *Am. J. Physiol. 110*:348 (with S. H. Brockett and M. A. Spiers).
1934 The respiratory quotient of muscle of depancreatized dogs, *Am. J. Physiol. 110*:352 (with W. Goldfarb, N. Rakieten, L. H. Nahum, and D. DuBois).
1934 A study of ketosis in the phlorhizinized rat, *J. Biol. Chem. 105*:283 (with W. Goldfarb and S. B. Barker).

1934   A study of ketosis in fasted and fat-fed rats, *J. Biol. Chem. 105*:287 (with W. Goldfarb and S. B. Barker).
1934   The metabolism of fever. With special reference to diabetic hyperpyrexia, *Bull. N.Y. Acad. Med. 10*:16.
1934   The effect of some compounds of barbituric acid and of urethane, *J. Pharmacol. Exp. Ther. 50*:328 (with N. Rakieten, L. H. Nahum, D. DuBois, and E. F. Gildea).
1934   Morphine acidosis, *J. Pharmacol. Exp. Ther. 52*:437 (with N. Rakieten and D. DuBois).
1935   Glucose excretion after exercise in experimental diabetes, *J. Biol. Chem. 108*:217 (with W. H. Chambers and M. A. Kennard).
1935   A comparative study of some of the changes produced by various types of drugs in schizophrenic patients, *Am. J. Psychiatry 91*:1289 (with E. F. Gildea, O. E. Hubbard, and J. F. Fazekas).
1935   Changes of the RQ following the injection of methylene blue, cysteine, or cystine, *Am. J. Physiol. 113*:51 (with W. Goldfarb).
1935   Effect of nicotine on oxidations in the brain, *Am. J. Physiol. 113*:63 (with J. F. Fazekas).
1935   The carriage of the blood gases and the acid–base equilibrium of the blood, in: *A Textbook of Biochemistry* (Harrow and Sherwin, eds.), pp. 441–461, Saunders, Philadelphia.
1935   Respiration and respiratory metabolism, in: *A Textbook of Biochemistry* (Harrow and Sherwin, eds.), pp. 462–489, Saunders, Philadelphia.
1935   Diabetic hyperpyrexia, in: *Problèmes d. Biol. et d. Méd.*, Volume jubilaire dédié au Prof. Lina Stern, pp. 377–385 (with J. F. Fazekas).
1936   The carbohydrate metabolism of the heart during pancreas diabetes, *Am. J. Physiol.) 114*:273 (with W. Goldfarb and J. F. Fazekas).
1936   Metabolic aspects of thyroid–adrenal interrelationship, *Am. J. Physiol. 115*:415 (with S. B. Barker and J. F. Fazekas).
1936   Effect of nicotine on the oxidations of the diabetic brain, *Am. J. Physiol. 116*:46 (with J. F. Fazekas).
1936   A mechanism of dehydration in diabetes, *Am. J. Physiol. 116*:75 (with J. F. Fazekas).
1936   The effect of methylene blue, cystine and cysteine on the metabolism of the intact animal, *Am. J. Physiol. 117*:631 (with W. Goldfarb and J. F. Fazekas).
1936   The effect of zinc and aluminum on the hypoglycemic action of insulin, *J. Pharmacol. Exp. Ther. 58*:260 (with J. F. Fazekas).
1936   Effect of methylene blue, cystine and cysteine on the metabolism of isolated brain tissue, *Am. J. Physiol. 117*:631 (with W. Goldfarb and J. F. Fazekas).
1936   Blood sugar in experimental diabetes, *Am. J. Physiol. 12*:284.
1936   Studies on sodium loss, *Proc. Soc. Exp. Biol. (N.Y.) 34*:450 (with J. F. Fazekas and M. A. Spiers).
1936   The effects of inhalation of carbon dioxide on the carbon dioxide capacity of arterial blood, *J. Biol. Chem. 113*:383 (with E. F. Gildea, N. Rakieten, and D. DuBois).
1936   Studies on the physiology of lactation. V. The induction of lactation in depancreatized dogs, *Anat. Rec. 66*:201 (with W. O. Nelson and J. F. Fazekas).
1937   The respiratory quotient of renal tissue of Houssay dogs, *Am. J. Physiol. 118*:297 (with J. F. Fazekas and E. H. Campbell).
1937   The formation of acetylcholine-like substances by excised tissues, *Am. J. Physiol. 119*:306 (with J. F. Fazekas).
1937   The effect of hypoglycemia on the metabolism of the brain, *Endocrinology 119*:335 (with J. F. Fazekas).
1937   Effect of metrazol convulsions on brain metabolism, *Proc. Soc. Exp. Biol. (N.Y.) 37*:359 (with K. M. Bowman, J. F. Fazekas, and L. L. Orenstein).

1937 Chronic adrenal insufficiency and pancreas diabetes, *Proc. Soc. Exp. Biol. (N.Y.)* *37*:361 (with J. F. Fazekas and S. J. Martin).

1937 Brain metabolism during the hypoglycemic treatment of schizophrenia, *Science 86*:271 (with K. M. Bowman, J. Wortis, and J. F. Fazekas).

1937 The effect of hypoglycemia on the metabolism of the brain, *Am. J. Physiol. 21*:800 (with J. F. Fazekas).

1937 Protamine-insulin and infection, *Am. J. Med. Sci. 194*:345 (with J. F. Fazekas).

1938 Carbohydrate oxidation in normal and diabetic cerebral tissues, *J. Biol. Chem. 125*:545 (with Z. Baker and J. F. Fazekas).

1938 Respiratory quotient of diabetic liver, *Proc. Soc. Exp. Biol. (N.Y.) 38*:137 (with J. F. Fazekas).

1938 Carbohydrate metabolism, *Annu. Rev. Biochem. 7*:143.

1938 Effect of adrenal vein ligation and pancreatectomy on metabolism of renal tissue, *Proc. Soc. Exp. Biol. (N.Y.) 38*:499 (with Z. Baker and J. F. Fazekas).

1938 Syndromes secondary to prolonged hypoglycemia, *Proc. Soc. Exp. Biol. (N.Y.) 39*:244 (with J. F. Fazekas, A. O. Bernstein, E. H. Campbell, and S. J. Martin).

1938 Effect of acute anoxia produced by breathing nitrogen on the course of schizophrenia, *Proc. Soc. Exp. Biol. (N.Y.) 39*:367 (with F. A. D. Alexander and B. Lipetz).

1938 The effect of ligation of the lumboadrenal veins on the course of experimental diabetes in cats and dogs, *Science 87*:144 (with J. F. Fazekas and S. J. Martin).

1938 Effect of nicotine on the oxidation of glucose, *Am. J. Physiol. 123*:6 (with Z. Baker).

1938 The oxidation of various substrates by the diabetic kidney, *Am. J. Physiol. 123*:62 (with J. F. Fazekas and Z. Baker).

1938 Metabolism of depancreatized dogs and cats following bilateral ligation of the lumboadrenal veins, *Am. J. Physiol. 123*:100 (with J. F. Fazekas and S. J. Martin).

1938 Syndromes produced in pancreatized cats and dogs as a result of bilateral ligation of the lumboadrenal veins, *Am. J. Physiol. 123*:142 (with S. J. Martin and J. F. Fazekas).

1938 The effect of bilateral ligation of the lumboadrenal veins on the course of pancreas diabetes, *Am. J. Physiol. 123*:725 (with J. F. Fazekas and S. J. Martin).

1939 The mechanism of the symptoms of insulin hypoglycemia, *Am. J. Psychiatry 96*:371 (with J. P. Frostig, J. F. Fazekas, and Z. Hadidian).

1939 Nitrogen inhalation therapy for schizophrenia. Preliminary report on technique, *Am. J. Psychiatry 96*:643 (with F. A. D. Alexander).

1939 Clinical electroencephalographic and biochemical changes during insulin hypoglycemia, *Proc. Soc. Exp. Biol. (N.Y.) 40*:401 (with J. P. Frostig, J. F. Fazekas, H. Hoagland, and Z. Hadidian).

1939 Effect of pyocyanin on cerebral metabolism, *Proc. Soc. Exp. Biol. (N.Y.) 42*:446 (with J. F. Fazekas, H. Colyer, and S. Nesin).

1939 Effect of cyanide on cerebral metabolism, *Proc. Soc. Exp. Biol. (N.Y.) 42*:496 (with J. F. Fazekas and H. Colyer).

1939 Effect of hypothermia on cerebral metabolism, *Proc. Soc. Exp. Biol. (N.Y.) 42*:537 (with J. F. Fazekas).

1939, 1940, 1941 Brain metabolism, *Trans. Kans. City Acad. Med,* presented at the Kansas City Academy of Medicine, November 17, 1939.

1939 Cerebral metabolism and electrical activity during insulin hypoglycemia in man, *Am. J. Physiol. 125*:578 (with Z. Hadidian, J. F. Fazekas, and H. Hoagland).

1939 The respiratory metabolism of infant brain, *Am. J. Physiol. 125*:601 (with Z. Baker and J. F. Fazekas).

1939 Nitrogen inhalation therapy for schizophrenia, *Am. J. Physiol. 126*:535 (with F. A. D. Alexander, B. Lipet, and J. F. Fazekas).

1939 Effect of hypoglycemia and pentobarbital sodium on the electrical activity of the dog cerebral cortex and hypothalamus, *Am. J. Physiol. 126*:536 (with H. Hoagland, E. H. Campbell, J. F. Fazekas, and Z. Hadidian).

1939   The formation of acetylcholine by tissues of the rat, *Am. J. Physiol. 127*:381 (with P. Sykowski and J. F. Fazekas).

1939   The glucose and lactic acid exchanges during hypoglycemia, *Am. J. Physiol. 127*:685 (with J. F. Fazekas and S. Nesin).

1939   Biochemical changes occurring in the cerebral blood during the insulin treatment of schizophrenia, *J. Nerv. Ment. Dis. 89*:273 (with K. M. Bowman, J. Wortis, and J. F. Fazekas).

1939   Metabolism of the brain during insulin and metrazol treatments of schizophrenia, *J. Am. Med. Assoc. 112*:1572 (with K. M. Bowman, J. Wortis, and J. F. Fazekas).

1939   Electrocardiographic changes during hypoglycemia and anoxemia, *Endocrinology 24*:536 (with S. J. Martin, F. A. D. Alexander, and J. F. Fazekas).

1939   Effects of hypoglycemia and pentobarbital sodium on electrical activity of cerebral cortex and hypothalamus (dogs), *J. Neurophysiol. 2*:276 (with H. Hoagland, E. H. Campbell, J. F. Fazekas, and Z. Hadidian).

1939   The effect of cocarboxylase upon metabolism and neuropsychiatric phenomena in pellagrins with beriberi, *Science, 90*:141 (with F. H. Lewy, J. P. Frostig, and T. D. Spies).

1939   Cerebral metabolism during fever, *Science 90*:398 (with K. M. Bowman, W. Goldfarb, and J. F. Fazekas).

1940   A study of the central action of metrazol, *Am. J. Psychiatry 973*:366 (with B. Libet and J. F. Fazekas).

1940   Oxygen consumption in the psychoses of the senium, *Am. J. Psychiatry 97*:566 (with D. E. Cameron, S. R. Rosen, and J. F. Fazekas).

1940   Changes in cerebral blood flow and arterio–venous oxygen difference during insulin hypoglycemia, *Proc. Soc. Exp. Biol. (N.Y.) 45*:468 (with K. M. Bowman, C. Daly, J. F. Fazekas, J. Wortis, and W. Goldfarb).

1940   Prolonged coma and cerebral metabolism, *Arch. Neurol. Psychiatry (Chicago) 44*:1098 (with K. M. Bowman and J. F. Fazekas).

1940   Cerebral carbohydrate metabolism during deficiency of various members of the vitamin B complex, *Amer. J. Med. Sci. 199*:849 (with T. D. Spies, J. F. Fazekas, and S. Nesin).

1940   Temperature and brain metabolism, *Am. J. Med. Sci. 200*:347 (with K. M. Bowman, J. F. Fazekas, and W. Goldfarb).

1940   Temperature and brain metabolism, *J. Physiol. USSR 29*:271 (with K. M. Bowman, W. Goldfarb, and J. F. Fazekas).

1940   Cerebral metabolism in mongolian idiocy and phenylpyruvic oligophrenia, *Arch. Neurol. Psychiatry (Chicago) 44*:1213 (with J. F. Fazekas).

1940   Brain metabolism in mongolian idiocy and phenylpyruvic oligophrenia, *Am. J. Ment. Defic. 45*:37 (with J. F. Fazekas and S. Nesin).

1940   The effects of alcohol and pentobarbital on metabolism of excised cerebral tissues of adult and infant rats, *Am. J. Physiol. 129*:382 (with P. Sykowski and J. F. Fazekas).

1940   Control of electrical and oxidative activity of brain by temperature, *Am. J. Physiol. 129*:404 (with B. Libet, J. F. Fazekas, A. M. Meirowsky, and E. H. Campbell).

1941   The electrical response of the kitten and adult cat brain to cerebral anemia and analeptics, *Am. J. Physiol. 132*:232 (with B. Libet and J. F. Fazekas).

1941   A comparative study of excised cerebral tissues of adult and infant rats, *Am. J. Physiol. 132*:293 (with P. Sykowski and J. F. Fazekas).

1941   Comparative studies of the metabolism of the brain of infant and adult dogs, *Am. J. Physiol. 132*:454 (with J. F. Fazekas).

1941   Cerebral blood flow and brain metabolism during insulin hypoglycemia, *Am. J. Physiol. 132*:640 (with K. M. Bowman, C. Daly, J. F. Fazekas, J. Wortis, and W. Goldfarb).

1941   Comparative effects of stimulants on infant and adult cerebral tissues, *Am. J. Physiol. 133*:325 (with H. C. Herrlich and J. F. Fazekas).

1941   Tolerance of the newborn to hypoxia and anoxia, *Am. J. Physiol. 133*:327 (with F. A. D. Alexander and J. F. Fazekas).

1941   Hypoglycemia in the infant rat, *Am. J. Physiol. 133*:328 (with J. F. Fazekas and F. A. D. Alexander).

1941   Tolerance of the newborn to anoxia, *Am. J. Physiol. 134*:281 (with J. F. Fazekas and F. A. D. Alexander).

1941   The significance of a pathway of carbohydrate breakdown not involving glycolysis, *J. Biol. Chem. 139*:971 (with J. F. Fazekas).

1941   Effects of cyanide and iodoacetate on survival period of infant rats, *Proc. Soc. Exp. Biol. (N.Y.) 46*:553 (with J. F. Fazekas and F. A. D. Alexander).

1941   Composition of the milk of the monkey *(M. Mulatta), Proc. Soc. Exp. Biol. (N.Y.) 48*:133 (with G. van Wagenen and H. R. Catchpole).

1941   Survival of infant and adult rats at high altitudes, *Proc. Soc. Exp. Biol. (N.Y.) 48*:446 (with H. C. Herrlich and J. F. Fazekas).

1941   Availability of lactic acid for brain oxidations, *J. Neurophysiol. 4*:243 (with J. Wortis, K. M. Bowman, W. Goledarb, and J. F. Fazekas).

1942   Action of insulin on pyruvate formation in depancreatized dogs, *Fed. Proc. Fed. Am. Soc. Exp. Biol. 1*:12 (with E. Bueding and J. F. Fazekas).

1942   Effect of insulin on pyruvic acid formation in depancreatized dogs, *Science 95*:282 (with E. Bueding, J. F. Fazekas, and H. C. Herrlich).

1942   A study of the comparative toxic effects of morphine on the fetal, newborn and adult rats, *J. Pharmacol. Exp. Ther. 75*:363 (with A Chesler and G. C. LaBelle).

1942   The relative effects of toxic doses of alcohol on fetal, newborn and adult rats, *Q. J. Stud. Alcohol 3*:1 (with A. Chesler and G. C. LaBelle).

1942   Brain metabolism and the mental deficiencies, *Am. J. Ment. Defic. 46*:302.

1942   Fundamental concepts in the treatment of diabetes mellitus and its complications. An interpretation of the smyptoms of hypoglycemia, No. 21 of series published by The New York Diabetes Association, 2 East 103rd St., New York City, May 1942.

1942   Hypoglycemic reactions, *Proc. Am. Diabetes Assoc. 2*:161.

1942   Mechanisms for the maintenance of life in the newborn during anoxia, *Am. J. Physiol. 135*:387 (with A. O. Bernstein, H. E. Herrlich, A. Chesler, and J. F. Fazekas).

1942   The metabolic effects of potassium, temperature, methylene blue and paraphenylenediamine on infant and adult brain, *Am. J. Physiol. 137*:327 (with A. O. Bernstein, J. F. Fazekas, H. C. Herrlich, and E. Rich).

1942   Effect of thyroid medication on brain metabolism of cretins, *Am. J. Psychiatry 98*:489 (with C. Daly, J. F. Fazekas, and H. C. Herrlich).

1942   Factor of hypoxia in the shock therapies of schizophrenia, *Arch. Neurol. Psychiatry 47*:800 (with J. F. Fazekas).

1942   Studies on the effects of adding carbon dioxide to oxygen-enriched atmospheres in low pressure chambers. II. The oxygen and carbon dioxide tensions of cerebral blood, *J. Aviat. Med. 13*:177 (with J. F. Fazekas, H. E. Herrlich, A. E. Johnson, and A. L. Barach).

1942   Effect of iodoacetate on survival period during hypoxia, *Fed. Proc. 1*:40 (with H. C. Herrlich, E. Rich, R. Barstow, and J. F. Fazekas).

1943   An evaluation of the factor of depression of brain metabolism in the treatment of schizophrenia, *Fed. Am. Soc. Exp. Biol. Psychiatr. Q. 17*:164 (with C. H. Bellinger, C. F. Terrence, and B. Lipet).

1943   Effect of insulin on pyruvic acid formation on depancreatized dogs, *J. Biol. Chem.* *148*:97 (with E. Bueding, J. F. Fazekas, and H. C. Herrlich).

1943   The glycogen content of various parts of the central nervous system of dogs and cats at different ages, *Arch. Biochem.* *2*:175 (with A. Chesler).

1943   Glycogen content of various parts of the central nervous system of dogs and cats, *Fed. Proc. Fed. Am. Soc. Exp. Biol.* *2*:6 (with A. Chesler).

1943   Effect of age on cerebral arterio-venous oxygen difference, *Fed. Proc. Fed. Am. Soc. Exp. Biol.* *2*:21 (with J. F. Fazekas).

1943   Effect of anoxia and hypoglycemia on survival period of adult rats, *Fed. Proc. Fed. Am. Soc. Exp. Biol.* *2*:23 (with E. Homburger).

1943   Comparative toxicity of pentobarbital in the newborn and adult rat, *J. Lab. Clin. Med.* *28*:706 (with B. Etsten and F. A. D. Alexander).

1943   Anaerobic survival of adult animals, *Am. J. Physiol.* *139*:366 (with J. F. Fazekas).

1943   Electroshock. A round table discussion, *Am. J. Psychiatry* *100*:361.

1943   The role of the vitamins in brain metabolism, *Res. Publ. Assoc. Res. Nerv. Ment. Dis.* *22*:33.

1943   Effect of neosynephrin on gaseous exchange of the brain, *Proc. Soc. Exp. Biol. (N.Y.)* *53*:78 (with C. Daly and J. F. Fazekas).

1943   Brain metabolism and mental deficiency, *Amer. J. Ment. Defic.* *48*:137 (with J. F. Fazekas).

1943   Cerebral arterio-venous oxygen difference. I. Effect of age and mental deficiency, *Arch. Neurol. Psychiatry* *50*:546 (with J. F. Fazekas).

1943   Effect of hypoglycemia and anoxia on the survival period of infant and adult rats and cats, *Endocrinology* *33*:96 (with J. F. Fazekas and E. Homburger).

1944   Carbohydrate metabolism in vitamin B_1 deficiency, *J. Biol. Chem.* *153*:219 (with A. Chesler and E. Homburger).

1944   A comparison of the relationship of lactic acid and pyruvic acid in the normal and diabetic dog, *J. Biol. Chem.* *155*:413 (with A. Chesler).

1944   Comparative studies of the rates of oxidation and glycolysis in the cerebral cortex and brain stem of the rat, *Am. J. Physiol.* *141*:513 (with A. Chesler).

1944   Glycolysis in the parts of the central nervous system of cats and dogs during growth, *Am. J. Physiol.* *142*:544 (with A. Chesler).

1944   The cerebral arterio-venous oxygen difference. II. Mental deficiency, *Arch. Neurol. Psychiatry* *51*:73 (with J. F. Fazekas).

1944   Effect of insulin hypoglycemia on glycogen content of parts of the central nervous system of the dog, *Arch. Neurol. Psychiatry* *52*:114 (with A. Chesler).

1944   The effects of insulin hypoglycemia on the glycogen content of the various parts of the central nervous system of the dog, *Fed. Proc. Fed. Am. Soc. Exp. Biol.* *3*:7 (with A. Chesler).

1944   Carbohydrate metabolism in vitamin B_1 deficiency, *Fed. Proc. Fed. Am. Soc. Exp. Biol.* *3*:93 (with A. Chesler and E. Homburger).

1944   The physiology of the "shock" therapies, *Psychiatr. Q.* *18*:357.

1944   A review of hypoglycemia, its physiology and pathology, symptomatology and treatment, *Am. J. Dig. Dis.* *11*:1.

1944   The oxygen content of cerebral blood in patients with acute symptomatic psychoses and acute destructive brain lesions, *Am. J. Psychiatry* *100*:648 (with J. F. Fazekas).

1945   Energy metabolism, *Annu. Rev. Physiol.* *7*:181.

1945   Cerebral metabolism in patients with depression, *Am. J. Psychiatry* *101*:453 (with D. E. Cameron, E. Homburger, and F. Feldman).

1945   Pyruvic acid cycle, *Fed. Proc. Fed. Am. Soc. Exp. Biol.* *4*:33 (with E. Homburger and W. A. Himwich).

1945   Chronic thiamin deficiency, *Fed. Proc. Fed. Am. Soc. Exp. Biol. 4*:155 (with W. A. Himwich).

1946   Stages and signs of pentothal anesthesia: Physiologic basis, *Anesthesiology 7*:536 (with B. Etsten).

1946   Similarity of cerebral arterio-venous oxygen differences in right and left sides of resting man, *Arch. Neurol. Psychiatry 55*:578 (with G. York and E. Homburger).

1946   Pattern of metabolic depression induced with pentothal sodium, *Arch. Neurol Psychiatry 56*:171 (with B. Etsten and G. York).

1946   The effect of hypoglycemia and age on the glycogen content of the various parts of the feline central nervous system, *Am. J. Physiol. 146*:389 (with S. Ferris).

1946   Effect of pentothal anesthesia on canine cerebral cortex, *Am. J. Physiol. 147*:343 (with E. Homburger, W. A. Himwich, B. Etsten, G. York, and R. Maresca).

1946   Criteria for the stages of pentothal anesthesia, *J. Nerv. Ment. Dis. 104*:407 (with B. Etsten).

1946   Pyruvic acid in exercising depancreatized dogs and diabetic patients, *J. Biol. Chem. 165*:513 (with W. A. Himwich).

1946   The effect of age on the hypoglycemic depletion of glycogen in the central nervous system, *Fed. Proc. Fed. Am. Soc. Exp. Biol. 5*:27 (with S. Ferris).

1946   Effect of pentothal anesthesia on canine cerebral cortex, *Fed. Proc. Fed. Am. Soc. Exp. Biol. 5*:47 (with E. Homburger, B. Etsten, R. Maresca, G. York, and W. A. Himwich).

1946   Organic phosphates and insulin, *Fed. Proc. Fed. Am. Soc. Exp. Biol. 5*:47 (with W. A. Himwich).

1946   Brain metabolism in unanesthetized and anesthetized man, *Fed. Proc. Fed. Am. Soc. Exp. Biol. 5*:47 (with W. A. Himwich, E. Homburger, and R. Maresca).

1946   Pyruvic acid exchange of the brain, *J. Neurophysiol. 9*:133 (with W. A. Himwich).

1947   The functional organization of the central nervous system as observed in pentothal anesthesia, in: *Abstracts of Communications of the Seventeenth International Physiological Congress,* Oxford.

1947   The influence of some organs on the pyruvate level in the blood, *Am. J. Physiol. 148*:323 (with W. A. Himwich).

1947   Brain metabolism in man: Unanesthetized and in pentothal narcosis, *Am. J. Psychiatry 103*:689 (with W. A. Himwich, E. Homburger, and R. Maresca).

1947   Factors influencing the susceptibility of rats to barbiturates, *Fed. Proc. Fed. Am. Soc. Exp. Biol. 6*:131 (with E. Homburger and B. Etsten).

1947   Some factors affecting the susceptibility of rats to various barbiturates, *J. Lab. Clin. Med. 32*:540 (with E. Homburger and B. Etsten).

1947   The influence of vitamin B_1 deficiency on the pyruvate exchange of the heart, *Am. Heart J. 33*:341 (with F. S. Randles, W. A. Himwich, and E. Homburger).

1948   Management of anoxia during pentothal anesthesia, *Am. J. Surg. 76*:268 (with B. Etsten).

1948   Anoxic survival and di-isopropyl fluorophosphate (DFP), *Science 108*:41 (with A. M. Freedman).

1948   Correlation between signs of toxicity and cholinesterase level of brain and blood during recovery from di-isopropyl fluorophosphate (DFP) poisoning, *Fed. Proc. Fed. Am. Soc. Exp. Biol. 7*:36 (with A. M. Freedman).

1948   The effect of size, sex and pregnancy on the lethality of di-isopropyl fluorophosphate (DFP), *Fed. Proc. Fed. Am. Soc. Exp. Biol. 7*:36 (with A. M. Freedman).

1948   Di-isopropyl fluorophosphate (DFP): Site of injection and variation in response, *Fed. Proc. Fed. Am. Soc. Exp. Biol. 7*:55 (with A. M. Freedman).

1948   Effect of age on lethality of di-isopropyl fluorophosphate, *Am. J. Physiol. 153*:121 (with A. M. Freedman).

1949   Experimental production of electrical major convulsive patterns, *Am. J. Physiol. 156*:117 (with A. M. Freedman, P. D. Bales, and Alice Willis).

1949   DFP: Site of injection and variation in response, *Am. J. Physiol. 156*:125 (with A. M. Freedman).

1949   Correlation between signs of toxicity and cholinesterase level of brain and blood during recovery from di-isopropyl fluorophosphate (DFP) poisoning, *Am. J. Physiol. 157*:80 (with A. M. Freedman and Alice Willis).

1949   Evidence for the evolution of the brain, *Humanist 8*:159.

1949   The brain and the symptomatology of the anoxias, *Anesthesiology 10*:663.

1949   Effects of di-isopropyl fluorophosphate (DFP) on electroencephalogram and cholinesterase activity, *Fed. Proc. Fed. Am. Soc. Exp. Biol. 8*:66 (with J. L. Hampson, C. F. Essig, and Alice Willis).

1949   Effect of tridione on convulsions caused by di-isopropyl fluorophosphate (DFP), *Fed. Proc. Fed. Am. Soc. Exp. Biol. 8*:75 (with C. F. Essig and J. L. Hampson).

1949   Cholinergic nature of the vestibular receptor mechanism: Forced circling movements, *Fed. Proc. Fed. Am. Soc. Exp. Biol. 8*: 75 (with C. F. Essig, J. L. Hampson, P. D. Bales, and A. M. Freedman).

1950   Effect of panparnit on brain wave changes induced by di-isopropyl fluorophosphate (DFP), *Science 111*:38 (with C. F. Essig, J. L. Hampson, P. D. Bales, and Alice Willis).

1950   An experimental analysis of biochemically induced circling behavior, *J. Neurophysiol. 13*:269 (with C. F. Essig, J. L. Hampson, and Alice McCauley).

1950   Effects of di-isopropyl fluorophosphate (DFP) on electroencephalogram and cholinesterase activity, *Electroencephalogr. Clin. Neurophysiol. 2*:41 (with J. L. Hampson, C. F. Essig, and Alice McCauley).

1950   Medical aspects of fat metabolism, *Cyclopedia of Medicine, Surgery, Specialties 9*:85.

1950   Some evidence on the functional organization of the brain, *Biochim. Biophys. Acta (Amsterdam) 4*:118.

1950   Effect of trimethadione (tridione) and other drugs on convulsions caused by di-isopropyl fluorophosphate (DFP), *Am. J. Psychiatry 106*:816 (with C. F. Essig, J. L. Hampson, P. D. Bales, and A. M. Freedman).

1950   A central action of some antihistamines. Correction of forced circling movements and of seizure brain waves produced by the intracarotid injection of di-isopropyl fluorophosphate (DFP), *Am. J. Psychiatry 107*:367 (with R. J. Johns).

1950   Forced circling movements (adversive syndrome), *Arch. Otolaryngol. 51*:672 (with M. Schiff and W. G. Esmond).

1951   The effects of DFP on the convulsant dose of theophylline, theophylline-ethylenediamine and 8-chlorotheophylline, *J. Pharmacol. Exp. Ther. 101*:237 (with R. J. Johns and P. D. Bales).

1952   Mechanism of seizures induced by di-isopropyl fluorophosphate (DFP), *Am. J. Psychiatry 108*:847 (with W. F. Bouzarth).

1952   Effect of shock therapies on the brain, in: *Biology of Mental Health and Disease*, pp. 548–561, Milbank Memorial Fund, Hoeber, New York.

1952   The functional organization of the central nervous system, an experimental analysis, *Proc. Inst. Med. Chicago 19*:115.

1952   Report of committee on research. III. Anticonvulsant and convulsant agents, *Epilepsia Third Ser. 1*:143.

1952   Comparative effects of antiepileptic and other drugs upon forced circling produced by the intracarotid injection of di-isopropyl fluorophosphate (DFP), *Fed. Proc. Fed. Am. Soc. Exp. Biol. 11*:70 (with I. H. Weiner, Alayne Coombs, and Edith Campbell).

1953 Biochemically induced circling behavior, *Confin. Neurol. (Basel) 13*:65 (with C. F. Essig and J. L. Hampson).

1953 General neurophysiology (biochemical aspects), in: *Progress in Neurology and Psychiatry*, Vol. VIII (E. A. Spiegel, ed.), pp. 14–39, Grune and Stratton, New York.

1953 Some effects of DFP (di-isopropyl fluorophosphate) and atropine on behavior, *Arzneim.-Forsch. 3*:228.

1954 Brain acetylcholinesterase activities in rabbits exhibiting three behavioral patterns following the intracarotid injection of di-isopropyl fluorophosphate, *Am. J. Physiol. 177*:175 (with M. H. Aprison and P. Nathan).

1954 Relationship between age and cholinesterase activity in several rabbit brain areas, *Am. J. Physiol. 179*:502 (with M. H. Aprison).

1954 A study of the relationship between asymmetric acetylcholinesterase activities in rabbit brain and three behavioral patterns, *Science 119*:158 (with M. H. Aprison and P. Nathan).

1955 Concentrations of a brain neurohormone, acetycholine, associated with a syndrome resembling the motor aura of an epileptic episode, American League against Epilepsy (Abstract), Dec. 8 (with M. H. Aprison and P. Nathan).

1955 Age and the water content of rabbit brain parts, *Am. J. Physiol. 180*:205 (with Juanita Graves).

1955 Basic research drugs used in psychiatry, in: *Proceedings of a Scientific Medical Conference, Marketing Conference*, pp. 48–53, American Pharmaceutical Manufacturers Association.

1955 General neurophysiology (biochemistry), in: *Progress in Neurology and Psychiatry*, Vol. X (E. A. Spiegel, ed.), pp. 16–56, Grune and Stratton, New York.

1955 The anatomy and physiology of the frontal lobes (metabolic considerations), in: *Clinical Neurosurgery* (Raymond K. Thompson, ed.), pp. 108–116, William and Wilkins, Baltimore.

1955 The new psychiatric drugs, *Sci. Am. 193*:80.

1955 The use of fluids and electrolytes in the management of the neurosurgical patient (the blood–brain barrier), in: *Clinical Neurosurgery* (Raymond K. Thompson, ed.), pp. 166–179, William and Wilkins, Baltimore.

1955 The permeability of the blood–brain barrier to glutamic acid in the developing rat, in: *Biochemistry of the Developing Nervous System* (H. Waelsch, ed.), pp.pp. 202–207, Academic Press, New York (with W. A. Himwich).

1955 The effect of age on cholinesterase activity of rabbit brain, in: *Biochemistry of the Developing Nervous System* (H. Waelsch, ed.), pp. 301–307, Academic Press, New York (with M. H. Aprison).

1955, 1956 An analysis of the activating system including its use for screening antiparkinson drugs, *Yale J. Biol. Med. 28*:308 (with F. Rinaldi).

1955 Some behavioral effects associated with feeding sodium glutamate to patients with psychiatric disorders, *J. Nerv. Ment. Dis. 121*:40 (with K. Wolff, A. L. Hunsicker, and W. A. Himwich).

1955 Prospects in psychopharmacology, *J. Nerv. Ment. Dis. 122*:413.

1955 The cerebral electrographic changes induced by LSD and mescaline are corrected by Frenquel, *J. Nerv. Ment. Dis. 122*:424 (with F. Rinaldi).

1955 A comparison of the effects of atropine with those of several central nervous system stimulants on rabbits exhibiting forced circling following the intracarotid injection of di-isopropyl fluorophosphate, *Confin. Neurol. (Basel) 15*:1 (with P. Nathan and M. H. Aprison.

1955 The site of action of antiparkinson drugs, *Confin. Neurol. (Basel) 15*:209 (with F. Rinaldi).

1955   Effect of some centrally acting drugs on convulsive circling, *Proc. Soc. Exp. Biol. (N.Y.) 90*:364 (with P. Nathan and M. H. Aprison).

1955   Therapeutic effects of Frenquel in psychotic patients: A comparison of high and low dosage, presented by Dr. H. E. Himwich at AAAS Meeting, December, Atlanta, Georgia (with R. Rinaldi, E. E. Haynes, and L. H. Rudy).

1955   A comparison of effects of reserpine and some barbitures on the electrical activity of cortical and subcortical structures of the brain of rabbits, *Ann. N.Y. Acad. Sci. 61*:27 (with F. Rinaldi).

1955   Alerting responses and actions of atropine and cholinergic drugs, *Arch. Neurol. Psychiatry 73*:387 (with F. Rinaldi).

1955   Cholinergic mechanism involved in function of mesodiencephalic activating system, *Arch. Neurol. Psychiatry 73*:396 (with F. Rinaldi).

1955   Drugs affecting psychotic behavior and the function of the mesodiencephalic activating system, *Dis. Nerv. Syst. 16*:3 (with F. Rinaldi).

1955   Frenquel corrects certain cerebral electrographic changes, *Science 122*:198 (with F. Rinaldi).

1955   The effect of meratran on twenty-five institutionalized mental patients, *Am. J. Psychiatry 111*:837 (with J. W. Schut).

1955   The use of Frenquel in the treatment of disturbed patients with psychoses of long duration, *Am. J. Psychiatry 112*:343 (with F. Rinaldi and L. H. Rudy).

1955   Comparative effects of Frenquel, reserpine and chlorpromazine on moderately disturbed patients with long histories of hospitalization, presented at the A.P.A. Midwest Regional Conference, September (with L. H. Rudy).

1956   A cholinergic mechanism of the brain involved in convulsive circling, *Am. J. Physiol. 184*:244 (with M. H. Aprison and P. Nathan).

1956   Alcohol and brain physiology, in: *Alcoholism* (George N. Thompson, ed.), pp. 291–408, Charles C. Thomas, Springfield, Illinois.

1956   The effect of Frenquel on EEG changes procuded by LSD-25 and mescaline, in: *Lysergic Acid Diethylamide and Mescaline in Experimental Psychiatry,* (Louis Cholden, ed.), pp. 19–26, Grune and Stratton, New York.

1956   Views of the etiology of alcoholism (the organic view), in: *Alcoholism as a Medical Problem* (H. D. Kruse, ed.), pp. 32–39, Hoeber–Harper, New York.

1956   Brain metabolism in relation to aging, *J. Chron. Dis. 3*:487 (with W. A. Himwich).

1956   An examination of phenothiazine derivatives with comparisons of their effects on the alerting reaction, chemical structure and therapeutic efficacy, *J. Nerv. Ment. Dis. 124*:53 (with F. Rinaldi and Dorothy Willis).

1956   Discussion of papers on basic observations of new psychopharmacological agents, *Psychiatr. Res. Rep. 4*:24.

1956   Comparative effects of azacyclonol, reserpine and chlorpromazine on moderately disturbed psychotic patients with long histories of hospitalization, *Psychiatr. Res. Rep. 4*:49 (with L. H. Rudy and F. Rinaldi).

1956   Therapeutic effects of azacyclonol in psychotic patients, *Psychiatr. Res. Rep. 4*:115 (with F. Rinaldi, E. E. Haynes, and L. H. Rudy).

1956   Clinical evaluation of azacyclonol, chlorpromazine and reserpine on a group of chronic and psychotic patients, *Am. J. Psychiatr. 112*:678 (with F. Rinaldi and L. H. Rudy).

1956   Clinical evaluation of Frenquel, chlorpromazine and reserpine on a group of chronic psychotic patients, *Am. J. Psychiatry 112*:678 (with F. Rinaldi and L. H. Rudy).

1956   Central and peripheral nervous effects of atropine sulfate and mepiperphenidol bromide (Darstine) on human subjects, *J. Appl. Physiol. 8*:635 (with R. P. White and F. Rinaldi).

1957   Some relationships between tranquilization, indollkylamines and brain structure, in:

Psychotropic Drugs (S. Garattini and V. Ghetti, eds.), pp. 21–25, Elsevier, Amsterdam (with E. Costa and F. Rinaldi).

1957 A comparative evaluation of two new central nervous system stimulants in severe psychoses, *J. Clin. Exp. Psychopathol. 18*:248 (with F. Hagenauer and L. H. Rudy).

1957 Evidence of interrelation among doctrines (from the organic approach), in: *Integrating the Approaches to Mental Disease* (H. D. Kruse, ed.), pp. 75–76, Hoeber, New York.

1957 *Alcoholism*, American Association for the Advancement of Science, Washington, D.C.

1957 Some recent advances in the physiology of alcohol and the treatment of acute and chronic alcoholism, in: *Alcoholism*, pp. 199–208, American Association for the Advancement of Science, Washington, D.C.

1957 The physiology of alcohol. *J. Am. Med. Assoc. 163*:545.

1957 *Tranquilizing Drugs*, American Association for the Advancement of Science, Washington, D.C.

1957 Analysis of the action of benztropine methanesulfonate against parkinsonism, in: *Tranquilizing Drugs* (H. E. Himwich, ed.), pp. 47–57, American Association for the Advancement of Science, Washington, D.C. (with F. Rinaldi).

1957 Viewpoints obtained from basic and clinical symposia on tranquilizing drugs, in: *Tranquilizing Drugs* (H. E. Himwich, ed.), pp. 183–192, American Association for the Advancement of Science, Washington, D.C.

1957 General neurophysiology (biochemistry), in: *Progress in Neurology and Psychiatry*, Vol. XII (E. A. Spiegel, ed.), pp. 18–42, Grune and Stratton, New York (with W. A. Himwich).

1957 The antiparkinson activity of benactyzine, *Arch. Int. Pharmacodyn. Ther. 110*:119 (with F. Rinaldi).

1957 The effect of drugs on the reticular system, in: *Brain Mechanisms and Drug Action* (W. W. Fields, ed.), pp. 15–43, Charles C. Thomas, Springfield, Illinois (with F. Rinaldi).

1957 Brain composition during the whole life span, *Geriatrics 12*:19 (with W. A. Himwich).

1957 A comparative study of two central nervous system stimulants, MER-22 and SKF 5, on chronic, blocked and withdrawn psychotic patients, *Am. J. Psychiatry 113*:840 (with F. Hagenauer and L. H. Rudy).

1957 Clinical evaluation of two phenothiazine compounds, promazine and mepazine, *Am. J. Psychiatry 113*:979 (with L. H. Rudy and D. C. Tasher).

1957 A clinical evaluation of l-glutavite in the treatment of elderly chronic deteriorated mental patients, *Ill. Med. J. 112*:121 (with T. T. Tourlentes and D. S. Huckins).

1957 Analysis of forced circling induced by DFP and ablation of cerebral structures, *Am. J. Physiol. 189*:513 (with R. P. White).

1957 Circus movements and excitation of striatal and mesodiencephalic centers in rabbits, *J. Neurophysiol. 20*:81 (with R. P. White).

1958 Book review of: *The Chemical Concepts of Psychosis* (Herman C. B. Denber, ed.), 485 pp., McDowell, Obolensky, New York.

1958 Designated discussion, in: *Reticular Formation of the Brain* (Herbert H. Jasper, ed.), pp. 169–176, Little, Brown, Boston.

1958 Introduction to the second round table discussion, in: *Neurological and Psychological Deficits of Asphyxia Neonatorum* (W. F. Windle, ed.), pp. 141–151, Charles C. Thomas, Springfield, Illinois.

1958 Prospects in psychopharmacology, in: *The New Chemotherapy in Mental Illness* (H. L. Gordon, ed.), pp. 23–35, Philosophical Library, New York.

1958 Psychopharmacological drugs, *Science 127*:59.

1958 Reticular formation of the brain, in: *International Symposium*, Henry Ford Hospital, pp. 169–173, Little, Brown, Boston.

1958   Clinical evaluation of BAS (benzyl analog of serotonin), a tranquilzing drug, *J. Nerv. Ment. Dis. 126*:284 (with L. H. Rudy, E. Costa, and F. Rinaldi.

1958   Brain disorders (trifluoperazine in mentally defective patients), in: *Trifluoperazine: Clinical and Pharmacological Aspects* (Henry Brill, ed.), pp. 169–172, Lea and Febiger, Philadelphia (with L. H. Rudy, E. Costa, and F. Rinaldi).

1958   A clinical evaluation of psychopharmacological agents in the management of disturbed mentally defective patients, *Amer. J. Ment. Defic. 62*:855 (with L. H. Rudy and F. Rinaldi).

1958   Triflupromazine and trifluoperazine: Two new tranquilizers, *Am. J. Psychiatry 114*:747 (with L. H. Rudy, F. Rinaldi, E. Costa, W. Tuteur, and J. Glotzer).

1958   Cortical and rhinencephalic electrical potentials during hypoglycemia, *Arch. Neurol. Psychiatry 80*:314 (with W. G. Van Meter and Helen F. Owens).

1959   Interactions of monoamine oxidase inhibitors with physiological and biochemical mechanisms in brain. A discussion of the paper by H. E. Himwich, E. Costa, G. R. Pscheidt, and W. G. Van Meter, *Ann. N.Y. Acad. Sci. 80*:614 (with B. B. Brodie, S. Spector, and P. A. Shore).

1959   Effect of reserpine on urinary tryptamine excretion in man, *Physiologist 2*:19 (with G. W. Brune).

1959   Brain serotonin metabolism in insulin hypoglycemia, in: *Biochemistry of the Central Nervous System, Vol. III* (O. Hoffman-Ostenhol, ed.), pp. 283–290, Pergamon Press, New York (with E. Costa).

1959   Behavioral changes following increases of neurohormonal content in selected brain area, *Fed. Proc. Fed. Am. Soc. Exp. Biol. 8*:379 (with E. Costa, W. A. Himwich, S. G. Goldstein, and R. G. Canham).

1959   Insulin hypoglycemia and rabbit brain norepinephrine, *Fed. Proc. Fed. Am. Soc. Exp. Biol. 18*:123 (with G. R. Pscheidt).

1959   Discussion of paper of Mayer-Gross: EEG interactions of LSD-25 and mescaline with tranquilizing drugs, in: *Neuro-Psychopharmacology* (P. B. Bradley, ed.), pp. 129–133, Elsevier, Amsterdam.

1959   Effects of injections of bufotenin into various arterial sites, in: *Neuro-Psychopharmacology* (P. B. Bradley, ed.), pp. 299–303, Elsevier, Amsterdam (with E. Costa and W. A. Himwich).

1959   An EEG analysis of psychotomimetic drugs, in: *Neuro-Psychopharmacology* (P. B. Bradley, ed.), pp. 329–333, Elsevier, Amsterdam (with W. G. Van Meter and Helen F. Owens).

1959   Biochemistry of the nervous system in relation to the process of aging, in: *The Process of Aging in the Nervous System* (J. E. Birren, H. A. Imus, and W. F. Windle, eds.), pp. 101–112, Charles C. Thomas, Springfield, Illinois.

1959   Some drugs used in the treatment of mental disorders, *Am. J. Psychiatry 115*:756.

1959   Book review of: *Neuropharmacology: Transactions of the Second Conference, Am. J. Psychiatry 116*:88.

1959   Book review of: *The Chemical Concepts of Psychosis, Am. J. Psychiatry 116*: 286.

1959   Stimulants, *Assoc. Res. Nerv. Dis. Proc. 37*:356.

1959   The functional organization of the brain, a reconsideration, read at Regional Research Conference of A.P.A., Chicago, June.

1959   Correlations between effects of iproniazid on brain activating system with brain neurohormones, in: *Biological Psychiatry* (Jules H. Masserman, ed.), pp. 2–16, Grune and Stratton, New York (with E. Costa, G. R. Pscheidt, and W. G. Van Meter).

1959   Drugs used in the treatment of the depressions, in: *Biological Psychiatry* (Jules H.

Masserman, ed.), pp. 27–52, Grune and Stratton, New York (with W. G. Van Meter and Helen F. Owens).

1959 Triflupromazine (Vesprin) in the treatment of psychotic patients, in: *Biological Psychiatry* (J. Masserman, ed.), pp. 292–305, Grune and Stratton, New York (with F. Rinaldi, E. Costa, L. H. Rudy, W. Tuteur, and J. Glotzer).

1959 Interaction of monoamine oxidase inhibitors with physiological and biochemical mechanisms in brains, *Ann. N.Y. Acad. Sci. 80*:614 (with E. Costa, G. R. Pscheidt, and W. G. Van Meter).

1959 Triflupromazine and trifluoperazine in the treatment of disturbed mentally defective patients, *Am. J. Ment. Defic. 64*:711 (with E. Costa, F. Rinaldi, and L. H. Rudy).

1959 General neurophysiology (biochemistry), in: *Progress in Neurology and Psychiatry* Vol. XIV (E. A. Spiegel, ed.), pp. 19–36, Grune and Stratton, New York (with W. A. Himwich).

1959 Neurochemistry of aging, in: *Handbook of Aging and the Individual* (James E. Birren, ed.), pp. 187–216, University of Chicago Press (with W. A. Himwich).

1959 *Insulin Treatment in Psychiatry*, 380 pp., Philosophical Library, New York (with M. Rinkel).

1959 Studies of the hypoglycemic brain. Amino acids, nucleic acids, total nitrogen, and side-group ionization of proteins in cat brain during insulin coma, *Arch. Neurol. Psychiatry 81*:458 (with F. E. Samson, Jr., D. R. Dahl, and Nancy Dahl).

1959 The effects of tofranil, an antidepressant drug, on electrical potentials of rabbit brain, *Can. Psychiatr. Assoc. J. 4, Special Suppl. S113* (with W. G. Van Meter and Helen F. Owens).

1960 Hemodynamic studies on the circle of Willis in dogs, in: *Transactions of the American Neurological Association* (Melvin D. Yahr, ed.), pp. 187–188, Springer-Verlag, New York (with G. F. Ayala and W. A. Himwich).

1960 Effects of reserpine on urinary tryptamine and indole-3-acetic acid excretion in mental deficiency schizophrenia and phenylpyruvic oligophrenia, reprinted from: *Acta of the International Meeting on the Techniques for the Study of Psychotropic Drugs,* Bologna, June 26–27 (with G. Brune).

1960 Technics for the study of behavior induced by drugs using injections into selected arterial sites in the brain, Reprinted from: *Acta of the International Meeting on the Techniques for the Study of Psychotropic Drugs,* Bologna, June 26–27 (with W. A. Himwich and E. Costa).

1960 Brain concentrations of biogenic amines and EEG patterns of rabbits, *J. Pharmacol. Exp. Ther. 130*:81 (with E. Costa, G. R. Pscheidt, and W. G. Van Meter).

1960 Biochemical and neurophysiological action of psychoactive drugs, in: *Drugs and Behavior* (L. Uhr and J. G. Miller, eds.), pp. 41–85, John Wiley and Sons, New York.

1960 Book review of: *Differential Treatment and Prognosis in Schizophrenia, Ment. Hyg. (N.Y.) 44*:593.

1960 Functional organization of the brain, past and present, *J. Nerv. Ment. Dis. 130*:505.

1960 Similarities between tranquilizers and antidepressants, in: *Memorial Research Monographs Naka,* pp. 125–142, Committee on the celebration of the 60th birthday of Professor S. Naka, Osaka, Japan.

1960 Some drugs useful in the treatment of emotional disorders. Physiology, indications and contra-indications, *Am. Pract. 11*:687.

1960 *Tranquilizers, barbiturates and the brain* (brochure), pp. 20.

1960 Neurochemistry of aging, in: *A Handbook of Aging and the Individual Psychological and Biological Aspects* (J. E. Birren, ed.) pp. 187–215, University of Chicago Press (with W. A. Himwich).

1960   Effect of therapeutic doses of psychotropic drugs on clinical symptomatology and urinary amines, *Physiologist 3*:126 (with G. R. Pscheidt and G. G. Brune).

1961   Carbohydrate metabolism in mental disease, in: *Chemical Pathology of the Nervous System* (J. Folch-Pi, ed.), pp. 470–496, Pergamon Press, New York.

1961   Study of the EEG convulsant activity of pentylenetetrazol injected arterially into restricted areas of the rabbit brain, *J. Neuropsychiatry 2*:138 (with G. F. Ayala and W. G. Van Meter).

1961   Effects of methaqualone, an experimental CNS depressant, on electrical potentials of rabbit brains, *Trans. Am. Neurol. Assoc. 192* (with D. A. Baylor).

1961   Biphasic action of reserpine and isocarboxazid on behavior and serotonin metabolism, *Science 133*:190 (with G. G. Brune).

1961   Effects of reserpine and isocarboxazid on behavior of mental patients and some urinary products, in: *Symposium on the Biology of Schizophrenia*, V.A. Hospital, Battle Creek, Michigan, March 16–17, pp. 22–34 (with G. G. Brune and G. R. Pscheidt).

1961   Discussion to the first symposium: The problem of antagonists to psychotropic drugs, in: *Neuropsychopharmacology*, Vol. 2 (E. Rothlin, ed.), pp. 32–33, Elsevier, Amsterdam.

1961   Correlations between behavior and urinary indole amines during treatment with reserpine and isocarboxazid, separately and together, in: *Neuropsychopharmacology*, Vol. 2, (E. Rothlin, ed.), pp. 465–474, Elsevier, Amsterdam (with G. G. Brune).

1961   5-HT content of brain structures of dogs given 5-HTP (5-hydroxytryptophan) compared with the degree of behavioral and neurological changes, in: *Neuropsychopharmacology*, Vol. 2 (E. Rothlin, ed.), pp. 475–478, Elsevier, Amsterdam (with E. Costa and W. A. Himwich).

1961   Brain serotonin in relation to imipramine interaction with a monoamine oxidase inhibitor, in: *Neuropsychopharmacology*, Vol. 2 (E. Rothlin, ed.), pp. 485–489, Elsevier, Amsterdam (with W. A. Himwich and E. Costa).

1961   A laboratory manual for general hospital psychiatry, in: *Frontiers in General Hospital Psychiatry* (L. Linn, ed.), pp. 449–474, International Universities Press, New York (with E. E. Haynes).

1961   Carbohydrate metabolism in mental disease. Part 1: Studies on oral glucose tolerance tests and some associated phenomena, in: *Chemical Pathology of the Nervous System* (J. Folch-Pi, ed.), pp. 470–496, Pergamon Press, New York.

1961   Clinical and basic analyses of the similarities and differences in the actions of tranquilizing and antidepressant drugs, in: *Symposium on the Biology of Schizophrenia*, V.A. Hospital, Battle Creek, Michigan, March 16–17, pp. 11–12.

1961   Drugs and the Kefauver bill, *Science 134*:1560.

1961   Uniform response of biogenic amines to psychotropic drugs in selected schizophrenic patients, *Fed. Proc. Fed. Am. Soc. Exp. Biol. 20*:305c (March) (with G. R. Pscheidt and G. G. Brune).

1961   Effects of hallucinogenic drugs in man: Introductory remarks, *Fed. Proc. Fed. Am. Soc. Exp. Biol. 20*:874.

1961   Book review of: *Handbook of Toxicology*, Vol. IV, Tranquilizers, *Psychosom. Med. 23*:90.

1961   Pavlovian conference on higher nervous activity. Discussion. Part II, *Ann. N.Y. Acad. Sci. 92*:978.

1961   Psychopharmacological aspects of the nervous system, in: *Neurochemistry*, 2nd Ed. (K. A. C. Elliott, I. H. Page, and J. H. Quastel, eds.), pp. 766–789, Charles C. Thomas, Springfield, Illinois.

1961 Research and its application to gerontology, *Medicine,* Proceedings of Joint Conference Cook County Community Aging, pp. 34–43.

1961 Similarities and dissimilarities between some tranquilizers and antidepressants, in: *Recent Advances in Biological Psychiatry,* Vol. 3 (Joseph Wortis, ed.), p. 77, Grune and Stratton, New York.

1961 Correlations between the behaviour of patients with mental disturbances and effects of psychoactive drugs on some urinary products, in: *The Third World Congress of Psychiatry 1*:111, presented at Montreal, Canada, June 4–10 (with G. G. Brune and G. R. Pscheidt).

1961 Correlations between amine metabolism and activity of psychosis in schizophrenic patients, in: *The Third World Congress of Psychiatry 1*:124 (abstract), presented at Montreal, Canada, June 4–10 (with G. G. Brune).

1961 Behavioral, EEG and biochemical variations after the administration of alpha-methyl-tryptamine (IT 403), in: *Recent Advances in Biological Psychiatry,* Vol. 3 (Joseph Wortis, ed.), pp. 166–177, Grune and Stratton, New York (with W. G. Van Meter, E. Costa, and G. F. Ayala).

1961 Failure of ethanol to lower brain stem concentration of biogenic amines, *Q. J. Stud. Alcohol 22*:550 (with G. R. Pscheidt and B. Issekutz Jr.).

1961 A pilot study of the effects of pathcole, a serotonin antimetabolite, on schizophrenic patients, *Am. J. Psychiatry, 117*:1121 (with G. Vassiliou, E. Costa, G. Brune, C. Morpurgo, G. Ayala, and V. Vassiliou).

1961 Psychological effects of isocarboxazid and nialamide on a group of depressed patients, *J. Clin. Psychol. 17*:319 (with V. Vassiliou).

1962 Effects of methionine loading on the behavior of schizophrenic patients, *J. Nerv. Ment. Dis. 134*:447 (with G. G. Brune).

1962 Indole metabolites in schizophrenic patients, *Arch. Gen. Psychiatry 6*:324 (with G. G. Brune).

1962 Relevance of drug-induced extrapyramidal reactions to behavioral changes during neuroleptic treatment. I. Treatment with trifluoperazine singly and in combination with trihexyphenidyl, *Compr. Psychiatry 3*:227 (with G. G. Brune, C. Morpurgo, A. Bielkus, T. Kobayashi, and T. T. Tourlentes).

1962 Relevance of drug-induced extrapyramidal reactions to behavioral changes during neuroleptic treatment. II. Combined treatment with trifluoperazine–mobarbital, *Compr. Psychiatry 3*:292 (with G. G. Brune, T. Kobayashi, C. Bull, and T. T. Tourlentes).

1962 Discussion, in: *Research Approaches to Psychiatric Problems* (T. T. Tourlentes, S. L. Pollack, and H. E. Himwich, eds.), pp. 69–73, Grune and Stratton, New York.

1962 Emotional aspects of mind: Clinical and neurophysiological analyses, in: *Theories of the Mind* (Jordan Scher, ed.), pp. 145–180, MacMillan, New York.

1962 H. E. Himwich: Finds 2 processes lead to progress, *Drug Trade News,* pp. 4–5 (Jan. 22 and Feb. 5).

1962 Questions and answers, *J. Am. Med. Assoc. 179*:476 (Feb. 10).

1962 Some specific effects of psychoactive drugs, in: *Specific and Non-specific Factors in Psychopharmacology* (Max Rinker, ed.), pp. 3–82, Philosophical Library, New York.

1962 Research in medical aspects of aging, *Geriartrics 17*:89.

1962 The reticular activating system—current concepts of function, in: *Psychosomatic Medicine* (John H. Nodine and John H. Moyer, eds.), pp. 211–220, Lea and Febiger, Philadelphia.

1962 Tranquilizers, barbiturates, and the brain, *Mod. Med. 109*: (Feb. 19).

1962   Tranquilizers, barbiturates and the brain, *J. Neuropsychiatry 3*:279.

1962   Drugs affecting rhinencephalic structures, *J. Neuropsychiatry, Suppl. 1, 3*:S15 (with A. Morillo and W. G. Steiner).

1962   Antagonists of serotonin action, *Fed. Proc. Fed. Am. Soc. Exp. Biol. 21*:336f (with W. A. Himwich and F. M. Knapp).

1962   An electrocorticographic study of changes in mouse brain with age, *Life Sci. 7*:343 (with T. Kobayashi).

1962   Central cholinolytic action of chlorpromazine, *Science 136*:873 (with W. G. Steiner).

1962   Anoxia and cerebral metabolism, *Int. J. Neurol. 3*:413–427 (with W. A. Himwich).

1963   Alcoholism, in: *Encyclopaedia Britannica,* pp. 547–551, William Benton, U.S.A.

1963   Reserpine, monoamine oxidase inhibitors and distribution of biogenic amines in monkey brain, *Biochem. Pharmacol. 12*:65 (with G. R. Pscheidt).

1963   The psychoactive drugs, in: *The Psychological Basis of Medical Practice* (H. I. Lief, V. F. Lief, and N. R. Lief, eds.), pp. 531–544, Hoeber Medical Division, Harper and Row, New York.

1963   Biogenic amines and behavior in schizophrenic patients, in: *Recent Advances in Biological Psychiatry,* Vol. 5 (J. Wortis, ed.), pp. 144–160, Plenum Press, New York (with G. G. Brune).

1963   A multidisciplinary study of changes in mouse brain with age, in: *Recent Advances in Biological Psychiatry,* Vol. 5 (J. Wortis, ed.), pp. 293–308, Plenum Press, New York (with T. Kobayashi, O. Inman, and W. Buno).

1963   An EEG and behavioral analysis of the anticonvulsant action of amphenidone in the rabbit, *Arch. Int. Pharmacodyn. Ther. 142*:1 (with W. G. Steiner).

1963   An electrographic study of psilocin and 4-methyl-alpha-methyl tryptamine (MP-809), *J. Pharmacol. Exp. Ther. 140*:8 (with J. F. Brodey and W. G. Steiner).

1963   Different responses of urinary tryptamine and of total catecholamines during treatment with reserpine and isocarboxazid in schizophrenic patients, *Int. J. Neuropharmacol. 2*:17 (with G. G. Brune and G. R. Pscheidt).

1963   Influence of methodology on electroencephalographic sleep and arousal: Studies with reserpine and etryptamine in rabbits, *Science 141*:53 (with W. G. Steiner and G. R. Pscheidt).

1963   Relevance of the *N,N*-dimethyl configuration to the pharmacological action of chlorpromazine, *Biochem. Pharmacol. 12*:679 (with G. G. Brune, H. H. Kohl, and W. G. Steiner).

1963   Chicken brain amines, with special reference to cerebellar norepinephrine, *Life Sci. 7*:524 (with G. R. Pscheidt).

1963   Alpha-ethyltryptamine (etryptamine): An electroencephalographic, behavioral and neurochemical analysis, *Psychopharmacologia 4*:354 (with W. G. Steiner, G. R. Pscheidt, and E. Costa).

1963   An electroencephalographic study of the blocking action of selected tranquilizers as a function of terminal methylamine group, *Biochem. Pharmacol. 12*:687 (with W. G. Steiner).

1963   Participants in psychiatric problems in non-psychiatric practice, *Ill. Med. J. 124*:217.

1963   Effects of antidepressant drugs on limbic structures of rabbit, *J. Nerv. Ment. Dis. 137*:277 (with W. G. Steiner).

1963   Alcohol and evoked potentials in the cat, *Nature (London) 200*:1328 (with A. R. Dravid, R. DiPerri, and A. Morillo).

1963   Dimethylamine configuration in chlorpromazine, *Fed. Proc. Fed. Am. Soc. Exp. Biol. 23*:2438 (with H. Kohl, G. Brune, and W. G. Steiner).

1963 Review of: *A Decade of Alcoholism Research; a Review of the Research Activities of the Alcoholism and Drug Addiction Research Foundation of Ontario, 1951–1961* (R. E. Popham and W. Schmidt, eds.), *Brookside Monogr. 3,* 64 pp., University of Toronto Press (reviewed in *J. Am. Med. Assoc. 183*:980).

1963 Effects of trifluoperazine on rabbit EEG, *J. Neuropsychiatry 5*:123–131 (with T. Kobayashi).

1963 Psychopharmacologic management of crisis, Tenth Annual Conference, Group Psychotherapy Association of Southern California, Inc., June 15.

1963 Psychiatric problems in non-psychiatric practice, *Ill. Med. J. 124*:207–222 (with T. T. Tourlentes, C. H. Hardin, J. H. Masserman, L. H. Rudy, D. Oken, R. Drye, and S. L. Pollack).

1963 Urinary excretion of bufotenin-like substance in psychotic patients, *J. Neuropsychiatry 5*:14–17 (with G. G. Brune and H. H. Kohl).

1964 Review of *Outline of Psychiatry* (L. Cammar, ed.), 338 pp., McGraw-Hill, New York *Am. J. Psychiatry 120*:718–719.

1964 A comparative study of chlorpromazine and its demethylated derivatives: Potency and tissue distribution, *Biochem. Pharmacol. 13*:539–541 (with H. H. Kohl and G. G. Brune).

1964 Endogenous metabolic factor in schizophrenic behavior, *Science.144*:311–313 (with H. H. Berlet, C. Bull, H. Kohl, K. Matsumoto, G. R. Pscheidt, J. Spaide, T. T. Tourlentes, and J. M. Valverde).

1964 Non-uniform response of urinary indole compounds to variations of tryptophan intake, *Fed. Proc. Fed. Am. Soc. Exp. Biol. 23*:279 (with H. H. Berlet, H. Kohl, and J. Spaide).

1964 A pharmacological study of terminal methyl groups in animals: (1) Electrophysiological analysis of chlorpromazine, imipramine, and amitriptyline, and their demethylated congeners; (2) Behavioral evaluations of chlorpromazine and its demethylated congeners in relation to brain concentrations of phenothiazines, in: *Recent Advances in Biological Psychiatry,* Vol. 6 (J. Wortis ed.), Chapt. 18, Plenum Press, New York (with G. G. Brune, W. G. Steiner, and H. H. Kohl).

1964 An electroencephalographic and chemical re-evaluation of the central action of reserpine in the rabbit, *J. Pharmacol. Exp. Ther. 144*:37–44 (with G. R. Pscheidt and W. G. Steiner).

1964 An electrographic study of bufotenin and 5-hydroxytryptophan, *J. Pharmacol. Exp. Ther. 144*:253–259 (with A. K. Schweigerdt).

1964 Neurohistological studies of developing mouse brain, in: *Progress in Brain Research,* Vol. 8, *Biogenic Amines* (H. E. Himwich and W. A. Himwich, eds.), pp. 87–88, Elsevier, New York and Amsterdam (with T. Kobayashi, O. R. Inman, and W. Buno).

1964 Summary, in: *Progress in Brain Research,* Vol. 8, *Biogenic Amines* (H. E. Himwich and W. A. Himwich, eds.), pp. 226–240, Elsevier, New York and Amsterdam.

1964 An electroencephalographic study of some structural aspects of D-amphetamine antagonism in phenothiazine and related compounds, *Int. J. Neuropharmacol. 2*:327–335 (with W. G. Steiner and K. Bost).

1964 Electroencephalographic changes following administration of *N*-dimethylacetamide and other antitumor agents to rabbits, *Int. J. Neuropharmacol. 3*:327–332 (with W. G. Steiner).

1964 Variations of urinary creatinine and its correlation to tryptamine excretion in schizophrenic patients, *Nature (London) 203*:1198–1199 (with H. H. Berlet, G. R. Pscheidt, and J. Spaide).

1964   Excretion of catecholamines and exacerbation of symptoms in schizophrenic patients, *J. Psychiatr. Res. 2*:163–168 (with G. R. Pscheidt, H. H. Berlet, C. Bull, and J. Spaide).

1964   Studies on norepinephrine and 5-hydroxytryptamine in various species. Regional distribution in the brain, response to monoamine oxidase inhibitors, comparison of chemical and biological assay methods for norepinephrine, in: *Comparative Neurochemistry* (D. Richter, ed.), pp. 401–412, Pergamon Press, London (with G. R. Pscheidt and C. Morpurgo).

1964   An electroencephalographic study of some structural aspects of D-amphetamine antagonism in phenothiazine and related compounds, *Int. J. Neuropharmacol. 2*:327–335 (with W. G. Steiner and K. Bost).

1964   Effects of psychotropic drug combinations on urinary constituents in the dog, *J. Neuropsychiatry 5*:502–508 (with G. R. Pscheidt, G. G. Brune, and W. A. Himwich).

1964   Hypertension with methionine in schizophrenic patients receiving tranylcypromine, *Am. J. Psychiatry 121*:381–382 (with C. Bull, J. M. Valverde, H. H. Berlet, J. K. Spaide, and T. T. Tourlentes).

1965   The place of psychoactive drugs in the eclectic therapy of disturbed children, in: *Medical Aspects of Mental Retardation* (C. H. Carter ed.), pp. 966–986, Charles C. Thomas, Springfield, Illinois.

1965   Psychoactive drugs, *Postgrad. Med. 37*:35–45.

1965   Effects of reduction of tryptophan and methionine intake on urinary indole compounds and schizophrenic behavior, *J. Nerv. Ment. Dis. 140*:297–304 (with H. H. Berlet, J. Spaide, H. Kohl, and C. Bull).

1965   Effects of some psychoactive drugs on electroencephalogram and brain amines of immature rabbits, *Life Sci. 4*:1333–1343 (with G. R. Pscheidt and A. Schweigerdt).

1965   Biochemical effects of psychoactive drugs in various vertebrate classes, *Neuro-Psychopharmacology* (D. Bente and P. B. Bradley, eds.), Vol. 4, pp. 38–42, Elsevier, Amsterdam (discussion—with G. R. Pscheidt).

1965   Anatomy and physiology of the emotions and their relation to psychoactive drugs, in: *The Scientific Basis of Drug Therapy in Psychiatry*, Proceedings of a Symposium at St. Bartholomew's Hospital, London, September 7–8, 1964, pp. 3–24, Pergamon Press, New York.

1965   Intake of tryptophan and methionine and excretion of urinary indoles in relation to exacerbations of symptoms in schizophrenic patients, in: *Neuro-Psychopharmacology* (D. Bente and P. B. Bradley, eds.), Vol. 4, pp. 295–298, Elsevier, Amsterdam (with H. H. Berlet, C. Bull, and J. K. Spaide).

1965   Functional studies of the circle of Willis: Vertebral artery pressure responses to carotid artery occulsion measured in the dog and in a model, in: *Transactions of the American Neurological Association* (M. D. Yahr, ed.), Vol. 90, pp. 254–256, Springer, New York (with M. E. Clark, B. Cucciniello, and W. A. Himwich).

1965   Chicken brain amines: Normal levels and effect of reserpine and monamine oxidase inhibitors, in: *Progress in Brain Research, Horizons in Neuropsychopharmacology* (W. A. Himwich and J. P. Schade, eds.), Vol. 16, pp. 245–249, Elsevier, Amsterdam (with G. R. Pscheidt).

1965   Comparative clinical and basic evaluations of various groups of psychotropic drugs, *Psychosomatics 6*:254–260.

1965   Loci of actions of psychotropic drugs in the brain, *Folia Psychiatr. Neurol. Jpn. 19*:217–244.

1965   Alcohol and evoked potentials in the cat, *Nature (London) 208*:688 (with A. K. Schweigerdt, A. R. Dravid, and A. H. Stewart).

1965 Mescaline, 3,4-dimethoxyphenylethylamine, and adrenaline: Sites of electroencephalographic arousal, *Science 150*:1309–1310 (with Y. Takeo).

1965 Biochemical correlates of behavior in schizophrenic patients, *Arch. Gen. Psychiatry 13*:521–531 (with H. H. Berlet, K. Matsumoto, G. R. Pscheidt, J. Spaide, and C. Bull).

1966 Variations of urinary creatinine and its correlation to excretion of indole metabolites in mental patients, *Clin. Chim. Acta 13*:228–234 (with G. R. Pscheidt, H. H. Berlet, and J. Spaide).

1966 An electrographic study of D-lysergic acid diethylamide and nine congeners, *J. Pharmacol. Exp. Ther. 151*:353–359 (with A. K. Schweigerdt and A. H. Stewart).

1966 Biogenic amines in various brain regions of growing cats, *Brain Res. 1*:363–368 (with G. R. Pscheidt).

1966 Excretion of 17-hydroxycorticosteroids and 17-ketosteroids in relation to schizophrenic symptoms, *J. Psychiatri. Res. 4*:1–12 (with K. Matsumoto, H. H. Berlet, and C. Bull).

1966 An EEG study of 2-phenyl-3-ethylaminobicyclo-(2,2,1)-heptane HCl (Fencamfamin hydrochloride), *Life Sci. 5*:299–308 (with J. R. Bueno).

1966 Comparative susceptibility to alcohol of the cortical area and midbrain reticular formation of the cat, *Psychosom. Med. 28*:458–463 (with R. DiPerri, A. Dravid, and A. Schweigerdt).

1966 Studies on the association of urinary tryptamine with the excretion of amino acids and 17-ketosteroid hormones in schizophrenic patients, in: *Amines and Schizophrenia* (H. E. Himwich, S. Kety, and J. R. Smythies, eds.), pp. 69–85, Pergamon Press, Oxford (with H. H. Berlet, J. K. Spaide, and K. Matsumoto).

1966 Comparative neurophysiological studies of psychotomimetic *N*-dimethylamines and *N*-diethylamines and their non-psychotomimetic congeners devoid of the *N*-dimethyl or *N*-diethyl configurations, in: *Amines and Schizophrenia* (H. E. Himwich, S. Kety, and J. R. Smythies, eds.), pp. 137–149, Pergamon Press, Oxford.

1966 Effect of diet on schizophrenic behavor, in: *Psychopathology of Schizophrenia* (P. Hoch and J. Zubin (eds.), pp. 425–452, Grune and Stratton, New York (with H. H. Berlet, C. Bull, H. Kohl, K. Matusomoto, G. R. Pscheidt, J. Spaide, T. T. Tourlentes, and J. M. Valverde).

1966 Relationship between indole metabolism and schizophrenic behavior, in: *Biological Treatment of Mental Illness* (M. Rinkel, ed.), pp. 284–302, L. C. Page and Co., New York (with G. G. Brune).

1966 Hyperactivity and EEG alerting with increases of brain serotonin, in: *Transactions of the American Neurological Association* (M. D. Yahr, ed.), Vol. 91, pp. 199–200, Springer, New York (with J. R. Bueno and G. R. Pscheidt).

1966 The effect of syrosingopine on spontaneous EEG and EEG arousal induced by external stimuli in rabbits, *Life Sci. 5*:1503–1508 (with Y. Takeo and G. R. Pscheidt).

1966 The influence of cortisone on tryptophan-induced increases in brain serotonin levels, *Brain News 3*:1–6 (with N. S. Shah).

1967 Schizophrenic behavior and urinary tryptophan metabolites associated with cysteine given with and without a monoamine oxidase inhibitor (Tranylcypromine), *Life Sci. 6*:551–560 (with J. Spaide, H. Tanimukai, R. Ginther, and J. Bueno).

1967 Comparative electroencephalographic study of phenylethylamines and their methoxy derivatives, *Arch. Int. Pharmacodyn. Ther. 166*:47–59 (with Y. Takeo).

1967 Comparative studies on development of biogenic amines in brains of growing rabbits and cats, in: *Regional Development of the Brain in Early Life* (M. Minkowski, ed.), pp. 273–296, Blackwell Scientific, Oxford (with G. R. Pscheidt and A. K. Schweigerdt).

1967 A dualistic approach to some biochemical problems in endogenous depressions, *Psychosomatics 8*:82–94 (with J. R. Bueno).

1967 Effect of physostigmine on the level of brain biogenic amines in rats and rabbits, *Biochem. Pharmacol. 16*:1132–1134 (with G. R. Pscheidt and Z. Votava).
1967 The significance of methyl groups in the electroencephalographic effects of indolealkylamines in the rabbit, *Biochem. Pharmacol. 16*:1013–1022 (with Y. Takeo).
1967 Occurrence of bufotenin (5-hydroxy-*N,N*-dimethyltryptamine) in urine of schizophrenic patients, *Life Sci. 6*:1697–1706 (with H. Tanimukai, R. Ginther, J. Spaide, and J. R. Bueno).
1967 Psychotomimetic indole compound in the urine of schizophrenics and mentally defective patients, *Nature (London) 216*:490–491 (with H. Tanimukai, R. Ginther, and J. Spaide).
1967 Behavioral reaction of rats pretreated with reserpine to LSD-25, *Int. J. Neuropharmacol. 6*:543–547 (with Z. Votava and S. N. Glisson).
1967 An examination of a possible cortical cholinergic link in the EEG arousal reaction, in: *Progress in Brain Research*, Vol. 28, *Anticholinergic Drugs* (P. B. Bradley and M. Fink, eds.), pp. 27–39, Elsevier, Amsterdam (with Z. Cuculic and K. Bost).
1967 Excretion of indoleamines in schizophrenia, *Int. J. Neurol. 6*:65–76 (with J. R. Bueno).
1967 Psychotropic drugs used in the management of schizophrenia, *Int. J. Neurol. 6*:77–93 (with J. R. Bueno).
1967 Review of: *Psychopharmacological Methods*, 1963 (Z. Votava, M. Horvath, and O. Vinar, eds.), Macmillan Company, New York (reviewed in *Electroencephalogr. Clin. Neurophysiol. 22*:594).
1968 Effect of chronic administration of cortisone on the tryptophan induced changes in amine levels in the rat brain, *Arch. Int. Phamacodyn. Ther. 171*:285–295 (with N. S. Shah and S. Stevens).
1968 Effects of alcohol on evoked potentials of various parts of the central nervous system of cat, *Q. J. Stud. Alcohol, 29*:20–37 (with R. DiPerri, A. Dravid, and A. Schweigerdt).
1968 The ontogeny of sleep in kittens and young rabbits, *Electroencephalogr. Clin. Neurophysiol. 24*:307–318 (with A. Shimizu).
1968 Metabolism and pharmacology of alcohol, in: *Alcoholism, The Total Treatment Approach* (R. J. Cantanzaro, ed.), pp. 26–38, Charles C. Thomas, Springfield, Illinois.
1968 Psychotogenic *N,N*-dimethylated indole amines and behavior in schizophrenic patients, in: *Recent Advances in Biological Psychiatry*, Vol. 10 (J. Wortis, ed.), pp. 6–15, Plenum Press, New York (with H. Tanimukai, R. Ginther, J. Spaide and J. R. Bueno).
1968 Effects of phenothiazine derivatives on the sleep–wakefulness cycle in growing kittens, in: *Recent Advances in Biological Psychiatry*, Vol. 10 (J. Wortis, ed.), p. 257, Plenum Press, New York (with A. Shimizu).
1968 Effects of chronic administration of some psychoactive drugs on EEG arousal on rabbit, *Int. J. Neuropharmacol. 7*:87–95 (with C. Doyle and A. Shimizu).
1968 Cerebral cortical structures and local anesthetic action, in: *Pain* (A. Soulairac, J. Cahn, and J. Charpentier, eds.), pp. 451–461, Academic Press, London (with Z. Cuculic).
1968 Behavioral and biochemical alterations in schizophrenic patients, *Arch. Gen. Psychiatry 18*:658–665 (with J. Spaide, H. Tanimukai, and J. R. Bueno).
1968 Effects of ethanol on EEG and blood pressure in the rabbit, *Q. J. Stud. Alcohol 29*:290–301 (with J. W. Kakolewski).
1968 Interactions of monoamine oxidase inhibitors and reserpine: An EEG, gross behavioral and biochemical analysis, *Psychopharmacologia (Berlin) 12*:400–413 (with J. R. Bueno and G. R. Pscheidt).
1968 The effects of amphetamine on the sleep-wakefulness cycle of developing kittens, *Psychopharmacologia (Berlin) 13*:161–169 (with A. Shimizu).

1968 Effect of LSD on the sleep cycle of the developing kitten, *Dev. Psychobiol. 1*:60–64 (with A. Shimizu).

1968 Electroencephalographic studies of haloperidol, *Int. Pharmacopsychiatry 1*:134–142 (with A. Shimizu and K. Bost).

1968 Electroencephalographic alerting sites of D-amphetamine and 2,5-dimethoxy-4-methyl-amphetamine, *Nature (London) 220*:491–494 (with M. Fujimori).

1968 Imipramine affects dopamine uptake by rat brain, *J. Pharm. Pharmacol. 20*:809–810 (with G. R. Pscheidt).

1968 Biochemistry and the schizophrenias, in: *Psychiatric Research in Our Changing World* (G. F. D. Heseltine, ed.), pp. 91–106, Excerpta Medica Foundation, Amsterdam.

1969 Neurophysiological correlates of psychotropic drug action: Animal studies, in: *Drugs and the Brain* (P. Black, ed.), pp. 75–92, Johns Hopkins Press, Baltimore (with A. Shimizu).

1969 Relationship between urinary constituents and exacerbations of behavior in schizophrenic patients, *The Future of the Brain Sciences* (S. Bogoch, ed.), pp. 473–484, Plenum Press, New York.

1969 An *in vitro* study of the effects of tricyclic antidepressant drugs on the accumulation of C^{14}-serotonin by rabbit brain, *Biol. Psychiatry 1*:81–85 (with H. S. Alpers).

1969 Methionine and tryptophan loading in schizophrenic patients receiving a MAO inhibitor: Correlation of behavioral and biochemical changes, *Biol. Psychiatry 1*:227–233 (with J. Spaide, L. Neveln, and J. Tolentino).

1969 Electroencephalographic analyses of amphetamine and its methoxy derivatives with reference to their sites of EEG alerting in the rabbit brain, *Int. J. Neuropharmacol. 8*:601–613 (with M. Fujimori).

1969 Effects of psychotropic drugs on the sleep–wakefulness cycle of the developing kitten, *Dev. Psychobiol. 2*:161–167 (with A. Shimizu).

1969 The acute effects of reserpine on the sleep–wakefulness cycle in rabbits, *Psychopharmacologia (Berlin) 16*:240–252 (with K. Tabushi).

1970 Comparative behavioral and biochemical effects of tranylcypromine and cysteine on normal controls and schizophrenic patients, *Life Sci. 9*:1021–1032 (with N. Narasimhachari, B. Heller, J. Spaide, L. Haskovec, M. Fujimori, and K. Tabushi).

1970 Detection of psychotomimetic *N,N*-dimethylated indoleamines in the urine of four schizophrenic patients, *Br. J. Psychiatry 117*:421–430 (with H. Tanimukai, R. Ginther, J. Spaide, and J. R. Bueno).

1970 Comparative behavioral and urinary studies on schizophrenics and normal controls, in: *Biochemistry of Brain and Behavior* (R. E. Bowman and S. P. Datta, eds.), pp. 207–221, Plenum Press, New York (with N. Narasimhachari, B. Heller, J. Spaide, L. Haskovec, M. Fujimori, and K. Tabushi).

1970 5-Hydroxytryptophan and the sleep–wakefulness cycle in rabbits, *Biol. Psychiatry 2*:183–188 (with K. Tabushi).

1970 EEG arousal reactions to amphetamine and 2,5-dimethoxy-4-methylamphetamine in reserpine-pretreated rabbits, *Biol. Psychiatry 2*:241–250 (with M. Fujimori).

1970 Psychopharmacology, in: *Annual Review of Pharmacology,* Vol. 10 (H. W. Elliott, W. C. Cutting, and R. H. Dreisbach, eds.), pp. 313–334, Annual Reviews, Palo Alto (with H. S. Alpers).

1970 *N*-Dimethylated indoleamines in blood of acute schizophrenics, *Separatum Experienta 26*:503 (with B. Heller, N. Narasimhachari, J. Spaide, and L. Haskovec).

1970 Biochemical changes in the schizophrenias with special reference to urinary products (indoleamines), in: *Modern Trends in Psychological Medicine,* Vol. 2 (J. H. Price, ed.), pp. 78–101, Butterworths, London (with H. Tanimukai).

1971   Indoleamines and the schizophrenias, in: *Biochemistry, Schizophrenias and Affective Illnesses* (H. E. Himwich, ed.), pp. 79–122, Williams and Wilkins Co., Baltimore.

1971   Indoleamines and the depressions, in: *Biochemistry, Schizophrenias and Affective Illnesses* (H. E. Himwich, ed.), pp. 230–282, Williams & Wilkins Co., Baltimore.

1971   EEG arousal sites of amphetamine and its psychotomimetic methoxy derivatives in rabbit brain, *Biol. Psychiatry 3*:367–377 (with M. Fujimori and K. L. Bost).

1971   Urinary studies of schizophrenics and controls, *Biol. Psychiatry 3*:9–20 (with N. Narasimhachari, B. Heller, J. Spaide, L. Haskovec, M. Fujimori, and K. Tabushi).

1971   The effects of aging on schizophrenic and mentally defective patients: Visual, auditory, and grip strength measurements, *J. Gerontol. 26*:137–145 (with D. A. Callison, H. F. Armstrong, L. Elam, R. L. Cannon, and C. B. Paisley).

1971   Plasma amino acids in schizophrenic patients with methionine or cysteine loading and a monoamine oxidase inhibitor, *Am. J. Clin. Nutr. 24*:1053–1059 (with J. K. Spaide and J. M. Davis).

1971   A comparative study of mescaline and 3,4-dimethoxyphenylethylamine in isolated brain mitochondria and brain homogenate, *Brain Res. 34*:163–170 (with N. S. Shah).

1971   Study with mescaline-8-C^{14} in mice: Effect of amine oxidase inhibitors on metabolism, *Neuropharmacology 10*:547–556 (with N. S. Shah).

1971   Electroencephalographic study of the effects of methysergide on sleep in the rabbit, *Electroencephalogr. Clin. Neurophysiol. 31*:491–497 (with K. Tabushi).

1971   Blocking of 5-methoxy-N-dimethyltryptamine-induces EEG alerting in the rabbit by previous administration of antiserum to this compound, *Biol. Psychiatry 3*:227–236 (with M. Strahilevitz, N. Narasimharchari, and M. Fujimori).

1971 N,N-Dimethylated indoleamines in blood, *Biol. Psychiatry 3*:21–23 (with N. Narasimhachari, B. Heller, J. Spaide, L. Haskovec, H. Meltzer, and M. Strahilevitz).

1971   Biochemical and behavioral comparisons between chronic schizophrenic patients and normal controls, *Excerpta Med. Int. Congr. Ser. No. 274, Psychiatry (Part I), Proceedings of the Vth World Congress of Psychiatry,* pp. 63–76 (with T. T. Tourlentes and N. Narasimhachari).

1972   Effects of tranylcypromine and L-cysteine on plasma amino acids in controls and schizophrenic patients, *Am. J. Clin. Nutr. 25*:302–310 (with J. M. Davis and J. K. Spaide).

1972   3:4-Dimethoxyphenylethylamine, a normal or abnormal metabolite?, *J. Psychiatr. Res. 9*:325–328 (with N. Narasimhachari and J. Plaut).

1972   Regional localization of 3,4-dimethoxyphenylethylamine-^{14}C (DMPEA-^{14}C) in rabbit brain: Effects of reserpine and iproniazid pretreatment, *J. Pharmacol. Exp. Ther. 180*:144–150 (with N. S. Shah and H. S. Alpers).

1972   The effects of chronic imipramine administration on rat brain levels of serotonin, 5-hydroxyindole-acetic acid, norepinephrine and dopamine, *J. Pharmacol. Exp. Ther. 180*:531–538 (with H. S. Alpers).

1972   Studies of drug-free schizophrenics and controls, *Biol. Psychiatry 5*:311–318 (with N. Narasimhachari, J. Avalos, and M. Fujimori).

1972   The determination of bufotenin in urine of schizophrenic patients and normal controls, *J. Psychiatr. Res. 9*:113–121 (with N. Narasimhachari).

1972   Indolethylamine-N-methyltransferase in serum samples of schizophrenics and normal controls, *Life Sci. (Part II) 11*:221–227 (with N. Narasimhachari and J. M. Plaut).

1972   A biochemical study of early infantile autism, *J. Autism Child. Schizophr. 2*:114–126 (with R. L. Jenkins, M. Fujimori, N. Narasimhachari, and M. Ebersole).

1973   Inhibition of indolethylamine-N-methyltransferase by S-adenosylhomocysteine, *Biochem. Biophys. Res. Commun. 54*:751–759 (with R. Lin and N. Narasimhachari).

1973 Δ^9-Tetrahydrocannabinol and the sleep–wakefulness cycle in rabbits, *Physiol. Behav.* *11*:291–295 (with M. Fujimori).

1973 Δ^9-Tetrahydrocannabinol: Electroencephalographic changes and autonomic responses in the rabbit, *Life Sci. (Part I)* *12*:553–563 (with M. Fujimori and D. M. Trusty).

1973   Early studies of the developing brain, in: *Biochemistry of the Developing Brain*, Vol. 1 (W. A. Himwich, ed.), pp. 1–53, Marcel Dekker, New York.

1973   Gas chromatographic–mass spectrometric identification of *N:N*-dimethyltryptamine in urine samples from drug-free chronic schizophrenic patients and its quantitation by the technique of single (selective) ion monitoring, *Biochem. Biophys. Res. Commun.* *55*:1064–1071 (with N. Narasimhachari).

1973   GC–MS identification of bufotenin in urine samples from patients with schizophrenia or infantile autism, (Part II) *Life Sci.* *12*:475–478 (with N. Narasimhachari).

1973   Biochemical approaches to the study of schizophrenia, in: *Chemical Modulation of Brain Function* (H. C. Sabelli, ed.), pp. 297–311, Raven Press, New York (with N. Narasimhachari, B. Heller, J. Spaide, L. Haskovec, M. Fujimori, and K. Tabushi).

1974   Comparative biochemical and behavioral studies of chronic schizophrenic patients and normals, in: *Neurohumoral Coding of Brain Function* (R. D. Myers and R. R. Drucker-Colin, eds.), pp. 313–330, Plenum Publishing, New York (with N. Narasimhachari).

1974   Inhibitor of indolethylamine *N*-methyltransferase in pineal extract, *Res. Commun. Chem. Pathol. Pharmacol.* *9*:375–378 (with N. Narasimhachari and R. L. Lin).

1975   Biochemical studies in early infantile autism, *Biol. Psychiatry* *10*:425–432 (with N. Narasimhachari).

1975   Summary of symposium: Recent advances in the field of early infantile autism, Boston, Massachusetts, June 7–10, 1974, *Biol. Psychiatry* *10*:453–458.

Index